TRANCE AND POSSESSION IN BALI

TRANCE AND POSSESSION IN BALI

A WINDOW ON WESTERN MULTIPLE PERSONALITY, POSSESSION DISORDER, AND SUICIDE

LUH KETUT SURYANI
GORDON D. JENSEN

KUALA LUMPUR
OXFORD UNIVERSITY PRESS
OXFORD SINGAPORE NEW YORK
1993

Oxford University Press

Oxford New York Toronto
Delhi Bombay Calcutta Madras Karachi
Kuala Lumpur Singapore Hong Kong Tokyo
Nairobi Dar es Salaam Cape Town
Melbourne Auckland Madrid

and associated companies in
Berlin Ibadan

Oxford is a trade mark of Oxford University Press

Published in the United States
by Oxford University Press, New York

First published 1993

British Library Cataloguing in Publication Data
Data available

Library of Congress Cataloging in Publication Data

Suryani, Luh Ketut, 1944–
Trance and possession in Bali: a window on Western multiple personality, possession disorder, and suicide/Luh Ketut Suryani, Gordon D. Jensen.
p. cm.
Includes bibliographical references and index.
ISBN 0–19–588610–0 (hard):
1. Bali Island (Indonesia)—Religion. 2. Trance—Indonesia—Bali Island. 3. Demoniac possession—Indonesia—Bali Island. 4. Spiritual healing—Indonesia—Bali Island. 5. Multiple personality—Cross-cultural studies. 6. Psychiatry and religion. I. Jensen, Gordon D. II. Title.
BL2120.B2S88 1993
154.4–dc20
93–20252
CIP

Typeset by Typeset Gallery Sdn. Bhd., Malaysia
Printed in Singapore by Kyodo Printing Co. (S) Pte. Ltd.
Published by Oxford University Press,
19–25, Jalan Kuchai Lama, 58200 Kuala Lumpur, Malaysia

Acknowledgements

THIS book would not have been possible without the help of many. We wish to acknowledge the encouragement and critiques of the following Americans: Ernest R. Hilgard, Emeritus Professor of Psychology, Stanford University; Eugene L. Bliss, Emeritus Professor of Psychiatry, University of Utah, School of Medicine; and Marlene Steinberg, Research Scientist, Department of Psychiatry, Yale University, School of Medicine. We also wish to record our deep appreciation of the warmth and kindness of the many Balinese who graciously invited us to observe both private and community ceremonies and who consented to personal interviews without thought of remuneration. Grateful thanks are also due to the many traditional healers (*balian*) for allowing us to interview them and to observe, photograph, and videotape their practices and to the Province of Bali Government (Pemerintah Daerah Tingkat I Bali) for granting us permission to study in the field. Dr Tjokorda Alit K. Adnyana, Lecturer in Pharmacology, Udayana University, was of great assistance in the logistics of our studies and also conducted some of the interviews. Last but not least, we are indebted to Jane Derry for taking most of the photographs, to Made Rapini Ari Hantana for helping with our correspondence, and to Jane Rachford for typing.

Denpasar, Bali
Davis, California
May 1992

LUH KETUT SURYANI
GORDON D. JENSEN

Contents

	Acknowledgements	*v*
	Tables	*x*
	Figure	*x*
	Plates	*xi*
	Introduction	*1*
Chapter 1	**Bali and Balinese Background**	*6*
	Social Systems That Bind	*8*
	Ceremonies	*11*
	Principal Hindu–Dharma Beliefs in Bali	*15*
	The Sibling Spirits	*16*
	Factors in Balance and Concepts of Illness	*16*
Chapter 2	**Trance and Possession**	*19*
	Dissociation	*20*
	'Hidden by the Evil Spirit'	*23*
	Latah	*24*
	Dissociation in Mental Disorders	*27*
	Trance/Hypnosis	*28*
	Possession and Trance-possession	*33*
	Leak	*40*
Chapter 3	**Trance and Trance-possession in Traditional Healers and Their Clients**	*49*
	Treatment of Grief or Bereavement by Trance-mediums	*51*
	A Trance-medium (*Balian Taksu*)	*61*
	Annotated Translation of a *Balian Taksu*'s Treatment	*69*

A *Balian* Who Treats by Physical Manipulation 71
A *Balian* Who Uses Trance, Chinese Coins, and *Lontar* 74
A *Balian* Who Extracts Bones from Clients 75
A *Balian* Who Uses Massage 77
Clients of *Balian* Who Fall into Trance-possession 78
A Balinese Physician's Personal Experience with *Balian* 82
Balian and Shamans: A Comparison 83
Western Channellers 85
Western Psychiatric Treatment of Balinese Patients 85

Chapter 4 **Mass Trance-possession in Ceremonies** 89
Mass Trance-possession at Timbrah 89
Mass Trance-possession at Kesiman 95
Mass Trance-possession at Jimbaran 98
Mass Trance-possession at Family Ceremonies 105

Chapter 5 **Trance-possession in Dance and Drama and Individual Trance-possession** 108
The Little Girl Trance-possession Dance (*Sang Hyang Dedari*) 109
The Fire/Hobby-horse Dance (*Sang Hyang Jaran*) 111
The *Kecak* Dance 113
A Combination of Modern Western and Balinese Dances 114
Individual Trance-possession 115

Chapter 6 **Self-hypnosis in Gamelan Musicians** 119
Selection and Interviews 120
Results of the Study 121
Conclusion: Trance with Spirituality 125

Chapter 7 **Dissociative Disorders, Trance-suicide, and Trance-possession Disorders** 129
Trance-suicide in Bali 130
The Trance-suicide Concept 136
Amok 143
Bebainan: A Trance-possession Disorder 146
Kasurupan: A Dissociative Disorder in Schoolchildren 152
Spirit Possession in Other Cultures 156

Chapter 8 **Meditation, Meditation Healing, and Hypnotherapy** *160*
Meditation *160*
Meditation Healing and Possession *163*
Hypnotherapy with Possession *167*
Yoga in Bali *169*

Chapter 9 **Conclusions and Implications of Trance and Possession for Western Concepts of Multiple Personality, Possession Disorder, Suicide, and Mental Health** *171*
Characteristics of Trance-possession *172*
The Dissociation Continua *177*
Professional Recognition of Possession *179*
Possession Disorders: Balinese and Western *181*
Diagnostic Criteria for Possession Disorders *183*
Differential Diagnosis of Possession Disorder *185*
Hallucinations: Normal and Abnormal *190*
Theories of Possession *191*
Multiple Personality Disorder (MPD) Conceptualized as a Trance-possession Process *196*
Therapeutic Implications of MPD as a Trance-possession Process *222*
Trance-suicide *229*
Trance-possession and Mental Health *230*

Glossary *238*
Bibliography *242*
Index *259*

Tables

7.1 Cases of Suicide Attempts Admitted to Hospitals in Bali in 1989 by Sex, Age, and Marital Status *131*
9.1 Characteristics of Auditory and Visual Hallucinations in the Balinese under Three Different Conditions *192*
9.2 Psychological Process Similarities and Differences in Trance-medium Possession and MPD Alter Personality *213*

Figure

9.1 Parallel Continua of Dissociative Phenomena *178*

Plates

Between pages 48 and 49

1 The usual Balinese household consists of five to seven pavilions. Two women are seated in front of the rice storage house which has sacred status. On the right is the kitchen, in the direction of the sea (*kelod*). In the centre rear is a pavilion for preparing food for family ceremonies. The sleeping pavilions (not pictured) are to the left and front of the rice storage house.

2 Each household has a temple containing shrines of its ancestors and of God. Each shrine is given due respect with periodic ceremonies and offerings. This low middle-class household has six shrines in their temple.

3 Shrines located throughout rice paddies are for the worship of the goddess of rice. Farmers regularly place offerings in these shrines.

4 Rice planting is done on an auspicious day, determined by consulting the Balinese calendar. The men work in the paddies between 3.00 a.m. and 9.00 a.m. and again in the afternoon. Rice farming involves a high degree of co-operation.

5 Rice, a dietary staple in Bali and a result of the gods' assistance, is grown on steep hillsides as well as on the plains. The goddess of rice presides over the irrigation system (*subak*), designed to deliver water to myriads of different levels of paddies.

6 In the Kintamani area, Mt. Batur is regarded as the holy mountain and place of the gods. The crater lake below, believed to be the home of a goddess of the lake, is considered to be holy as well. These examples illustrate the Balinese Hindu belief in the religious aspect of nature.

7 Banyan trees, considered to be the dwelling-places of the gods, are often planted in temple grounds. The Balinese respect every aspect of the non-human environment.

8 Cocks raised for fighting are seen in every village. This old man is tending to the daily feeding of rice and corn. Ceremonial cock-fights have religious significance: spilled blood from the fight appeases the evil spirits who live near the ground. Most cock-fights function primarily as arenas for betting and associated social interaction of men.

9 Each child has a special ceremony at six months of age, in this case presided over by the high priest, who is shown holding the offerings over the head of the birthday child. This ceremony signifies that the spirit of the reincarnated ancestor has left the holy child and the child has now become a person. Following this, the child is allowed to touch the ground for the first time. In this instance, four generations of the family are represented and the child is being carried by the great-grandmother.

10 A child who was born on a bad day (*wuku wayang*) attends a special ceremony to promote a good personality in him. At midnight, after a shadow puppet performance (*wayang kulit*), he is purified by holy water from a sacred puppet.

11 The tooth-filing ceremony, usually held in adolescence, is a very important rite of passage and signifies the expulsion of undesirable, naturally inborn feelings such as jealousy and anger. It is presided over by a priest (left) with the extended family in attendance. The filing of the canines to make them even with the incisors is now slight and symbolic rather than complete and painful as in years past.

12 Every *galungun* (210 days by the Balinese calendar), each household places a *penjor* in front of its house. This is a bamboo pole decorated with symbols to give thanks to the gods for providing the household with products such as rice and coconut. A small bamboo shrine at the base is for offerings.

13 At many crossroads, bridges, and stream or river crossings stands one or more stone-carved gods whose purpose is to ensure safe travel. This four-sided monument in the centre of the capital city of Denpasar is huge with a body and face looking towards each of the four directions. It stands on a lotus blossom, the holy flower.

14 Men of a village in the plains working together to prepare decorations and furnishings for a village ceremony at their temple.

15 Daily offerings are given to the gods and spirits. This young woman is shown setting small offerings of rice, onion, and salt—prepared in the morning before the family has eaten any of these—on a banana leaf on the ground in front of her household gate. Such offerings are also placed at many locations in the household.

16 On ceremonial days, beautifully arranged offerings of fruits, rice, and chicken are prepared in special ways. One member of each family is chosen to bring the offering for the gods to the temple where it will be blessed by the priest and subsequently taken back home for consumption by the family.

17 At a yearly ceremony, in this instance at the village of Jimbaran near Denpasar, an elaborate and artistic offering made of fried pigskin and the pig's head and feet is provided for the gods at the village temple.

18 Women carrying offerings on their heads for a temple ceremony (*odalan*) through the split gate of a village temple in Bangli.

19 Carved stone statues adorn every temple. This statue in Pura Dalem, in the monkey forest at Ubud, depicts the queen of the witches, the evil Rangda. She is in the act of eating her food—a baby held in her arms.

20 Stone carvings at Balinese temples are ornate and graphic. The temple at Ubud features the evil goddess Druga, with pendulous breasts and a 1-metre-long tongue. Behind her is a gate with a typical carved stone symbol of Boma above the doorway, which is believed to help ward off evil spirits.

21 The brightly coloured, mirror-glistening Barong at a ceremony at the mountain village of Kintamani. The holy Barong is a welcome part of many regular ceremonies.

22 The closed temple gate at Kesiman on a non-ceremonial day.

23 Inside the most sacred part of the temple at Kesiman on a non-ceremonial day.

24 A woman with *latah* at the point of surprise stimulation by the person seated next to her (hand visible on the right).

25 The woman in Plate 24, still in the *latah* state, performing a dance suggested by the person who startled her.

26 A 65-year-old woman who has had *latah* for many years sits quietly and calmly, responding to Suryani's questions.

27 The woman in Plate 26 behaving mechanically in a state of *latah* after being startled by a family member.

Between pages 128 and 129

28 A carved stone statue of a *balian* using the smoke technique to treat a client in front of the Mental Hospital in Bangli. The client is shown leaning over a brazier. *Balian* do not treat patients at this hospital.

29 A *balian* trance-medium residing in the Sukawati area poses, seated at her altar, prior to a healing seance. Her face is calm and characteristic of her usual appearance when not in trance-possession. On the left, in front, is incense which is lighted before each seance. In the centre is a tray of offerings. On the right is holy water. The cans in front contain herbal medicaments for clients.

30 The *balian* in Plate 29 in a trance-possession state, in which she assumes the behaviour of the client's ancestor's spirit who possesses her. In trance-possession her eyes are always closed and she speaks animatedly and articulately at a rapid rate.

31 A *balian* trance-medium in Denpasar seated at her altar prior to entering trance-possession to treat her client.

32 The shrine of the trance-medium in Plate 31 contains a Barong mask and several small statues. The statues on top represent her gods. On the lower levels are the gods' helpers, offerings, and a jug of holy water.

33 A client's tray of offerings for the gods of the trance-medium in Plate 31 containing a coconut, rice, an egg, money, and *banten*. Offerings of other clients are strewn on the right. The offering has to suit the type of help needed.

34 In trance-possession, the *balian* in Plate 31 speaks to her client with her eyes open. *Balian* experienced in possession states do not show any of the facial changes seen in ceremonial participants who are less experienced in the trance-possession state.

35 A *balian* trance-medium in Denpasar prior to entering the trance-possession state.

36 The *balian* in Plate 35 in trance-possession, with eyes closed and eyelids fluttering, is shown advising her client.

37 A client in trance-possession while under treatment by a *balian* shows some flattening of the facial muscles and expresses

pain, which is believed to be caused by black magic being extruded during treatment.

38 The client in Plate 37 showing her normal facial appearance immediately following treatment.

39 A *balian usada* living near Klungkung who specializes in the management of black magic spirit possession. Clients often enter into trance during his treatment. In front of him is a client's offering of money.

40 Paraphernalia used by the *balian* in Plate 39 to test for evil spirit possession. The pewter cylinder (centre) is held against the client's forehead for several minutes and if the client falls into trance, black magic is indicated. Black magic is also deemed to be the cause of problems if patients fall into trance at the sight of the ring.

41 This small wooden stick placed between the fingers of a client by the *balian* in Plate 39 causes severe pain if the client suffers from black magic. Otherwise it has no effect.

42 A *balian* in Denpasar who uses Chinese coins to discern his client's problem is shown 'reading' advice from a blank *lontar*.

43 Chinese coins offered by the *balian* in Plate 42 and selected by his client were distributed on a plate by the *balian* in order to determine the reason for the client's visit and the nature of his problem.

44 This masked dancer at the mass trance-possession ceremony at Jimbaran is a companion of Rangda, who acts against the benevolent Barong and his followers. The Jimbaran ceremony, a high point in the life of the village, is held to protect the villagers against disaster and illness and to promote success for everyone.

45 A trancer at the mass trance-possession ceremony at Jimbaran being guided confidently and carefully by two men who are not in trance. On awakening, this man could not recall his behaviour in the trance-possession state.

46 An unconscious trancer at the mass trance-possession ceremony at Timbrah being assisted calmly by two villagers. Following the ceremony, he was amnesic with regard to his trance-possession state.

47 Another unconscious trancer, this time at the mass trance-possession ceremony at Kesiman, being assisted by a villager on each side of him. After being guided into the sacred part of

the temple, he was brought out of trance by the sprinkling of holy water.

48 A villager possessed by a god at the Timbrah mass trance-possession ceremony dancing with a small live chicken in his mouth. He will later swallow the chicken's blood, in imitation of what is believed to be an act of the god possessing him.

49 An unconscious trancer at the Timbrah mass trance-possession ceremony being carried into the sacred part of the temple where he will be revived by holy water.

50 Men in trance-possession performing kris stabbing at the Jimbaran mass trance-possession ceremony. Considerable force is applied to the dagger, but no harm is sustained when the men are in a trance state.

51 The little girl trance-possession dance (*Sang Hyang Dedari*) performed in unison for tourists.

52 The fire/hobby-horse dance (*Sang Hyang Jaran*) performed for tourists at Bona. The fire dancer is able to touch and stand on the hot coals for several seconds without sustaining burns because of a change in sensibility caused by his trance-possession state.

53 In the *kecak* dance, some men in the circular chorus enter trance-possession, as is evident in the two on the right. The female dancer is not in trance-possession.

54 Gamelan musicians before a performance exhibiting facial expressions characteristic of their usual state of consciousness.

55 The gamelan musicians in Plate 54 playing traditional (ceremonial) music and showing the flattened facial expressions characteristic of a trance state.

56 One of the schoolgirls who experienced trance-possession is shown in an unconscious state which lasted about 15 minutes.

57 The same girl in Plate 56 immediately after coming out of trance-possession. She remained confused and appeared to be in an altered state of consciousness for about 10 minutes.

58 Suryani sitting in a meditation state which lasted about 10 minutes. Her facial musculature appears flattened compared with that of her usual state of consciousness.

Introduction

TRANCE in Bali was first studied over 50 years ago by Belo, an American anthropologist and artist. Her book *Trance in Bali* (1960) provided detailed descriptions of many of the ceremonial dances and healers who were possessed and in trance. At about the same time, Bateson and Mead (1942), two of the most famous anthropologists of this century, came to Bali and were fascinated by the people in trance and possession who performed in dramas and dances. They recognized trance in Bali as being essentially the same phenomenon as hypnosis but did not recognize possession. They produced a classic film—still used in college courses in anthropology—of the popular Barong dance in which dancers in trance and possessed by gods stab themselves with krises (daggers). Trance and possession in these forms and many others continue to occur in Bali and may be witnessed by visitors to the island.

At the outset it is helpful to distinguish between the terms 'trance' and 'possession', although these two phenomena are described in detail in Chapter 2. Both are states in which the consciousness of the individual is different from that of his or her usual state. They are traditionally called altered states of consciousness (ASC). The state of trance is essentially and phenomenologically the same as the state of hypnosis. Both can be manifested at varying levels from light to deep. Possession is an ASC distinguished from trance because it is characterized by the experience of being taken over by a power, spirit, or god which then acts through the person, causing the person to behave automatically or without self-control. In the Balinese, a state of trance generally precedes the manifestation of possession and then the two states coexist. In contrast to people in trance, persons possessed are often amnesic for part of or throughout the entire episode. The term 'trancer' may be used to designate a person in a state of trance or trance-possession.

Reading the reports of what was referred to as trance-ceremonies by Belo (1960),[1] one wonders whether some of those ceremonies still take place and if so, how much they have remained the same. As in other countries, Balinese culture is a living system that is continually evolving. However, it is the authors' view that in spite of superficial changes, the basic beliefs, customs (including religious dances and trance-possession ceremonies), as well as the character of the Balinese are essentially as they have been for at least five decades (Jensen and Suryani, 1992). Several other observers have formed similar opinions. Belo (1960) felt that Balinese rituals and character had changed very little between 1935 and 1960. Belo's (1960) and De Zoete and Spies's (1970) descriptions of Balinese dances of the 1930s are strikingly similar to current descriptions, including Jensen and Suryani's (1992), of the same dances and ceremonies. Covarrubias (1937) concluded that the Balinese assimilate new and foreign ideas into their traditional forms, thus enabling them 'to create new styles constantly, to inject new life steadily into their culture, which at the same time never loses its Balinese characteristics'. More recently, Ramseyer (1986) stated that the Balinese absorbed material culture without a break in tradition and that 'the basic values shaped by religious and communal social interactions have remained remarkably intact'.

Whereas the trance-possession ceremonies of Bali have remained essentially unchanged over the years, scientific knowledge about hypnotic phenomena has increased tremendously and the field of psychiatric study has advanced to the point where further study of trance and possession phenomena in Bali can only lead to a better understanding of such processes and their relationship with other unusual psychic activity and psychopathology.

Hypnotherapy, defined as the psychotherapeutic treatment of behavioural and mental problems and disorders by hypnosis, is experiencing a revival or renaissance—the first since the wave of popularity among psychiatrists about 100 years ago (Erikson, 1970). The most famous of the early medical practitioners utilizing hypnotherapy was Charcot in France and his renowned pupil, Sigmund Freud.[2] The current surge of scientific interest in hypnotherapy and its use suggests that it has become better understood, particularly with regard to its functions. Nevertheless, although a great deal has been learned about psychotherapy, which is integral to hypnotherapy, there remain glaring gaps in knowledge about the hypnotic process itself. For example, it is still not known what happens neurophysiologically in the brain to account for the marvellous and often fantastic changes that hypnosis brings about. The answers to such questions may be found in studies of naturally occurring non-therapist induced states of hypnosis or trance.

Trance is but one of what has been popularly called the altered states of consciousness (ASC). Other examples of ASC include meditation and possession. The phenomenon of possession, which has been described in a number of cultures (Oesterreich, 1974) and studied by several scholars of Balinese culture (Bateson and Mead, 1942; Belo, 1960), is well known to the Balinese people. However, Western medicine has paid scant attention to possession and little attempt has been made to explain how it works in terms of Western concepts of psychology and neuropsychophysiology.

Possession usually occurs with trance in Bali and has been woven into its customs since pre-Hindu and prehistoric times, as evidenced by possession in dances that date from those early periods, such as the little girl trance dance, *Sang Hyang Dedari* (Bandem, 1990). The spiritual, ethereal, mystifying, and spectacular manifestations of trance and possession have long fascinated Western travellers and scholars. At times, the concept of possession had led to the unfortunate deaths of innocent individuals, as seen in the persecution of 'witches' in the seventeenth and eighteenth centuries (Hansen, 1969; Oesterreich, 1974).[3] In contrast, possession to the Balinese is rarely a sinister happening; rather, it is in most instances a pleasurable and valued experience. Furthermore, possession in a religious context is regarded as a privilege to the possessed person and it is believed to give some traditional healers special powers which can help heal the inseparable mind and body.

Jensen and Suryani's interest in investigating trance and possession in Bali stemmed from their individual clinical experiences in psychiatry. Suryani discovered that Balinese who tried to commit suicide described experiences during the attempt that indicated that they were in trance. This finding helped to explain the occurrence of suicide in a culture whose religious customs and beliefs forbid the taking of one's own life. Jensen's observations of patients with multiple personality disorder (MPD) in California suggested that the basic process of this disorder might be the same as possession and he recognized that Bali would be an ideal culture in which to study possession phenomena. After a 6-year study of Balinese customs and character (Jensen and Suryani, 1992), the authors were ready to focus on trance and possession in Bali, combining both Balinese and Western approaches and viewpoints and using a common base of knowledge in Western psychiatry.

In this book the authors have brought together a number of studies of normal Balinese in various trance and possession activities and of patients whose problems involved ASC. The data reported were derived from interviews of more than 175 Balinese, conducted in their native language, either Indonesian or Balinese. Although most of the interviews and observations were carried out from 1988, in total they spanned a 16-year period.

Often a great deal of questioning of individual Balinese, as well as of corroborative sources, was required in order to obtain accurate data. Different villagers sometimes gave conflicting information about the meanings of similar ceremonies. For example, at the Jimbaran ceremonies, it was necessary to ask specific questions not only of individual participants but also of the priest who presided at the ceremonies. Several of the village ceremonies reported on were videotaped, as were most of the traditional healers treating their clients. This enhanced the accuracy of hand-rendered interview data and enabled updated observations of events.

Bali offers a particularly rich source for the study of trance and possession because these occur in many aspects of daily life (Jensen and Suryani, 1992). For these reasons and because the two authors are psychiatrists using hypnotherapy both in Bali and America, they elected to study trance and possession in Bali in order to gather information for a more thorough understanding of trance/hypnosis phenomena, possession, hypnotherapy, and dissociative disorders[4] that occur in both Bali and Western cultures. The authors believe that it is useful for Western mental health professionals, including hypnotherapists, to become knowledgeable about possession states because they are aspects of some emotional disorders which are also encountered in Western society, such as cases of patients professing to be possessed and persons believed to be possessed and subjected to exorcism rituals by the Catholic Church.

Trance and possession in Bali are fascinating topics and merit psychologic and psychiatric study in themselves. At the least, such studies would describe trance/hypnosis and possession in a culture currently attracting increasing interest among travellers, scholars, and scientists. There is no country in the world more beautiful and culturally rich in which to observe these phenomena. The legacy of such studies could be the recognition by Western psychology and psychiatry of what has been called the possession syndrome in normal individuals and the roles that trance and possession play in the mental conditions and disorders of Westerners.

1. Although Belo (1960) used the word 'trance' and did not distinguish between trance and possession in terminology, she described trance phenomena as the gods coming down, entering the persons, and speaking through them, which is tantamount to possession.

2. Early in his career, Freud abandoned hypnosis as a technique of therapy in favour of free association because he did not feel he was a skilful enough hypnotist and because patients were not generally hypnotizable. Later in his career, however, he wrote an essay on occult phenomena (Jones, 1953) and noted in a letter, 'If I had my life to live over again, I would study psychical states instead of psychoanalysis.'

3. In New England, 300 years ago, an epidemic of trance and possession disorders resulted in the hanging of more than a dozen persons, mostly women, a result of the notorious Salem (Massachusetts) witch trials. While most persons convicted or suspected of witchcraft in that era in both America and Europe were women, Aldous Huxley described in *The Devils of London* the case of a man convicted of practising witchcraft on a nun in order to possess her and make her become infatuated with him. He was burned at the stake in 1634 (Lewis, 1971).

4. 'Dissociative disorders' is the term used by psychiatry to designate a number of mental disorders, including fugue states, psychogenic amnesia, and multiple personality disorder. All have in common the psychological mechanism of dissociation, defined as a mental separation or split of thoughts, feelings, and actions from the person's usual state of consciousness and current situation (see Chapter 2).

Chapter 1
Bali and Balinese Background*

BALI as a nation has experienced several major political changes over the centuries. It was first colonized by the Hindus who left Java in the fourteenth century and established their kingdoms and religion on the island. Then the Dutch began their colonization with the conquest of North Bali in 1846, followed by that of South Bali in 1908. The Dutch were noted for allowing Balinese culture to continue with relatively little interference or reshaping in their image. After the Dutch came the Japanese who invaded and occupied Bali until their defeat in 1945. In 1946, Bali became a province of the newly independent Indonesian republic; its capital is the city of Denpasar.

The island of Bali is geographically located about 8 degrees south of the equator and about 18 degrees north of the western end of Australia. It is a relatively small island, one of about 13,000 that make up the archipelago of Indonesia, often unrecognized as the fifth largest nation in the world. Bali extends over 5 633 square kilometres and is about twice as long as it is wide. A range of high volcanic mountains divides it into northern and southern portions. For the Balinese Hindu, the mountains are the palaces of the gods. The highest mountain, Gunung Agung (2 900 metres), located in Karangasem district, is sacred to the Balinese Hindus; on its slope stands the oldest and biggest temple in Bali, the mother temple, Pura Besakih.

The population of Bali in 1989 was 2,644,127, with about equal numbers of males and females. This represents less than 2 per cent of the total population of Indonesia, but Bali is the destination

*The content of this chapter is based on *The Balinese People: A Reinvestigation of Character* (Jensen and Suryani, 1992). A knowledge of the fundamental concepts held by the Balinese people, particularly their religious practices and ceremonies, is essential to an understanding of their use of trance and possession.

of more than 50 per cent of tourists visiting Indonesia.

Approximately ninety-three per cent of the Balinese are Hindu. About 5 per cent are Muslim, and the remainder are Buddhist, Protestant, and Catholic. Occupations include farmers (animal husbandry, cultivation of paddy and other crops), foresters, and fishermen, 50.74 per cent; government officers and public services, 15.33 per cent; tradesmen, hotel staff, and restaurant employees, 14.52 per cent; industrial workers, 9.84 per cent; and builders, 4.82 per cent.

Earlier books on Bali (Krause, 1988; Powell, 1930) pictured and described the island at the beginning of this century as a paradise in terms of the beauty of its lush tropical landscape and the grace of its people, often with an unreal emphasis on lovely young women bathing nude under falling water. The former is still very much in evidence, but the latter is uncommon. Although the land is much more densely populated now than it was a half century ago, it remains incredibly beautiful with vistas of terraced rice paddies, some deep green, some brown, mirroring mountains, clouds, and palm trees, set against backdrops of palms, bamboo groves, and an occasional house with a grass roof. A rice harvest is always going on somewhere owing to non-synchronous planting; rice is harvested in the traditional, rather primitive way, with groups of people, predominantly women, cutting the rice plants by hand and carrying them on their heads to another spot where the rice plants are threshed against a board.

There are eight districts (*kabupaten*) in Bali. The villages (*desa*) are made up of organizational units called *banjar*. The total number of *banjar* is about 4,200. These governing and social groups form the basis of much of the communal life of Balinese society. *Banjar* are a major institution in the community. They are the main link with the central government and they transmit directives, as well as co-ordinate the customs of religion. Like the family, they are of critical importance in everyday life. Traditional *banjar* also deal with work, dances, music, and other arts. The *banjar* meeting hall, centrally located in every village, is an open pavilion, serving as a local clubhouse and gathering place day and night. Gamelan clubs often practise at various *banjar*, attracting a few villagers who gather around, chatting and watching. *Banjar* activities can draw large crowds, creating a festive atmosphere occasionally resembling that at temples during major ceremonies.

Members of the *banjar* are obliged to help one another perform a number of duties, especially in religious ceremonies such as the burial of a *desa* citizen and the construction and maintenance of buildings necessary for the functions of the *banjar*. These are obligatory activities for *banjar* members and take precedence over regular jobs and duties, regardless of whether such members are employed by state institutions or private enterprise. A man may need to leave his job without notice and without pay for days, or even weeks, in order to work for his *banjar*. One function of the *banjar* is to interpret the written and unwritten laws of the country and the *banjar* in order to ensure the security and peace of the *desa* and to uphold the honour and good name of *banjar* and *desa*. When problems arise, the mechanisms of the *banjar*, rather than lawyers and courts, settle disputes and mete out punishment. For example, if a *desa* member violates the decorum of the community, breaks its rules, or fails in his duties for the *banjar*, a sacred oath-taking ceremony (*mecor*) witnessed by the men of the *banjar* is held to determine his guilt or innocence. It is understood by all that if the decision is in error and fails to punish the guilty, the gods will do so. A guilty person is sanctioned, fined, or, if convicted of a very serious offence, isolated from the community. The latter punishment is indeed severe because it means that no one in the community will talk to him/her (*puik*) or help him/her to perform religious ceremonies, and the person so punished may not take part in the activities of the *banjar*. An awareness of these sanctions motivates the people to strive faithfully to execute all their *banjar* duties and follow the village rules which are clearly known to all.

Social Systems That Bind

Four social systems bind the Balinese together: the clan system (*dadia*), the stratification system (*kasta*), the community system (*banjar*), and the interest and working group system (*seka*). The *dadia* system encompasses the combined extended families and all the ancestors. In this relationship, family members periodically band together in one place for ceremonies dedicated to the worship of God: at the house shrine (*sanggah* or *mrajan*) for the immediate family or at the temple (*pura*) for the extended family. Besides strengthening the family bond, these ceremonies foster the feeling of devotion to or respect for elders; for example, at the ceremony of death (*nyumbah*), family members eat food which had been offered earlier to their ancestors (*nyurud*).

The family, ancestors, and community are tightly enmeshed and interdependent. No one, except the wanderer or mentally ill, can function without being part of all three. Every Balinese Hindu is imbued with a sense of this trilateral force from birth and this early structuring of reality, with regular and frequent reinforcement, lasts throughout this life and the lives thereafter.

The divisions of caste, originally of Hindu origin, were based on their functions in the community: Brahmana (the highest caste comprising high priests) were responsible for religious ceremonies; Ksatria had roles in the government; Wesia were involved in business and activities involving public welfare; and Sudra were farmers who performed tasks for the other castes as well. There has never been an untouchable or outcast group as in Hindu India. Beginning in the 1920s, some members of the lowest caste, Sudra, objected to the social implications of the caste terminology and changed it to Catur Wangsa (meaning 'four inheritances') or Catur Warna (meaning 'four colours'); they also changed Sudra to Jaba. In Bali, caste is determined by inheritance at birth, but it is no longer significant for an individual's function in society or in an occupation. Today caste is functional only for social status and inheritance. The priestly roles in ceremonies are carried out not only by the high priest but also by priests from the lower castes; in fact, most priests come from the lowest caste. In practice, many people of the Jaba caste regard priests from their caste as having high status, similar to that of the high priests from the Brahmana.

Each community is made up of many groups, each group consisting of individuals who come together for co-operative activities involving specific interests. Such groups are called clubs or *seka*. Each has a specific name according to its activity. There are working groups such as *seka manyi* for cutting rice and *seka numbeg* for cultivating; and there are groups which pursue an interest in the arts and even in palm wine drinking such as *seka gong gamelan* (orchestra), *seka drama* (theatre), *seka barong* (responsible for the care and dances of the *barong*), *kecak* (a dance), and *seka tuak* (palm wine). Young people, e.g. unmarried adolescents, are also members of their own special group called *seka truna-truni*. Equality and co-operation of members are the primary rules of these clubs.

The irrigation groups (*subak*) (Covarrubias, 1937), presided over by the high priest and the goddess of rice, are made up of representatives from villages affected by the regional irrigation systems. They control the distribution of irrigation water that flows from the mountains to the sea and make decisions about planting crops. These complex networks of streams, canals, and ditches, so essential to life, bind large portions of the island together. Allocation of water is up to the *subak*. Villages hold elaborate ceremonies in honour of the rice goddess who protects the rice planting, makes crops flourish, and ensures that rice storage houses in individual homes are full. The last-mentioned custom has recently dropped out since the introduction of new strains of rice which are not suitable for long-term storage, unlike the old traditional rice. *Subak* may be considered a system of the larger community and an expression of long-standing collaborative action on a grand inter-community scale.

Per capita income is relatively low in Bali, currently averaging less than the equivalent of US$500.00 per year. However, poverty is not evident in the way that it is in other developing countries such as India, Mexico, and certain South American countries. There are very few beggars or homeless people, even in the capital city of Denpasar, and even fewer in the countryside. There are no shanty towns. Even the poorest can afford or manage to obtain clothes, shelter, and food. In some villages, Western-type medical care is marginal. However, public health clinics exist even in remote areas.

Bali has no seasons in terms of temperature or planting, only a rainy season from December through March and a dry season. During the rainy season it usually seems hotter because of higher humidity. In the mountain areas it rains more than on plains and along the shores. Water is not a problem (except in the desolate western part of the island); it flows through the rice paddies, and in the streams, rivers, and ditches that run alongside the roads where people still bath themselves and their cows daily. These streams appear dirty from soil they pick up along the way and sometimes from refuse.

Of course, food is a critical aspect of life in Bali. People of all ages tend to be thin and obesity is very unusual. No one goes hungry because of the low cost of food, the availability of natural fruit, the food served at the frequent festivals, and family sharing. Rice is a staple (two or three times a day), but vegetables, meat (beef, pork, and chicken), and seafood (less in the mountains) are also consumed. The food is spicy and often hot with chopped peppers. Spice Islands, a historical name for Indonesia, remains apt.

Each village has its market-place and some of the larger ones draw people from several villages in the area. One can buy all sorts of foods and things: dried fish, live chickens, snacks, refreshments, imported items for homes, kitchen articles, incense, perfume oil from fresh blossoms, thongs, toys, woven mats, and hats. It is a place to meet, to socialize, or to just while away time in a busy, festive atmosphere.

Ceremonies

Religious ceremonies, which are integral to the thinking and attitudes of the Balinese, continue as frequently and as importantly as ever, and remain relatively unchanged over the years in spite of modernization trends. Children are excused from school and adults from work in order to participate in these ceremonies.

Balinese regularly perform a multitude of ceremonies which occupy a relatively large portion of their time and effort, consume a substantial portion of their savings, and are of great significance to their lives. A number of scholars have described many of these in detail (Belo, 1953; Boon, 1977; Covarrubias, 1937; Hooykaas, 1977; and Moerdowo, 1973). Ceremonies usually involve the extended family, one's own *banjar*, or the entire *desa*. Some, such as *panca wali krama* at the mother temple, involve all of Bali: during one month in every 10 years, cars, trucks, and buses bring people of all ages to pray and make offerings. Almost all ceremonies involve the participation of many people. Generally, both men and women take part and their roles are separate. For example, women make the *banten* and other offerings, and help prepare and serve food. Men prepare much of the food to be cooked for feasts, organize and arrange the procedure for the ceremony, attend to the construction of all effigies and special buildings for the occasion, make costumes for the dances, arrange and repair orchestral instruments, and manage the logistical problems which must be dealt with in order to ensure success.

Most ceremonies and dances take place in and around the temple structures, as is strikingly evident to visitors to Bali. There are more then 10,000 temples in Bali, all of which serve a variety of purposes (including those of the family, the state, rice fields, cemeteries, and the sea). The village temples are large enough to accommodate almost the whole community at a single ceremony. Temples are walled-in, open-air areas containing several small pavilions and shrines. Persons of all status, including the poorest families, are free to participate in community festivals and temple ceremonies.

An important group of ceremonies relate to the individual's life cycle (*manusa yadnya*). Each milestone in this cycle is marked by a ceremony, the purpose of which is to expiate past wrong deeds and thereby achieve greater perfection in this life, as well as in future lives. These ceremonies are conducted at birth, at the separation and burial of the placenta, at seven days of age, at one month, at one month and seven days, at three months, at six months, and at birthday celebrations every six months thereafter (*otonan*). Other milestone ceremonies occur at the loss of deciduous teeth, at menarche, at adolescence (e.g. tooth filing, now a token filing procedure to bring the upper teeth into a straight line in order to diminish the six evil qualities of human nature: anger, desire, greed, jealousy, irresoluteness, and intoxication), at marriage and death (e.g. *ngaben*, which includes cremation and *ngrorasin*, which is held twelve days after death), and at unification with God (*ngukur* or *mligia*). An elective milestone in life is the preparation (culminating in the *pawintenan* ceremony) to become a holy person: one who vows celibacy, is instructed in a certain diet (e.g. vegetarian), and participates in other rituals in order to remove bad thinking and better serve God and the gods. This preparation is not the same as that for a priest.

There are many general ceremonies related to time according to the Balinese calendar (e.g. *galungan* and *kuningan*). In a six-month period there are at least five *tumpek* ceremonies. The purpose of *tumpek landep* is to give thanks for all material things made from metal; *tumpek uduh*, for plants, *tumpek andang* or *tumpek uye*, for animals; *tumpek wayang*, for puppets; and *tumpek kuningan*, for the well-being of the world and its contents.

In addition there is the full moon ceremony (*purnama*), as well as the 'dark moon' ceremony (*tilem*); *kajeng kliwon*, which comes every fifteen days, is a potentially fearful time because on this day the evil spirits abound and persons with bad intentions may easily be possessed and, in turn, disturb others. Persons with mental illness generally date the onset of their symptoms to this day.

The ceremony of *nyepi* marks the new year, according to the Balinese Isaka calendar and occurs approximately every 364 days, usually in March. At *nyepi* all fires are extinguished, both literally in the real world and figuratively in hearts that are malevolent. By participating in this day of silence, the Balinese hope to restore inner peace. The day preceding *nyepi* is even more important. Exorcistic rituals of great power are conducted, and these are made more serious by the Balinese notion that for the past five months there have been an unusual number of dangerous demons roaming the villages causing illness, crop failure, and other disasters. The *mecaru* ceremony is performed with offerings and sacrifices (such as a chicken, duck, or cow) to placate the demon deities (*buta-kala*). The *ngrupuk* ceremony is held to appease all evil spirits which surround their homes, family, and members of the *banjar* and *desa* so that they will leave and peace will again prevail.

The ceremonies of *galungan* (every 210 days) and *kuningan* (the tenth day after *galungan*) are major events celebrating man's victory over evil such as anger, jealousy, thievery, and violence. On these festive occasions, there are many colourful ceremonies throughout the island which are easy for the visitor to encounter and attend because they are marked by processions of brightly clothed, traditionally dressed people, accompanied by gamelan orchestras, walking along the road or crowding around roadside temples.

The ceremony of Saraswati is held to thank the goddess of knowledge; Pagerwesi, to make offerings to God for providing welfare and giving happiness to the world and all its contents; and Siwalatri, to give thanks to Siwa for the dissolution of sins, such as being angry at a parent or failing to make an offering to the gods.[1]

Offerings to the gods and God are a part of every ceremony. They usually contain flowers and betel-nut arranged in a small tray made of woven young palm leaf (*banten*) along with incense smoke (*dupa*), and holy water (*tirta*), accompanied by a high priest's *mantera* (i.e. holy chanting to call the gods and God). Other offerings for ceremonies include not only *banten* but also aesthetically arranged baskets or stacks of fruit, eggs, chicken, or duck, which women usually carry on their heads to the temple.

In addition to the general community-wide and individual ceremonies, there are many other ceremonies such as those at home, at a *banjar*, at an anniversary of the construction or repair of a local temple, and even at a specific temple on the grounds of the mother temple at Besakih.

Mead (Bateson and Mead, 1942) has successfully captured the flavour of ceremonial days:

> But at the New Year, these same roads are empty, stretching up and down the frequent hills, between terraced fields holding green rice, to another district where the rice is golden, on to a third where the rice is so young that the flooded beds seem filled mostly with reflections from the sky. The air on every other day of the year is filled with sound, high staccato voices shouting the clipped ambiguous words of familiar speech or artificially prolonging the syllables of polite address, quips of passers-by to the vendor girls who make a professional art of repartee, babies squalling on

hips of their child nurses; over and above and behind all these human sounds, the air on other days carries music from practicing orchestras, from an individual idly tapping a single metallophone, from children with jew's-harps, and from whirring musical windmills set on narrow standards high against the sky. On feast days, the roads are crowded with processions of people in silks and brocades, walking in easily broken lines behind their orchestras and their gods; gods represented by temporary minute images seated in small sedan chairs; gods represented by images made of leaves and flowers; gods which are masks or bits of old relics. With the processions mingle groups of people grimed from work, hurrying lightly beneath heavy loads; and theatrical troupes, their paint and fine costumes tucked away in little bundles, trudge wearily behind the two-man mask, the patron dragon (Barong) who walks quietly with covered face.

To this may be added the heady images of a roadside procession comprising a group of 30 or more men in chorus singing long melodious chords, interspersed with a band of body-resonating giant gongs, throbbing drums, and cymbals; a small forest of coloured tassel-rimmed parasols high above the crowds; long lines of women carrying intricately arranged offerings stacked on their heads, with one occasionally appearing to go spontaneously into trance and possession by the gods while still miraculously maintaining the balance of the offering on her head; people sitting on the temple grounds raising their hands in prayer as the priest casts holy water over them; crowds of people milling about in the gathering darkness, lit only by lantern and moonlight; all seemingly happening at once, raising the emotions to a heightened and sustained level.

Trance rituals and ceremonies play a significant and enduring role in dealing with evil spirits and witchcraft (Belo, 1960). In some villages, almost the whole populace can go into trance at certain ceremonies. However, there are individuals who do not experience trance. Trance and possession states in ritual and dance are socially approved, facilitated, and controlled. McPhee (1946), an observer of trance and possession phenomena in the 1930s that exist today in the same manner and form, vividly described one such occurrence:

While, from the shadows, there came the sound of animated music from the *gamelan*, a group of women stepped forth to dance the *gabor*, the presentation of offerings of wine, oil, incense. Their shoulders were bare, their breasts bound with woven scarves, and in their hair were crowded orchids, jasmine, gardenias. I recognized Nyoman's two wives among them as they danced, seriously, tranquilly, as though in their sleep. In and out of the shrines they wove, disappearing in the shadows, emerging into the moonlight, until at last they paused before the altars, where a priestess stood, to fan the essence of the offerings in the direction of the gods.

It was close to dawn when, in the now almost deserted courtyard, the priestess fell once more in trance. In a hoarse, exhausted voice she announced the presence of the god. It was the god now speaking. There was a pause. The god called attention to the poor condition of the temple. It was in need of repair. Another pause. The priest now asked advice about certain village affairs. What must the offerings be for the next feast? Back and forth the voices went, until at last the priestess grew silent and would talk no more. In the dim light of early morning she woke, looked dazedly around, and we knew the gods had left.

Principal Hindu–Dharma Beliefs in Bali

The Balinese Hindu religion, which is of critical importance to an understanding of the Balinese (Geertz and Geertz, 1975), is unique. It has its roots in India but was developed largely in Java. It has been influenced by Buddhism, by the original Balinese (aboriginal) culture, and by Balinese pre-Hindu animistic and ancestral cults. The five principal beliefs (*panca srada*) are: (1) the existence of a Supreme God (Sang Hyang Widi Wasa); (2) the existence of an eternal soul (*atman*); (3) the conviction that every deed has a reward (*karma pala*); (4) reincarnation (*punarbawa*); and (5) eventual unity with God (*moksa*).

Punarbawa is repeated rebirth into the world until one attains the perfect life, at which point rebirth ends because one has become unified with God. *Punarbawa* is not only a belief but a prominent aspect of daily life. The Balinese believe that the events of a person's current life are caused, in part and often, by deeds in a previous life. One's present life is oriented to expiate past undesirable deeds and work towards a better future life.

In order for families to know what their reborn infant is like, they take him to a spiritual specialist (*balian matuun*) to find out which ancestor's soul is in the child and to find out the nature of that personality. As Mead put it, the body is the clothing for the soul. The *balian* becomes possessed by the soul of the ancestor, which tells the family what it needs in order to carry out its new life; for example, there may be promises that were not fulfilled in a previous life, such as holding a ceremonial puppet performance or offering a roasted pig to expiate a sin. The purpose of this visit is to strengthen the family's hope that their infant's present life will be a success.

The people of Bali believe that it is bad to be born on certain days. For example, *tumpek wayang* (a particular Saturday, *wuku wayang* by the Balinese calendar) is considered inauspicious and a person born on this day is destined to suffer from emotional distress and cause trouble to others. To counteract the consequences of this unfortunate situation, the Balinese perform a special ceremony of atonement in the hope that the gods will confer good fortune on the child and ensure that the unfortunate birthday circumstance will not adversely affect his future development.

The Sibling Spirits

Four spiritual forces which interact to form part of a person's personality are called the 'four siblings' (*kanda mpat*) (Connor, 1982). Their physical manifestations at birth are blood, amniotic fluid, placenta, and the vernix caseosa (the soft cheesy-like material that covers the newborn's skin). They are given respect and offerings by the person concerned; failure to do so could result in their working against that person and causing illness.

Factors in Balance and Concepts of Illness

The Balinese believe that three factors are crucial to a person's well-being, happiness, and health: (1) the microcosmos (*buana alit*), which is the individual or the soul[2] and is a manifestation of God, (2) the macrocosmos (*buana agung*), which is the universe; and (3) God (Sang Hyang Widi Wasa). In their daily lives, at home, in the market, or at the office, the Balinese strive to keep these three factors in equilibrium, a concept called *tri hita karana*. All living and working places have small temples to enable the people to make offerings and pray; for example, one could pray for safe automobile travel by calling on God to preserve the balance of vehicles on the street (the macrocosmos) so that a collision will be avoided and one's soul will not be jeopardized.

The practice of harmony and balance from the Balinese Hindu principles (*tri hita karana*) results in not showing too much vigour of emotional expression of any type and relates to the concept of a centre for all things. *Kaja* (towards the mountain) leads towards the sacred; *kelod* (towards the sea) leads to demons or evil; and the middle world, secular and without special forces, is where the people live. The house is located between the house shrine and the refuse pit (Bandem and deBoer, 1981). There is a middle colour made by mixing all colours, called *brumbum*, which is the symbol of the god Siwa. The village has three temples to protect the people—Pura Puseh (symbol of the god Brahma, the creator of all natural aspects of the world); Pura Desa (symbol of the god Wisnu, who maintains the natural world); and Pura Dalem (located at the local cemetery and symbolizing the power of the god Siwa, who is responsible for destroying life). Centre, harmony, and balance for all are unconsciously striven for in many aspects of thought, emotion, and behaviour in daily living.

The microcosmos (the soul) also interacts with the sibling spirits. To the authors' knowledge, the three factors (microcosmos, macrocosmos, and God) and their 'balance' are more influential in daily life than are the sibling spirits. Peace is attained by doing good deeds and by maintaining balance. Balance determines a person's well-being and imbalance causes symptoms such as anxiety or depression, other mental disorders, and physical illness.

The Balinese believe that one's soul is involved in illness and that they will become vulnerable to illness if the three factors are not in equilibrium. They believe that both natural factors (e.g. fractures and infections) and supernatural factors (e.g. evil spirits, mistakes in ceremonies, and sins of their ancestors) cause illnesses. They regard the traditional healer (*balian*) as being able to understand and treat problems arising from both supernatural and natural causes, and thus able to restore equilibrium of the three factors. They are of the opinion that doctors are able to treat only diseases caused by natural factors. For this reason, if a family member has a mental disorder, the Balinese generally go first to the *balian*. However, whether they go to a *balian* or a doctor, or both, family members also attend ceremonies to help ensure balance and equilibrium of the family and the individual (Connor, 1984).

Traditional healers (*balian*) are of several different types (Connor, 1982, 1986; see also Chapter 3) and they use a variety of techniques, including trance (of the healer and/or client), white magic (to counteract black magic), holy water, medicinal concoctions, meditation, massage, and smoke treatment. Smoke treatment, used for both physical and mental disorders, consists of the client sitting for about 30 minutes in a closed, small tent made of woven palm leaf mats with a smouldering sandalwood fire at the feet (Leimena and Thong, 1983). This is a method to rid the body of black magic or evil spirits.

The range of disorders for which *balian* are successful is wide but not unlimited. They treat disorders caused by natural causes, including fractures and infections, as well as those which Western physicians would regard as primarily psychogenic and psychiatrists would regard as mental disorders. *Balian* are often able to recognize mental and physical illnesses outside their scope of care and may refer their clients to practitioners of Western medicine.

* * *

The island of Bali has retained much of its natural scenic beauty in spite of pressure from a major tourist industry and a rapid infusion of modern technology. More strikingly, the Balinese people have maintained their fundamental customs of centuries past. This stable culture has nurtured a society remarkable for its gentleness and an extraordinarily low prevalence of Western scourges such as child abuse, alcohol and drug addiction, homelessness, and violence. Several Balinese Hindu beliefs are central to the culture and provide the key to the cognitive sets of the people: the Supreme God; the eternal soul; karma; reincarnation; and eventual unity with God. Spirituality is further extended to include all natural things, an extensive world of ancestors, and social systems that bind the people together. The Balinese believe that the microcosmos or soul, the macrocosmos or universe, and God are basic to health and they strive to keep these three factors in balance because lack of balance can result in illness or problems for the individual or the community. Traditional healers (*balian*) utilize a number of techniques to cure illness through restoring balance.

1. God spelled with a capital G means the supreme God. Gods spelled with a small g refer to lesser gods of the Hindu religion or ancestor gods which are manifestations of God or holy ancestors who have become gods.

2. In Bali all kinds of mental activity, including thoughts, emotions, behaviour, and personality, are determined by the soul, while physical activity is a function of the soul. In contrast, Westerners regard mental activity as primarily a function of the psyche or as a mental process, such as cognition.

Chapter 2
Trance and Possession

MOST Westerners know about hypnosis although there are many popular misconceptions. Since it is not usually taught in medical school curricula, the majority of physicians are little more knowledgeable about hypnosis than the general public. To many people, trance seems to be more mysterious than hypnosis because the term is largely associated with the occult or foreign cultures. Possession is equally strange to Westerners since not only is it rarely observed in the West but it is generally associated with bizarre happenings portrayed in the media as part of the religious rites of cults, 'primitive' cultures, or voodoo. Most Western hypnotists are unfamiliar with possession, and few have seen an example of it. People from non-Western cultures, however, tend to have different experiences and views. The Balinese are a case in point. In contrast to Westerners, they regard Western hypnosis as a means to affect a person negatively, not positively. They are familiar with possession (*kalinggihan*) and regard it as an everyday event which can be positive or occasionally negative, depending on the spirit possessed.

Bali offers Western scholars a multitude of opportunities to study the nature of possession. An understanding of the subject is of considerable significance to Western medicine and psychology because possession phenomena also occur in the West. It is important to be able to recognize when they exist in a normal form, such as in certain religious groups, and when they are symptoms of abnormal mental states, including possession disorder (see Chapter 9).

Dissociation

understand trance and possession, one needs to under- ociation. Unfortunately, there is lack of clarity about dissociation because of its many manifestations and the lack of a precise definition (Frankel, 1990). Dissociation is a psychological mechanism which operates in the everyday life of normal people and in abnormal mental states as well. Psychiatry has defined it as an unconscious 'defence'[1] mechanism through which emotional significance and affects (feelings) are split off, separated, or detached from an idea, situation, object, or person (APA, 1984). With some types of dissociation, aspects of experience are not consciously perceived or embedded in one's consciousness. Dissociation is also considered to be a disconnectedness or lack of normal integration of knowledge, thoughts, identity, memory, and control (Frankel, 1990) into the stream of consciousness (Bernstein and Putnam, 1986). There is a disruption of the usual integrative function (Nemiah, 1980) so that for a period of time, certain information is not associated or integrated with other information as it normally or logically would be (West, 1967: 890). Another definition is 'a structured separation of mental processes (e.g. thoughts, emotions, cognition, memory, and identity) that are ordinarily integrated' (Spiegel and Cardeña, 1991). 'Clinically, dissociation involves a fragmentation of consciousness and automaticity, usually for [psychologically] defensive purposes.' (D. Spiegel, 1990: 139.)

In the aggregate, these definitions and descriptions are consistent; they convey the quality of the mechanism and relate to the purposes which dissociation serves. It is common for psychiatry to regard dissociation as a 'defence' against anxiety or awareness of events for which the individual has no voluntary escape (Spiegel, Hunt, and Dondershine, 1988). As Spiegel, Hunt, and Dondershine (1988) put it:

> . . . while dissociation serves the function of defending consciousness from the immediate experience of painful events—physical pain, fear, anxiety, and helplessness—it then becomes an entrenched part of the overall view of self. Once the self is divided in a powerful way, the experience of unity becomes problematic, since ordinary self-consciousness is no longer synonymous with the entirety of self and personal history. Rather, it becomes associated with the awareness of some warded-off tragedy, the moment of humiliation and fear, the act of cowardice, the sense of having been degraded.

However, dissociation is also utilized as part of everyday activities in which one becomes absorbed. E. R. Hilgard (1977), emphasizing the normal aspects of dissociation, formulated dissociation as an extension of normal cognitive functioning.

Normal dissociative phenomena are depicted in famous children's poems such as those in *A Child's Garden of Verses* by Robert Louis Stevenson (1928)[2] and in children's stories such as the fairy-tales of Hans Christian Andersen and *Alice in Wonderland* by Lewis Carroll. These depict the innocent fantasies of being in magical or special places where one experiences perceptions and feelings different from those in the ordinary world.

Alice's adventures and escape into a world of wonder and magic represented or can be seen in part as Carroll's personal escape from his conflictual real world. This is a common dissociative pattern utilized by abused children as well as those capable of rich fantasy. Carroll's depiction of Alice's body shrinking and expanding in size illustrates changes in body schema which may occur when transiting from one state of consciousness to another, or during the dissociative phenomenon of depersonalization. According to one of his biographers (R. Wallace, 1990: 192), Lewis Carroll probably experienced sexual abuse as a child in boarding school and his conflicts of morality in adulthood were consistent with the interpretation that he led a personal life similar to that of the dissociated Jekyll and Hyde (R. Wallace, 1990: 154, 168; see Chapter 9). It is notable that Hans Christian Andersen also experienced significant neglect and loneliness as a child.

It is quite normal for people to dissociate in the activities of daily life. Examples include (1) driving a car and arriving at one's destination without being aware of familiar landmarks, (2) reading a book and ignoring events which one would ordinarily have noticed, and (3) watching a movie and being totally oblivious to one's surroundings. Such situations in which the person becomes so absorbed by certain thoughts or stimuli that he appears to lose touch with what is going on around him can stretch over relatively long periods of time. Many types of behaviour which are considered automatic or absent-minded, such as putting bananas in the wrong dish or placing a warm cup of coffee in a refrigerator in the morning and then forgetting where it was placed, may be attributed to dissociation.[3] A proverbial 'absent-minded professor' demonstrates dissociation, not memory problems. The husband who is so absorbed in the morning paper that he totally ignores his wife is probably dissociating. A high frequency of dissociative experiences has been noted in adolescents (Bernstein and Putnam, 1986) and college students (Myers and Grant, 1970; Sedman, 1966). Dreams are a form of dissociation in which one's thoughts are separated from normal consciousness and take different forms. When awakening from a dream, one may feel briefly that the events were real; however, on returning to a normal conscious state, one realizes that what has happened is only a dream. Dreams, like hypnotic states and unconscious thinking, follow non-logical patterns of thought and images. This pattern in some aspects of hypnosis has been called trance-logic (Brown and Fromm, 1986). Trance clearly involves the 'defence' mechanism of dissociation.

Ludwig (1983) pointed out that the mechanisms of dissociation have great individual and species survival value in that they provide (1) an escape from overwhelming reality, (2) a cathartic discharge of feelings, (3) a resolution of irreconcilable conflicts, (4) an ability to perform some behaviours automatically thereby permitting simultaneous conscious engagement in other behaviours, and (5) a beneficial enhancement of the 'herd sense', i.e. the human inclination to be affiliated with people engaged in similar activities.

Dissociation plays a predominant part in normal behaviour and sometimes in problematic sexual behaviour as well. For example, in their studies of the treatment of sexual disorders, Masters and Johnson (1970: 65–6) discovered that dissociation is a common aspect of male impotence.

They described the 'spectator role' or 'spectatoring': the patient behaves as if he is visualizing his lovemaking outside of himself or as if he is viewing his own sexual behaviour from a corner of the room. This phenomenon involves depersonalization and possibly the hidden observer effect of hypnosis, both of which are forms of dissociation.

The Balinese recognize a pattern of behaviour called *ngramang sawang* which literally means 'absent thinking' or 'no emotions'. It is characterized by an absence of thoughts, a staring or vacant-like facial expression, and inactivity, usually brief but lasting for about 1–5 minutes. Generally, *ngramang sawang* is brought on by a problem, such as a recent disagreement, or by frustration, disappointment, or simply fatigue. It is not seen very frequently. It often evokes the sympathy and interpersonal supportive behaviour of a friend or family member. *Ngramang sawang* tends to terminate rather abruptly. It appears that this behaviour is a form of dissociation which may be likened to meditation or self-hypnosis at a shallow level.

The many kinds of perceptions and experiences that typify dissociation can be measured quantitatively by using the Dissociative Experiences Scale or DES (Bernstein and Putnam, 1986). It enumerates 28 dissociative behaviours and serves as an index of the various kinds of behaviour, as well as a gauge of how frequently they occur.[4] Studies of dissociation using the DES in normal subjects revealed that over 25 per cent reported a substantial number of dissociative experiences (Ross, Joshi, and Currie, 1990). Bernstein and Putnam (1986) did not find any difference between males and females in their capacity to dissociate. Of all the dissociative disorders, multiple personality disorder (MPD) scores highest on the scale—40–50 per cent—in terms of frequency and intensity of experiencing the behaviour measured, which is far above the normal range. Persons with post-traumatic stress disorder (PTSD) score lower than those with MPD but their scores are also abnormally high (Carlson and Rosser-Hogan, 1991). The instrument can be helpful clinically in clarifying the diagnosis of dissociative disorders.

'Hidden by the Evil Spirit'

A unique form of dissociation called 'hidden by the evil spirit' (*engkebang memedi*) occurs in Bali. This condition is seen commonly in normal persons and also occasionally in psychotic individuals. While serving in the psychiatric unit of a hospital in Bali in 1976, Suryani observed *engkebang memedi* in two normal individuals and in six psychotic patients, all males. In all eight cases, the person concerned disappeared for a period of 7–30 days. The disappearance was considered to have been caused by an evil spirit who had hidden the person because he loved him. The Balinese believe that this evil spirit is small, has red hair, and lives in bamboo groves.

When a Balinese disappears, the first thing his family does is to approach a traditional healer who will usually say that the person has been hidden by an evil spirit. In an attempt to drive away the evil spirit, the family members walk through the village making a gong-like sound by striking a rod on a piece of iron. In most cases, when the missing person is found—in a cemetery, in a market-place, or near bamboo trees—he appears confused and has difficulty talking. He may recount such experiences as having gone to a beautiful home where he was treated like a king, where a beautiful woman offered to marry him, or where he was asked to stay and not go home. When confronted by his family with the real situation—e.g. being found in the cemetery or the market-place—the person is incredulous; as one afflicted person insisted, 'But I saw a palace here!' After the family conducts a purification ceremony to bring the person back into the real world, he returns to his normal state. A person suffering from *engkebang memedi* is rarely taken to psychiatrists and thus rarely hospitalized since the condition is not regarded as a mental disorder in Bali. By contrast, if such behaviour had occurred in a Western culture, it would likely have been regarded as abnormal and dysfunctional and classified as a type of dissociative disorder.

There is no condition reported in either Western or Eastern literature that corresponds to *engkebang memedi*. It resembles a fugue state in only a few respects.[5] No information is available on what actually happens to the afflicted person during his disappearance. The condition is a dissociative phenomenon.

Latah

To observe *latah* is to be struck by an exciting, dramatic, and puzzling condition (H. Geertz, 1968). *Latah* is basically an uncontrollable behaviour reaction occurring in certain individuals when startled by others. Kenny (1985) described it as a

> reduction in powers of self-control caused by sudden fright or startle reaction which leads to involuntary and normally inappropriate acts which may include one or more of the following: (a) mimicry; (b) compulsive obedience to commands; and (c) the utterance of affect-laden words generally pertaining to sexuality.

He also referred to it as 'startle', which leads to temporary dissociation accompanied by compulsive obscenity and/or mimicry. Because spectators are amused by the behaviour, they often intentionally provoke the reaction in persons with a known history of *latah*.

In the literature, *latah* has been called a culture-bound syndrome (Simons, 1985b) and even a mental disorder. It was originally discovered in Malaysians, but subsequently found in Indonesians (H. Geertz, 1968) and eventually in a number of other cultures widely distributed throughout the world,[6] although this is the first report of it in Bali.

A number of studies have attempted to explain the nature and mechanism of *latah*. A controversy exists between psychiatrists and anthropologists as to whether its origin is biologically (Simons, 1985b) or culturally (Kenny, 1985) based. Simons (1985b: 41) proposed that *latah* 'is best understood as a culture-specific elaboration of the potential startle reflex' inherent in all persons. *Latah* is included in this book because, in the authors' view, it is fundamentally a dissociative condition. Two case-studies of *latah* are given below.

Case 1

This man of high caste (Wesia) is a respected teacher at the high school. He is 48 years old and married. Jovial and friendly, he was happy to talk about his experience of *latah* and willing to give a demonstration. He explained that if someone unexpectedly stimulates him, such as by sticking him in the ribs, he becomes uncontrollable, automatically making sounds to indicate that he wishes to avoid further stimulation; at the same time, he directs his attention to the causal stimulus and focuses on it, unaware of the people around him. Although he appears to be laughing and enjoying himself, he is not. Immediately after he stops the uncontrollable laughing, he becomes aware of his environment again. The first time he experienced *latah* was in 1963, when he was at college in Surabaya. At that time, if his peers continued to stimulate him intermittently, the uncontrollable movements and expressions could go on for 30 minutes or more and he would feel tired afterwards.

According to this person, the reaction may be set off initially by someone touching him, but it can be continued simply by a similar threatening gesture. During the demonstration, he laughed very vigorously as he motioned and moved his arms and body about, as if to avoid any further touching. He shouted, '*De, de, de, Ai*' (No, don't do it! Ah!) repeatedly. When he was moving about in this manner, he was unaware of his surroundings and felt as if he was being 'pushed' by someone. This man's sister also suffers from *latah*, as do some members of his extended family. Neither he nor his sister has ever had any experiences with trance or possession. The *latah* reaction experienced by him and his sister has remained the same up to the present day. Neither one has any personality disorder; they are perfectly normal and have no symptoms of hypomania. He denied that *latah* ever concerned him or that it ever produced any embarrassment. On the contrary, he regarded it as an enjoyable situation in which the people around him laughed and enjoyed themselves as well. His sister described her reaction similarly, including the automatic behaviour. Neither she nor her brother has ever had any amnesia regarding the event.

Case 2

This 50-year-old unmarried woman of high caste (Wesia) was interviewed in the presence of a number of family members at her house. Her first *latah* experience was at the age of 30. Speaking cheerfully and animatedly, she informed us that when she is stimulated by surprise, she repeats words that people speak to her and says some obscene words. This state lasts for about 5 minutes without repeat stimulation, but longer if the stimulation is repeated. She does not always recall what she has said, and she has partial amnesia especially if the episode lasts for 30 minutes or more. During the episode, her behaviour is not under her control and she answers questions incoherently. For example, in response to the question why she behaved that way, she answered, 'Corpse'. The obscene words she used spontaneously in the episode observed by the authors were 'fuck' (*bangsat*), 'corpse' (*bangke*), and 'vagina' (*teli*). She also repeated short sentences or words spoken to her. *Latah* never strikes her spontaneously. She feels no embarrassment over it and acknowledges that the people around her enjoy the episode as much as she does. Her personality is regarded as normal and she does not have any mental symptoms or disorder.

Latah is an Indonesian word; the Balinese word for it is *gegean*. The condition is accepted in the Balinese culture in the same way that trance and possession are accepted. Far from considering it to be a source of unkind teasing, the Balinese look upon *latah* as being rather entertaining.

The descriptions of *latah* in the two case-studies above illustrate several points about the condition:

1. It is not a mental disorder in Bali, as persons with the condition never seek help for it from either psychiatrists or traditional healers.
2. It probably has a partial genetic basis as illustrated in its tendency to run in families[7] with an abrupt onset in full-blown form at a particular point in the life cycle of the individual (usually young adulthood).[8]
3. It presents as a constellation of behaviours in Bali as well as in a variety of characteristic diverse cultures.
4. The mechanism is fundamentally dissociation.[9]

Factors that support the dissociation hypothesis are abrupt onset and termination, the individual's loss of awareness of his immediate environment, attention focused only on the stimulus, automatic behaviour not in the stream of normal consciousness, and amnesia (partial or complete) concerning the episode. When the process or mechanism of *latah* is viewed as a dissociative reaction or condition, it seems more understandable. It can be interpreted as a basically psychobiological response with specific patterns of behaviour acquired by operant conditioning of the individual and shaped by expectations of the particular culture in which it occurs. It need not be seen as either a biologically or a culturally determined phenomenon but rather as one involving both factors. A genetic basis is further supported by the fact that not all persons are capable of the response. In this respect, it resembles trance and possession.

It may seem striking to a Westerner that most Balinese individuals manifesting *latah* do not experience embarrassment or shame, given that they exhibit sometimes shocking and totally out of character behaviour, individually and culturally, including the use of obscene language.[10] This characteristic of *latah* also points to dissociation as the basic mechanism. *Latah* behaviour of the Balinese, like that in a state of trance-possession, may be totally out of keeping with the person's usual behaviour. It may be even highly critical or insulting of individuals in the family or outside but it is never considered negatively by the audience. Because *latah* is not considered abnormal or symptomatic by the Balinese, the term 'syndrome', which signifies symptoms, and the term 'disorder', are not entirely appropriate; consequently the term 'condition' has been used in this book.

Dissociation in Mental Disorders

The Western definition of a dissociative disorder is a partial or complete loss of (1) the normal integration between memories of the past, (2) the awareness of identity and immediate sensations, and the control of bodily movements (WHO, 1992). Some dissociative disorders may involve trance and possession, as described in Chapters 8 and 9.

The dissociative phenomena manifest in mental disorders take multiple forms but can be defined clinically in terms of constellations of five core symptoms (Steinberg, 1991b): (1) amnesia, i.e. a specific and significant segment of time that is unavailable to memory

(Steinberg, Howland, and Cicchetti, 1986; Steinberg, Rounsaville, and Cicchetti, 1990); (2) depersonalization, i.e. a sense of detachment from self (Mayer-Gross, 1935; Steinberg 1991b); (3) derealization, i.e. a sense that one's surroundings are unreal (Steinberg, 1991b); (4) identity confusion, i.e. a feeling of confusion, uncertainty, or puzzlement regarding one's identity (Steinberg, 1991b); (5) identity alteration, i.e. objective behaviour that indicates a change in identity (Steinberg, Howland, and Cicchetti, 1986; Steinberg, Rounsaville, and Cicchetti, 1990). All or some of these symptoms occur in the various types of dissociative disorders (e.g. MPD and PTSD).

Trance/Hypnosis

Trance is an altered state of consciousness (ASC) characterized by changes in cognition, perceptions, and/or physiologically based sensibilities. In these aspects it is identical to hypnosis, which produces a state in which cognition and perception are altered (Frankel, 1976). Brown and Fromm (1986) have stated that 'dissociation is part of many hypnotic experiences'.

Hypnosis is generally brought on or induced by another person, the hypnotist, and involves a relationship between the two (Brown and Fromm, 1986). Hypnosis induced by the individual herself/himself is called self-hypnosis. Trance states in most cultures do not involve intentional induction by another individual but occur spontaneously, often in association with music, chanting, singing, or verbal encouragement (Rouget, 1985). Mind-altering or hallucinogenic plants or drugs are used in association with trance ceremonies in some cultures and these may also have supernatural significance.[11] The Balinese do not use 'mind-altering' substances or drugs in connection with trance. (In fact, they use very little alcohol and few psychoactive substances except betel-nut.) The *balian* usually lights incense sticks at the beginning of each treatment session and some smoke is inhaled. The ASC of trance and hypnosis can be induced in a variety of circumstances, including solitude, in groups, in ceremonies, and in therapy. The terms 'trance' and 'hypnosis' overlap and can be used interchangeably to refer to the same biopsychological state. Both show similar aspects of ASC.

Trance/hypnosis has both subjective and objective manifestations. Subjectively, the individual recognizes and can often describe changes in perceptions and feelings, such as a sensation of darkness or a sense of the body floating. There is a constriction of attention with consequent loss of awareness of much of the surrounding environment (Brown and Fromm, 1986). Trancers may also experience hallucinations. They often describe a richness or vividness of normal thought or visualization (generally with their eyes closed). Objective signs of trance/hypnosis include fluttering and slowly closing eyelids (indicating a state of light trance); abnormal postures (e.g. the arm rising slowly, but automatically, and held steadily and comfortably in a raised position for a prolonged period of time); decreased sensitivity to painful stimuli (e.g. walking on hot coals without feeling any pain); changes in physiological response to heat, cold, or piercing the skin (e.g. no blistering after touching hot objects); little bleeding when cut, as in surgery or tooth extraction; and increased sensitivity to stimuli (e.g. perception of pain when the hypnotist suggests that a pencil eraser is burning hot). It is important to note that all of these manifestations, including hallucinations and 'messages from spirits' while in trance states, also occur in normal, asymptomatic, non-mentally ill people.

The 'psychological set' of the trance/hypnosis subject is characterized by feelings of trust and a desire to allow oneself to enter and go freely into the state. Orne pointed out that 'the skills of the hypnotist consist largely in creating a context where the patient can feel comfortable, trusting and willing to allow himself or herself to respond' (Soskis, 1986). Jensen and Suryani (1992) hypothesized that the strong sense of trust-belief in the Balinese personality facilitates trance induction. This trust-belief is derived not only from a prolonged period (by Western standards) spent in the company of supportive and loving parents and caretakers in infancy and early childhood, but also from the closeness and security imparted by one's family, ancestors, and sibling spirits throughout life. Jensen and Suryani (1992) also identified hypnotizability or hypnotic susceptibility, meaning an inherent facility in a majority of the population to enter trance easily, as another trait of the Balinese.

It has been commonly believed that under hypnosis, people will not do what they would not want to do when in their non-hypnotic state; i.e. their morals and ethics are maintained in the trance state. The case of suicide while in trance may be an exception to this general rule (see Chapter 7).

E. R. Hilgard (1977) discovered that under hypnosis people can experience events as if they are observing their own behaviour and are cognizant of what is happening to them. For example, a hypnotized subject is told to be insensitive to pain. After immersing his hand for several minutes in ice water, the person may be asked by the hypnotist to touch that isolated part of himself that can feel the pain. The hypnotized or dissociated pain response can be activitated by invoking a type of mental function known as the 'hidden observer'. This 'hidden observer' is aware of the pain and says something to this effect: 'I know it is painful but it does not trouble me and I can endure it further.' A similar phenomenon probably occurs in Balinese in trance states who observe their own behaviour performed by the god or spirit possessing them (see 'Individual Trance-possession' in Chapter 5).

After coming out of hypnosis or trance, the persons affected may or may not recall what happened to them during the hypnotic or trance state. Subjects waking up from light trance states can usually recall the events during trance. If a hypnotist suggests to his hypnotized subjects that they will not recall something on 'awakening', they will not be able to recall it.

Whether experiences during trance or hypnosis are recalled post-hypnotically or not, they often have a profound psychological impact on the individual. For example, a hypnotist's suggestion to a subject that he/she is in control of his/her own body (only one among many statements made) may be regarded by the subject as being particularly meaningful. This is one illustration of the potential therapeutic impact of hypnotherapy. In Bali, it is quite common for a person's entire lifestyle or career to be changed as a result of a single trance experience in which a god told him/her to become a *balian*.

There is a contagious nature of trance (Chapters 4 and 9) and what has been called a 'field effect' of the ASC of meditation, i.e. the effects on others in the vicinity (Chapter 8). Contagion and after-effects of trance in the audience of shaman were described in the Eskimo Tungus culture by Shirokogoroff (1935: 53):

> The rhythmic music and singing and later the dancing of the shaman gradually involve every participant more and more in a collective action. When the audience begins to repeat the refrains together with the assistants, only those who are defective fail to join the chorus. The tempo of the action increases, the shaman with a spirit is not more an ordinary man or relative, but is a 'placing' (i.e. incarnation of the spirit); the spirit acts together with the audience, and this is felt by everyone. The state of many participants is now near to that of the shaman himself and only a strong belief that when the shaman is there the spirit may only enter him, restrains the participants from being possessed in mass by the spirit. This

is a very important condition of shamanizing which does not however reduce mass susceptibility to the suggestion, hallucinations, and unconscious acts produced in a state of mass ecstasy. When the shaman feels that the audience is with him and follows him he becomes still more active and this effect is transmitted to his audience. After shamanizing, the audience recollects various moments of the performance, their great psychophysiological emotion and the hallucinations of sight and hearing which they have experienced. They then have a deep satisfaction—much greater than that from emotions produced by theatrical and musical performances, literature and general artistic phenomena of the European complex, because in shamanizing the audience at the same time acts and participates.

One type of trance in Bali may be termed self-hypnosis: this is often seen in musicians playing traditional gamelan music (described in Chapter 6). Unlike most trances in Bali, this state is not associated with possession.

There is evidence of brain wave changes in hypnosis, although these have not yet been confirmed. In experimental studies of religious trance, Goodman (1972) reported a predominance of theta (5–7 cycles per second) waves on EEG (electroencephalogram) tracings. Beta-endorphin blood levels were also elevated on the conclusion of the experiments which could account for the euphoria often reported following religious trance experiences. The very deep hypnotic state was correlated with reductions in EEG amplitude.

The capacity to experience trance has been regarded as a psychobiological heritage of mankind (Bourguignon, 1973: 11). This is supported by an extensive literature on hypnosis in animals which suggests that hypnosis or dissociation may be a primitive psychobiological mechanism of self-defence, evolutionarily acquired in a number of species, with genetic components (Gallup, 1975; Gallup and Maser, 1977; Herzog, 1978; Klemm, 1966). Several species of animals, including monkeys, have been observed to engage in sudden changes in behaviour, such as resorting to immobility, as defence reactions against harm from other animals in situations of attack, fear, and terror. This behaviour, also called tonic immobility, consists of a virtual absence of movement (apart from falling) and a degree of muscle rigidity. The state can be provoked experimentally in birds, chickens, and cats by subjecting them to restraint and forced immobility. It occurs in natural situations, sometimes in cock-fights, and in Balinese ceremonies in which cocks are forcefully restrained as they are carried on poles.

Darwin proposed that feigning death might protect against predators reluctant to eat dead meat. Physiological concomitants of the condition include increased autonomic and EEG arousal patterns, described as 'EEG-behavioural dissociation' (i.e. EEG arousal along with behavioural 'sedation'). The neurotransmitter serotonin has been implicated in the neurophysiologic mechanism of tonic immobility (Wallanau and Gallup, 1977).

If trance and dissociation are evolutionarily acquired biopsychological mechanisms of man, they may be expected to be evident in some form in chimpanzees, man's closest evolutionary predecessors. The following pattern, usually termed a 'display', may in fact represent a dissociative phenomenon. Wild chimpanzees occasionally engage in episodes of apparently unprovoked explosive, aggressive-like behaviour while in the presence of other animals or humans; they suddenly charge through the forest or clearing for distances of up to about 50 metres, move their arms wildly about, and hoot loudly with a characteristic vocalization but do not directly attack other chimps or humans sitting or standing within a few feet of their path (van Lawick-Goodall, 1967).[12] Jensen's study of wild chimpanzees at Gambe Stream Reserve in Tanzania in 1974 showed that this charging behaviour, like dissociation, had an abrupt onset and termination and was relatively brief, mechanical, and stereotyped. It appeared as though the chimpanzee had briefly entered an ASC, possibly in an attempt to cope with or to discharge an inner state of tension. This behaviour of the chimpanzees is similar to some human dissociative behaviours, particularly those which have arisen as a means to cope with situations of anxiety and fear (see Chapter 9).

The theoretical concepts of dissociation and repression as discussed in the literature with regard to hypnosis can be confusing. As E. R. Hilgard (1977) pointed out, 'In clinical settings it may be expected that some dissociative phenomena and some repressive phenomena will be found together, and sharp distinctions between dissociative and repressive interpretations may be inappropriate.' Strictly speaking, dissociation involves a separation of thought from consciousness, which can be accessed if amnesia is overcome. Material regarded as repressed in the unconscious may be expressed symbolically or illogically and is often revealed only by inference, e.g. the interpretation of the symbolic content of dreams. So-called repressed material is also expressed during possession. E. R. Hilgard (1977) distinguished two kinds of repression: in the first one, the contents are concealed and have to be inferred; in the second, conflictual material arising from the earlier stages of development and impulses are inadequately translated into verbal symbols. A third kind of repression could perhaps be identified in the repressed impulses and ideas expressed by possessed Balinese in certain ceremonials or by *balian*, in which the contents are clearly and logically revealed. It is probable that what Freud originally referred to as repression is the amnesia of hypnotic states.[13] While the concept of repression is prominent in psychiatry and particularly in psychoanalysis, Holmes (1990) noted that 60 years of research has not produced any controlled laboratory evidence supporting it. Frankel (1990) argued that 'the concept of dissociation increasingly preempts repression and other defense mechanisms' but nevertheless cautioned restraint in too broad use of the concept of dissociation.

Possession and Trance-possession

In many cultures throughout the world, possession commonly occurs with the trance state. In a survey of 488 societies worldwide, 90 per cent had institutionalized some form of altered states of consciousness and 52 per cent associated these states with possession (Bourguignon, 1973). Bourguignon (1976) felt that these figures probably represented an under-reporting of the phenomenon. The common pattern described is given below:

> An individual suddenly seems to lose his identity and become another person. His physiognomy changes and shows a striking resemblance to the individual of whom he is, supposedly, the incarnation. With an altered voice, he pronounces words corresponding to the personality of the new individual. (Ellenberger, 1970: 13.)

Possession has a long history dating at least to the New Testament.[14] An early work by Oesterreich (1974), a German philosopher, reviewed in detail many historical documentations of possession from the second century to the nineteenth century in Greece, Mesopotamia, Western civilizations, and 'primitive' cultures throughout the world. He noted the uniformity of the reported phenomena, including observable manifestations (e.g. a typical physiognomy) and subjective manifestations. Except for possession in the shaman, almost all instances he reported were associated with religious entities (i.e. devils and demons) and involved unwanted, symptomatic, maladaptive, negative states in the individual and his society. A more current view of possession states in diverse cultures, indicates that most instances are not maladaptive, negative, ...omatic (Bourguignon, 1976).

...esterreich distinguished 'somnambulist' possession in which the subject loses consciousness from 'lucid' possession in which the subject does not lose consciousness and is not amnesic. The majority of cases involved treatment by exorcism. While he noted that a number of cases appeared to be identical to 'divided personality', the documentation provided was insufficient to make a clear determination. He pointed out that during possession, most cases took on a totally different personality.

In cases of possession, Oesterreich (1974) emphasized the critical role of belief in spirits and demons, for the most part negative but sometimes positive. He stated that possession usually produced an impression of horror and something sinister. On the other hand, spirits, alleged to speak through the possessed, afforded 'primitive' people a means for obtaining revelations, a value he felt was insufficiently appreciated by academic ethnology. As he put it:

> By the artificial provocation of possession primitive man has, moreover, to a certain degree had it in his power to procure voluntarily at a set time the conscious presence of the metaphysical, and the desire to enjoy that consciousness of the divine presence offers a strong incentive to cultivate states of possession quite apart from the need to ask advice and guidance from the spirits. (Oesterreich, 1974: 377.)

Oesterreich (1974: 378) went on to say that possession began to disappear among 'civilized races' as belief in such spirits lost its power.

The majority of indigenous American societies practised a phenomenon that anthropologists have called the 'guardian spirit complex' (Benedict, 1923). In some tribes, it was the practice for an adolescent to obtain a lifelong supernatural helper from whom he would gain for himself a name, as well as power through a visionary experience. In the Pacific North-west Coast area, the Kwakuitl tribe once staged a dramatic performance of spirit vision and possession during a secret society initiation (Jilck, 1982: 10). In the Pacific North-west Salish culture, an intimate relationship existed between shamanism and the guardian spirit doctrine (Benedict, 1923: 67). Shamans may obtain their powers from several spirits. Experienced Salish spirit dancers were able to exercise some control over their spirits and to determine to a certain extent the time of possession (Wick, 1941). Observations of the Vancouver Island Salish have revealed the 'comatose' state of new dancers possessed by their spirits' power and the automatic singing and barking of the possessed dancers.

Psychological and anthropological accounts of possession (Cardeña 1989; Bourguignon, 1968; Frigerio, 1989; Goodman, 1988; Linton, 1956) rarely contain detailed descriptions of the subjective experiences of the possessed person. An exception is Wick's (1941) record of a dancer's experience of possession: 'When you sing, your breath starts shaking. After a while, it goes into you. You try to sing, your jaws start to shake, then you sing out, "Get over it. When I dance, I don't act. Just follow your power; just follow the way of your power."'

Although possession has been studied by ethnologists for many years, relatively little attention has been paid to it by psychiatrists and psychologists. Janet (1898) was familiar with the literature on spiritualism and had discussed how the phenomena of the mediums of the era, as well as 'devil possessions' of an earlier age, reflected the same mechanisms of dissociation that he found in his hysterical patients. Freud (1950) devoted one paper to an analysis of a case of demoniacal possession which occurred in the seventeenth century. He called it a neurosis, attributing it to the inner life of the patient, and believed it to be caused by rejected and repressed culturally evil wishes.

Linton (1956), an anthropologist at Yale University, reviewed the known world-wide instances of possession, various forms of which he referred to as hysterias. These included the classic so-called culture-bound syndromes of *amok*, *latah*, Arctic hysteria, soul loss, and the 'hysteria of shamanism'. Curiously, he noted that possession was extremely rare in American Indians. The Algonquin tribe and other northern Indian tribes had a form of 'intermittent possession' in which one's soul would make demands on an individual through dreams. For instance, if one had an overwhelming desire, and it was essential to satisfy this need, the soul would bring about temporary changes in one's personality. Linton (1956: 121) cited the following example:

> A woman would occasionally dream that she wanted unlimited intercourse. Since this was regarded as a demand of her soul, it did not interfere with her social status as a respectable woman. She could, therefore pick out a whole collection of men anywhere (from 10 to 20) and could proceed to have intercourse with one after another until her soul (and presumably her body) was satisfied.

According to Linton (1956: 123), spirit possession is a means to provide a temporary physical body for supernatural beings:

> The supernatural being can become *pro tem*, a contemporary member of the society, so that people can deal with him, ask him questions, ask him for favors, get him to use clairvoyance to tell them what is happening at a

distance, and so on. Since there is a demand for these things, the individual who shows the capacity for such seizures will be encouraged and rewarded by the society.

This statement fits possession in Bali except for the implication of a true 'seizure'.

Linton (1956: 131) further described mediumistic hysterias as falling somewhere between regular possession by spirits and the mystic experience:

The idea behind this is that there is a need for complete passivity, and complete withdrawal, in order to encourage the controls, who either speak through the body of the subject or else draw upon his body energy or ectoplasm, which they can shape in various ways. Such mediumistic phenomena are widespread but are usually demonstrated only by minor practitioners. Although they rarely are the center of organized religion, they do flourish at least on the outskirts of our culture' [and it is an interesting fact that] the stories which are told about psychic phenomena are curiously uniform all over the world.

Linton (1956: 132) concluded that

hysterical phenomena are everywhere, very decidedly culturally patterned. In fact if one knows the culture, one can predict what form hysterias are going to take in that society—or pretty nearly so. This is the strongest possible argument in favor of the thesis that, whatever the etiology and dynamics of hysteria may be, its symptoms are extensively and intensively shaped by culture.

Cardeña (1989), a psychologist, and Frigerio (1989), an anthropologist, both proposed that there should be a range of possession experiences rather than a unitary state of consciousness in which the individual is totally amnesic for the events of the possession. Cardeña's proposal includes (1) 'transitional possession' with occasional changes in depth of involvement rather than a fixed state of consciousness or what some may call partial possession with a conscious awareness and changes in body sensations; (2) 'alternate identity possession' in which an alternate identity, human or otherwise, takes over the usual identity of the individual and there may be co-occurrence of the usual identity of the individual along with the alternate one which stabilizes the transitional possession into a stable state of consciousness with precise limits as defined by the spirit or force and the ritual context; and (3) 'transcendent possession' in which the individual is totally immersed or 'surrendered' and the individual does not perform the acts, songs, or movement but becomes 'him/herself, the act, the song and movement'. In this dimension, the individual may experience a sense of enormous energy. 'There is full absorption into an experience where inner and outer are indistinguishable' and the individual may not fully remember the events transpiring. Common manifestations found in various cultures include unusual vocalizations and movements, shaking, apparent immunity from damage, unfocused or fixed gaze, and eyes rolling upward. The individual may maintain intermittent contact with the social/physical context. According to Cardeña (1989), it is difficult to induce this condition at will.

Frigerio (1989) also proposed three stages with three levels of awareness as reported by Afro-Brazilian religious groups observed in Argentina: (1) the individual is aware of and later remembers everything that happened during possession; (2) the individual only remembers certain things; and (3) the individual remembers nothing. Frigerio referred to the first stage as 'irradiation', where some of the entities' energy is reaching the medium but does not have full control over his body. The medium may experience strange sensations in certain body parts or may have intuitions about certain problems but he is still 'basically himself'. The second stage is termed 'being beside', and here 'the spirit is leaning against the medium, is by his side, is touching him and in this way controlling his body'. It may also cause the medium to forget some of what he is witnessing. This stage and stage 1 are sometimes referred to as half-way possession. The third stage, known as 'incorporation', is that in which 'the entity has fully entered the body of the medium and he is therefore completely possessed'.

Different types of trance-possession in Bali could fit some of the three stages of experiences described by both Cardeña and Frigerio. For example, the people in communal trance-possession who are unconscious and amnesic (Chapter 4), the dancers in trance (Chapter 5), and some trance-mediums (Chapter 3) could be experiencing the third stage of possession. The individual trance-possession reports (Chapter 5) are comparable to the description of possession in the second stage, while the possession experience of Suryani (Chapter 8) appears to fit the first stage. However, because of the wide variability of the trance-possession experience in the same individual, or in the same situation, or under the same conditions, and the relative lack of knowledge of the basic psychophysiology of the states involved, there may be little heuristic value in dividing trance-possession into such types. Given the variability of the trance-possession states in Bali with respect to both degree of amnesia and type of possession, it is more useful to categorize them according to purposes served (e.g. healing) or to contexts relevant to the culture (e.g. ceremonials).

To the Balinese, trance-possession is a condition or state brought about at the behest of a god or spirit in which the god or spirit 'comes down' and acts through the person, i.e. possesses him or her. The Balinese have a number of different words for the phenomenon of trance-possession, including *kalinggihan*, *karauhan*, *kasurupan*, *ngadeg*, and *katakson*. The particular term used depends on village custom. Although the Balinese do not recognize or have a word for trance without possession, this condition does occur among them, e.g. in gamelan musicians (Chapter 6) and in some patients treated by *balian* (Chapter 3).

During prayer, a Balinese may become spontaneously possessed. Usually, the person desirous of possession prays that the gods will honour him and enter his body, but he and the society believe that the decision belongs wholly and solely to the gods. When possession occurs, the individual feels pleased and grateful. People who witness the individual's changed behaviour attribute it to the god who had possessed him; hence, if the behaviour is violent, abusive, unruly, or wildly emotional, they will say the person is not being himself and will thus not sanction or condemn him. More than one god or spirit may possess a trancer at the same time or sequentially. Two possessed spirits may talk with each other or a spirit may carry on a dialogue or discussion with others, as well as with the individual who is in trance-possession (Belo, 1960: 33).

The trance state can vary in depth from light to deep and most possession states appear to occur in deep trance. In one type of trance-possession, the trancers may become unconscious, fall, or tremble and move as if having a form of generalized convulsion or they may perform unusual feats such as dancing on hot coals, stuffing hot coals into their mouths, or walking on fire without suffering burns.[15] After coming out of trance, the trancers may report that they did not feel the heat of the fire that they danced on or that they felt the fire was cold. In trance-possession little girls can dance on the shoulders of men (Bateson and Mead, 1942; Belo, 1960) and people can exhibit incredible strength or perform amazing stunts. Men possessed by a monkey god can climb up to treetops, execute extraordinary acrobatic feats, and jump down on all fours (Forman, Mazek, and Forman, 1983: 98). Some possessed men may effortlessly scale a 2-metre concrete wall.

Trance-possession in Bali is usually terminated by a priest sprinkling holy water on the individual. Following most types of trance-possession, the majority of Balinese experience pleasant feelings which they call peace, health, and calmness; these feelings may last for 1–3 days and the individual sometimes experiences changes in consciousness which last a week or more and which are terminated by the conclusion of the lengthy village ceremonial. Trancers who have indulged in extraordinary physical exertions while in trance, evidenced by profuse sweating, do not recall being fatigued during their trance-possession state but they may feel tired afterwards.

Varying degrees of amnesia occur during the trance-possession state in the Balinese. Subjects who enter into light trance states are usually able to recall the events of the trance. Those who stab themselves with krises in ceremonies and in the Barong drama and many traditional healers or trance-mediums recall very little, if any, of their trance-possession experiences. Individuals who become unconscious during trance-possession usually have little or no recall of the events that occurred while in trance (see Chapter 4). The Balinese schoolchildren who suffered from trance-possession attacks had complete recall and were able to describe their hallucinatory experiences (see Chapter 7).

The majority of Balinese find it difficult to express the feelings that they experience during trance-possession. On being first questioned, most of them say 'I don't remember' or 'nothing happened'[16] but after further questioning, many are able to recall some of their feelings and sensations. However, the words they use to describe their experiences are often not readily or easily translated into English. Most of those who have entered into trance-possession find it impossible or difficult to verbalize their feelings and experiences. Generally, the Balinese answer interview questions with short sentences; they seldom explain fully or in detail. Their common response to questions, 'I don't remember' or 'I have forgotten' is a way of avoiding saying they are unable to explain. 'I have forgotten' does not mean a specific memory loss; rather it means that they are unable to control themselves or that God or another spirit is responsible for their actions. However, under skilful questioning, most are able to convey their feelings and experiences during trance-possession and indicate that they are not actually amnesic or unconscious of everything that happened. They often recall changed sensibilities and perceptions, such as hearing only the sound of the singers, or experiencing feelings of floating or the sensation that they were in another world, or sensing that they were possessed by a power which moved them, or feeling that they moved automatically rather than of their own volition. This is in contrast to some reports (Bourguignon, 1968) which indicated that the possessed are always amnesic with regard to the events of the trance experience.

In some areas of Bali, such as the city of Gianyar, many people do not readily believe a person's claims that he is possessed. In order to be sure, these people may test the individual by touching him with a hot object such as a lit cigarette or even fire to see if he cries out in pain. If he does, they believe that the person is lying and is not in a real trance. This kind of testing is not done in the Denpasar area and other localities where people readily accept the belief in possession.

Leak[17]

To a Balinese, the world is filled with gods and spirits. It is primarily the supernatural phenomena that are at the core of many activities of daily life, including ceremonies, rituals, dances, plays, possession, physical and mental illnesses, and healing. These supernatural phenomena include demons, witchcraft or black magic, and *leak* (spirits). Evil spirits are often present. For example, one should not start a journey at high noon or at dusk (about 6 p.m.) because it is believed that evil spirits come out then and are more likely to disturb, capture, or possess one at these times. These spirits are the focus of exorcistic treatment by *balian*. Physicians and psychiatrists in Bali who practise Western techniques need to know about the supernatural and the work of the *balian* in order to be effective.

Leak (pronounced, 'lay ack' and often spelled *leyak* or *lejak*) are witch-like spirits or creatures that are transformations of real people who live in the community.[18] People who have the ability to become *leak* can change themselves into other things, such as an animal, a light, or the wind, depending on their power, and they can travel anywhere. The wind is considered to be the highest or strongest type of *leak*. Some individuals who become *leak* are believed to derive their ability from an amulet purchased from a sorcerer. Some persons in a village are generally regarded as *leak* while others are believed to be *leak* by certain individuals. Almost any disliked acquaintance presents a potential danger because of the possibility that he/she may be transformed into a *leak* at any time. People who have special perception can recognize *leak* even when they change their forms. *Leak* can practise black magic and thereby initiate illness of all kinds, and they can disturb people to the point of causing death. They generally come out at night and are likely to frequent cemeteries. According to the beliefs of the people, Halloween-like activities occur: the goddess of death meets at midnight to dance and feast on the living blood of the dead brought back to life; entrails hang in trees, cauldrons catch dripping blood, and the roots of trees wind in and out of the skulls and bones (McPhee, 1946).

McPhee (1946) described one of his experiences thus:

It was perhaps a week later that I awoke again, late in the night, with the same strange feeling that someone had called. It was an unusually warm night, and I went outside on to the veranda. I could not believe my eyes.

Across the valley, halfway down the hillside, a row of lights glowed with a soft pure brilliance. They seemed to move ever so slightly, floating up and down as though anchored. Suddenly they went out, as suddenly went on again, but now to shine in a perpendicular line, one above the other. They merged slowly, until only the central one remained, which now began to float slowly up the valley. All at once it vanished. But within a minute the lights were shining in a row once more, far to the north.

I went to rouse Durus and Sampih, who were sleeping in the next room. Look! I said. What lights can these possibly be? They are too pale for lamps, and besides, there are no paths where they are moving.

The *léyaks*, said Durus, softly, almost inaudibly. They must be from Bangkasa [the village across the valley] . . . or from somewhere in the north, he added after a while.

We stood silently watching this magic display. The lights glowed and died, came close together, spread rapidly out in a long line. Slowly they floated back once more to where I had first seen them. One by one they went out, until only a single light remained. But all at once it was gone. The valley was in darkness.

All next day I was haunted by the weird beauty of the scene I had witnessed the night before. It was as if the stars had descended. If it had not been for Durus and Sampih I should have been unable to believe it had not been part of a dream. But when I mentioned it to Chokorda Rahi, and later to the *perbekel* in Pliatan, they were not surprised. Had I awoken out of an uneasy sleep? With a feeling of suffocation? There was only one explanation. Sorcery was in the air once more. It had only begun, and no one knew what was to follow.

Such experiences are reminiscent of Westerners' reports of UFOs.

Another of McPhee's (1946) experiences illustrates other types of *leak* phenomena:

No one was surprised, then, when all at once things began to go wrong in the house. Misfortunes occurred, one after another, and as they accumulated everyone began to have a worried, hunted look. Rantun the cook, slipped on the kitchen floor and broke her arm. Pugig stepped on a thumbtack and got an infected foot. The cat fell off the roof, actually fell, for no reason at all, and was killed, while Kesyur and Sampih declared the garage was haunted. Night after night they would wake, they said, unaccountably rigid, jaws clenched, unable to make a sound. They heard the bicycle bells of Durus and Pugig ring out in the darkness, although there was no one else with them in the garage. Voices called their names from outside, but they opened the doors to find no one. And late one night, as Kesyur walked up the road alone to the garage, he saw, sitting silently among the bamboos, a great bird, large as a horse.

This, however, was not all.

In the morning, as Pugig brought up the coffee, he would point to drops of blood that ran in an unbroken line all around the outside floor of the sleeping-house. A fight between two *tokés,* the great lizards that now hid and croaked in the thatch, I suggested; but Pugig did not agree, for he would wash the spots away, only to find them again the following morning. One night I awoke to hear the loud ticking of a clock almost in my ear. It was rapid and metallic, like an alarm clock, and seemed to come from outside the wall. As I reached for my flashlight it began to travel quickly around the four walls of the room. I ran outside, but there was no trace of anything at all.

Everyone agreed, as I related the experience in the morning, that all this was the work of *léyaks*.

These are excellent examples of how Westerners and Balinese perceive and interpret phenomena differently because of their different belief systems. The Westerner was startled and puzzled by what he saw. The Balinese interpreted the events as commonplace and readily understandable.

Suryani has personally seen *leak* a number of times in her life. When she was 10 years old, she saw a monkey *leak* on the wall of her compound. At the age of 14, on three separate occasions, when she was riding her bicycle home past a temple in an area with big trees considered to be magic, she saw red, yellow, and blue coloured lights. This frightened her and she rode swiftly home. Suryani's neighbours once reported a non-existent light in the backyard of Suryani's home. At the age of 15, when she was lying in her room and could hear her family's voices outside, a woman with blood on her hair appeared and wanted to kill her. She prayed to God for help and after a few minutes, the woman disappeared.

The following example of *leak* may be considered an instance of euthanasia by the husband of a dying woman with the assistance of a *balian.* A 50-year-old woman who suffered a haemorrhagic stroke and was comatose for a month had to be kept alive by tube feeding and intravenous fluids. She developed bedsores and was severely emaciated. She showed no improvement, and her husband felt increasingly hopeless about the situation. He went to the *balian* and asked what her problem was. The healer told him that his wife had become a *leak*—one at a very high level; he also said her body was dead, but her *leak* remained alive and because of this he (the husband) must help her leave the world.[19] He advised the husband to stand at the head of his wife's bed at midnight, take off all his clothes, and recite a mantra. The man did it, and a few minutes later his wife died. The nursing staff was puzzled over the event and reported it to Suryani. The husband said that he was sad to see her suffering; he did not want her to go on in this manner and he felt that this was a good way to help her be near God more quickly.

As mentioned earlier, *leak* may present themselves in various forms—a monkey, a human figure, light, or wind—depending on the degree of ability of the *leak*. It is believed that a small proportion of the people who can see, hear, and speak with *leak* are more vulnerable to their harm. Seeing a *leak* can evoke fear. Individuals who are regarded as being 'warm' humans are deemed to have no power or natural ability to see *leak* and do not have to worry about them; people who are considered 'cold' humans are able to see and hear *leak*. Such visions and auditory phenomena are distinguishable but similar to hallucinations manifest as symptoms in psychotic persons in Western cultures (see Chapter 9). In Bali, normal persons can experience hallucinations in their usual state of consciousness or in a state of meditation.[20] People are not concerned with *leak* most of the time; they take ordinary, semi-automatic precautions to be safe, comparable to the Western practice of washing hands before eating.

Two Western psychological concepts may explain the apparent hallucinatory aspects of *leak* phenomena. First, some of the sights and sounds could be illusions, i.e. perceptual misinterpretations of a real external stimulus (Kaplan, Freedman, and Saddock, 1980). Secondly, these sights and sounds could be hallucinations associated with dissociation and trance or self-hypnosis. The contagious aspect of trance is often involved, and the cultural beliefs also play a central role in the form and context of *leak* phenomena.

A similar phenomenon, Western encounters with UFOs, is structured on current Western beliefs. The following report of a UFO is remarkably similar to some *leak* phenomena:

The UFO came close to her car one evening she says, and stayed above her, silent, telephone-pole high. It had four lights on each side. She stopped the car and got out so that she could see it better. While she watched, the lights began to flow around the perimeter of the craft, the way they do on a marquee, and music played inside her head. After a few minutes she got back into her car. The craft followed for a while, the lights now back in their original position. Over an arroyo it 'disengaged', the lights blinked off, and it disappeared. (Gordon, 1991.)

UFO encounters are experienced for the most part by normal, non-mentally ill persons. Persons who report UFOs tend to regard them as 'real' or an experience of ordinary consciousness. Very few consider the experience to be a hallucination associated with self-hypnosis or trance.

Suryani found that Balinese patients are easily hypnotized[21] and under hypnosis, about 25 per cent become possessed. This possession is normally associated with a deep hypnotic state (see Chapter 8).

There are a number of similarities and differences in trance and possession between the West and Bali. Hypnosis in Westerners, sometimes also referred to as trance, is generally induced, controlled, and terminated by a hypnotist; the gods, prayer, and the supernatural are usually not involved. Westerners under hypnosis experience changes in perception similar to these of Balinese in trance. In the West, trance is rarely accompanied by possession, whereas in Bali, it generally is. Trance-possession in Bali usually occurs in public or in the presence of family members. Trance in these two vastly different cultures, the Western and the Balinese, have important features in common: a trusting, willing subject, and a dissociative state. One is induced by the hypnotist, the other by environmental stimuli, prayer, gods, or spirits. Trance-possession in the Balinese often occurs in the presence of singing or music. The biggest difference between possession in the West and that in Bali is the highly positive, reinforcing, encouraging, expectant, and socially controlling environment in Bali.

The majority of trance-possession experiences in the Balinese are accepted as normal behaviour, but there are occasions when trance-possession is considered to be abnormal, such as in trance-suicide, *amok*, *bebainan*, and *kasurupan* (see Chapter 7).

Amok has been described in a number of cultures, particularly in Malaysia (Arboledo-Florez, 1985). It is a condition in which the affected individual suddenly becomes aggressive and violent (usually caused by some provocation), sometimes killing people in a wild, uncontrolled spree. *Amok* has been known to occur in otherwise placid, non-aggressive Balinese (see Chapter 7). Whittkower (1970) correctly regarded it as a dissociative state. This kind of aggressive behaviour differs from the violent and uncontrolled behaviour of persons in trance-possession during religious ceremonies (see Chapter 4).

Dissociation, regardless of whether it occurs in a normal conscious state, in trance/hypnosis, or in a range of disorders, including hysterical paralysis and multiple personality disorder (MPD), is basically a type of psychological mechanism or 'defence'. To accommodate this range of behaviour and conditions, the various forms may be conceptualized as representing points on two continua: (1) normal states ranging from normal, through trance, to possession; and (2) abnormal states ranging from the dissociative disorders to MPD at the extreme end (see Chapter 9). The dissociation of MPD appears to be qualitatively different from that of trance, pointing to the possibility of psychophysiological differences between the two. This is further supported by the sharply different characteristics of the two phenomena and by the fact that a much higher percentage of people are capable of being hypnotized than of being possessed.

* * *

Dissociation is a basic psychological process or mechanism, operative not only in normal behaviours which do not involve ASC, but also in the ASC of hypnosis/trance, possession, and certain conditions labelled as mental disorders, such as multiple personality. The Balinese manifest a unique dissociative condition called 'hidden by the evil spirit'. Dissociation is a primitive psychological mechanism or 'defence', probably acquired through evolution, which has value from the survival point of view. Several animal species, including non-human primates, demonstrate a comparable state called animal hypnosis or tonic immobility. Trance/hypnosis in the West is generally induced by a hypnotist; self-hypnosis is self-induced. In most cultures trance usually occurs spontaneously, whether in a public or a religious context, and it is associated with music, often with a strong repetitious rhythm. Trance is probably pan-cultural. The apparent hallucinatory phenomenon of the Balinese involving *leak* (witch-like spirits) occurs in normal Balinese and may represent, in Western terms, self-hypnosis. In states of deep trance, possession may occur.

Possession is an experience of being taken over, psychologically and behaviourally, by forces, variably sensed as a power, God, an identified god, a spirit, or the soul. In Bali ritual possession is common, controlled, desirable, socially useful, highly valued, positively reinforced by the society, and individually satisfying. Ritual trance-possession is terminated by standard techniques, including the sprinkling of holy water by a priest. In the case of trance-mediums, the trance or trance-possession state can be terminated at will by the individual. In the West, possession is relatively rare, socially isolated, generally conceived (even by those who have not experienced it) as unwanted, uncontrolled, mysterious, evil, and the work of demons or devils. It is negatively regarded except in a few small religious groups and in the phenomenon of speaking in tongues. A few examples of trance-possession in Bali, such as *amok* and *bebainan*, represent mental disorders.

1. The concept of defence, meaning a process for dealing with anxiety, originated in psychoanalysis. It can be misleading to conceive of dissociation as a defence mechanism in abnormal circumstances because it can also operate as a normal process.

2. The following verses by Stevenson (1928) are illustrative of dissociation:

When children are playing alone on the green,
In comes the playmate that never was seen.
When children are happy and lonely and good,
The Friend of the Children comes out of the wood. (p. 171)

When at home alone I sit
And am very tired of it,
I have just to shut my eyes
To go sailing through the skies—
To go sailing far away
To the pleasant Land of Play;
To the fairy land afar
Where the Little People are. . . . (p. 87)

3. Many of the behaviours described by Freud (1901) in 'The Psychopathology of Everyday Life', which he formulated as directed by repressed thoughts in the unconscious, are probably more correctly interpreted as examples of dissociation (E. R. Hilgard, 1977).

4. The first two questions on the scale give us an idea of the types of dissociative behaviour measured by the DES:

(1) Some people have the experience of driving a car and suddenly realizing that they do not remember what has happened during all or part of the trip. Mark the line to show what percentage of the time this happens to you.

0% |________________________________| 100%

(2) Some people find that sometimes when listening to someone talk they suddenly realize that they have not heard part or all of what has just been said. Mark the line to show what percentage of the time this happens to you.

0% |________________________________| 100%

5. In fugue, a person travels to another place, assumes a different identity, and is amnesic about his real identity.

6. *Latah* has been reported in Burma, Thailand, the Philippines (Yap, 1969), Siberia (Czaplicka, 1914), South-West Africa (Gilmour, 1902), Lapland (Collinder, 1949), the Ainu of Japan (Nakagawa, 1973), and in French Canadians living in Maine (Kunkle, 1967).

7. Evidence of the hereditability of hypnotic susceptibility supports the idea of a genetic factor in *latah* (Morgan, 1973). This does not exclude factors of learning and identification.

8. A genetic component to *latah* does not discount the factor of learning in a family setting.

9. In the earliest observation on *latah*, Clifford (1898: 189) noted that it resembled hypnosis (a dissociative phenomenon) in many respects but it did not depend on an original voluntary surrender of willpower. More recently, Murphy (1976) remarked on the resemblance between some *latah* states and hypnotic states. Suggestibility, a cognitive change related to hypnosis (Cardeña and Spiegel, 1991), should also be considered as a factor in the mechanism of *latah*. Against this is the fact that *latah* is not communicable, as is trance.

10. Murphy (1976) reported that many of the females expressing coprolalia were embarrassed by the behaviour. Presumably he was referring to Malaysians.

11. A naturally occurring psychedelic substance called ibogaine, derived from the root of an African plant, has a long history of tribal use in Africa. It has hallucinogenic effects but is used by the indigenous people to induce an altered state in which they 'go back and visit their ancestors'. In this respect it has effects similar to those of age regression in hypnotherapy. 'The Bouitis of Africa employ the drug in rites of passage. Participants often describe visions of ancestors and past lives.' (Anon., 1992: 89.) These effects are similar to those of *balian* acting in states of trance or trance-possession while not under the influence of any drug.

12. By contrast, a wildly charging, silent chimpanzee may attack any animal or person in its path.

13. For a discussion of the history and relationship between repression and dissociation, see Kihlstrom and Hoyt (1990: 99–202), who claimed that the two terms were used erratically by investigators.

14. In Matthew (10: 19–20), Jesus tells his disciples not to worry about what to say when they are arrested: 'When the time comes, the words you need will be given you; for it is not you who will be speaking, it will be the Spirit of your Father speaking in you.' In the Gospel of John, Jesus said that the Advocate, the spirit of truth, would speak through his disciples (Hastings, 1991: 186).

15. Examples of fire-walking were described by Gaddis (1967).

16. Frigerio (1989) also found that informants tended to report that they could not remember what happened during possession.

17. A large part of this section on *leak* is reproduced from *The Balinese People: A Reinvestigation of Character* (Jensen and Suryani, 1992: 85–8).

18. For detailed descriptions of *leak*, see Covarrubias (1937: 322–5).

19. The Balinese believe that when *leak* die, they can pass on their *leak* ability to whomever they wish.

20. Psychotic Balinese also have auditory and visual hallucinations but these are not as brief or transient as those of *leak*; they are associated with other signs and symptoms of psychosocial decompensation, and are not characteristic of, or identified by the culture as, *leak* (see Chapter 9).

21. Suryani's technique of induction involves little verbalization in contrast to the common induction techniques used by Western hypnotists. She first asks the client to

feel his or her breath travelling through the nose and passing out through the feet, and then with the next inspiration, passing from the feet up through the fontanelle of the head. About 50 per cent of her clients fall into trance at the first trial. For those who do not, the procedure is repeated several times. About 85 per cent fall into trance by the third or fourth trial.

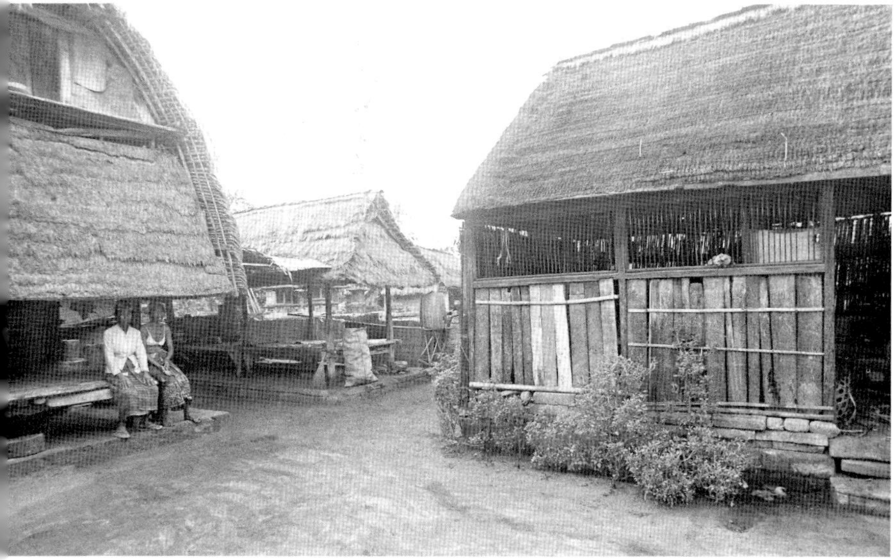

1 The usual Balinese household consists of five to seven pavilions. Two women are seated in front of the rice storage house which has sacred status. On the right is the kitchen, in the direction of the sea (*kelod*). In the centre rear is a pavilion for preparing food for family ceremonies. The sleeping pavilions (not pictured) are to the left and front of the rice storage house.

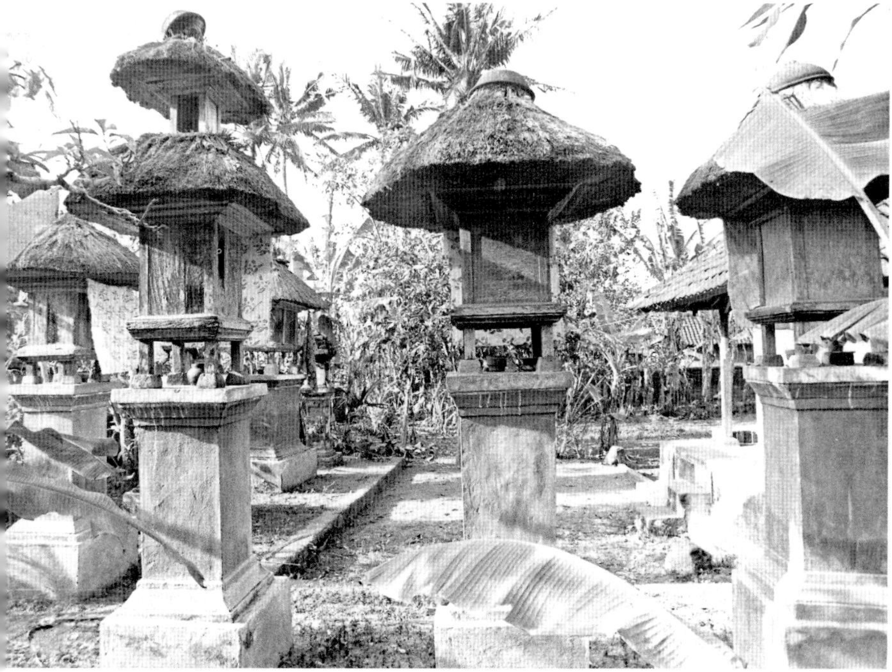

2 Each household has a temple containing shrines of its ancestors and of God. Each shrine is given due respect with periodic ceremonies and offerings. This low middle-class household has six shrines in its temple.

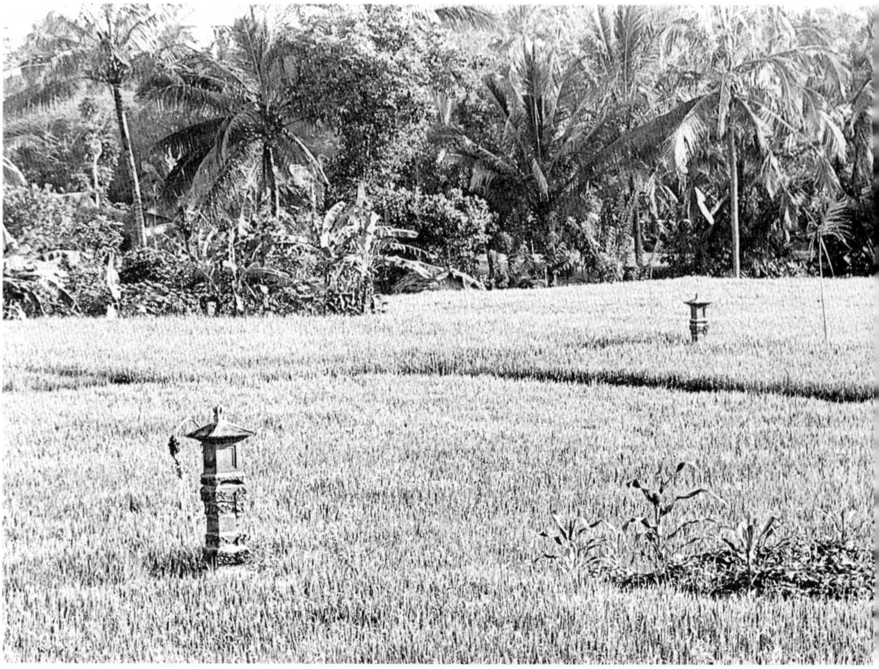

3 Shrines located throughout rice paddies are for the worship of the goddess of rice. Farmers regularly place offerings in these shrines.

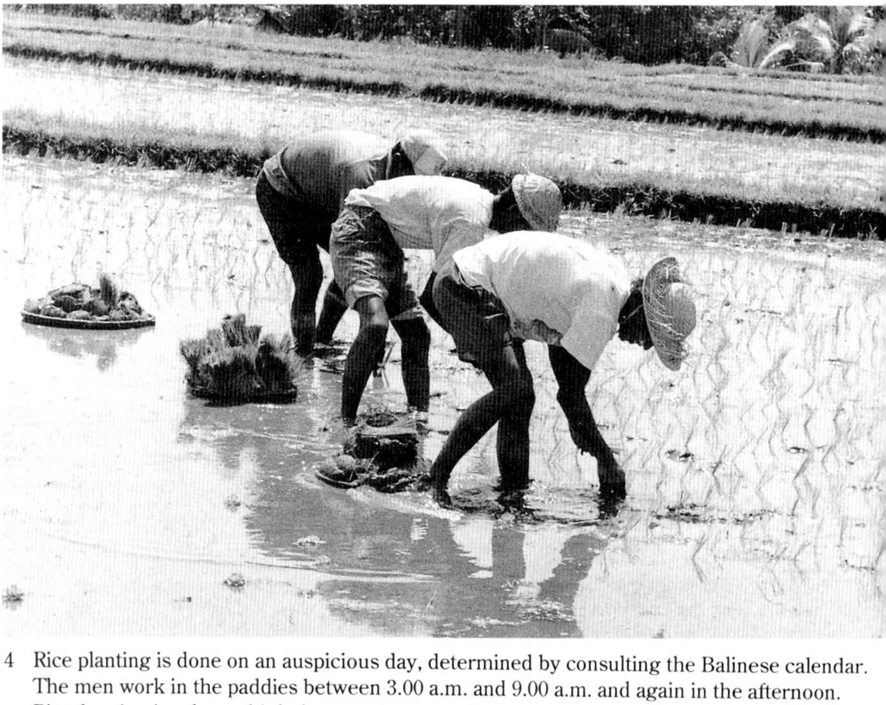

4 Rice planting is done on an auspicious day, determined by consulting the Balinese calendar. The men work in the paddies between 3.00 a.m. and 9.00 a.m. and again in the afternoon. Rice farming involves a high degree of co-operation.

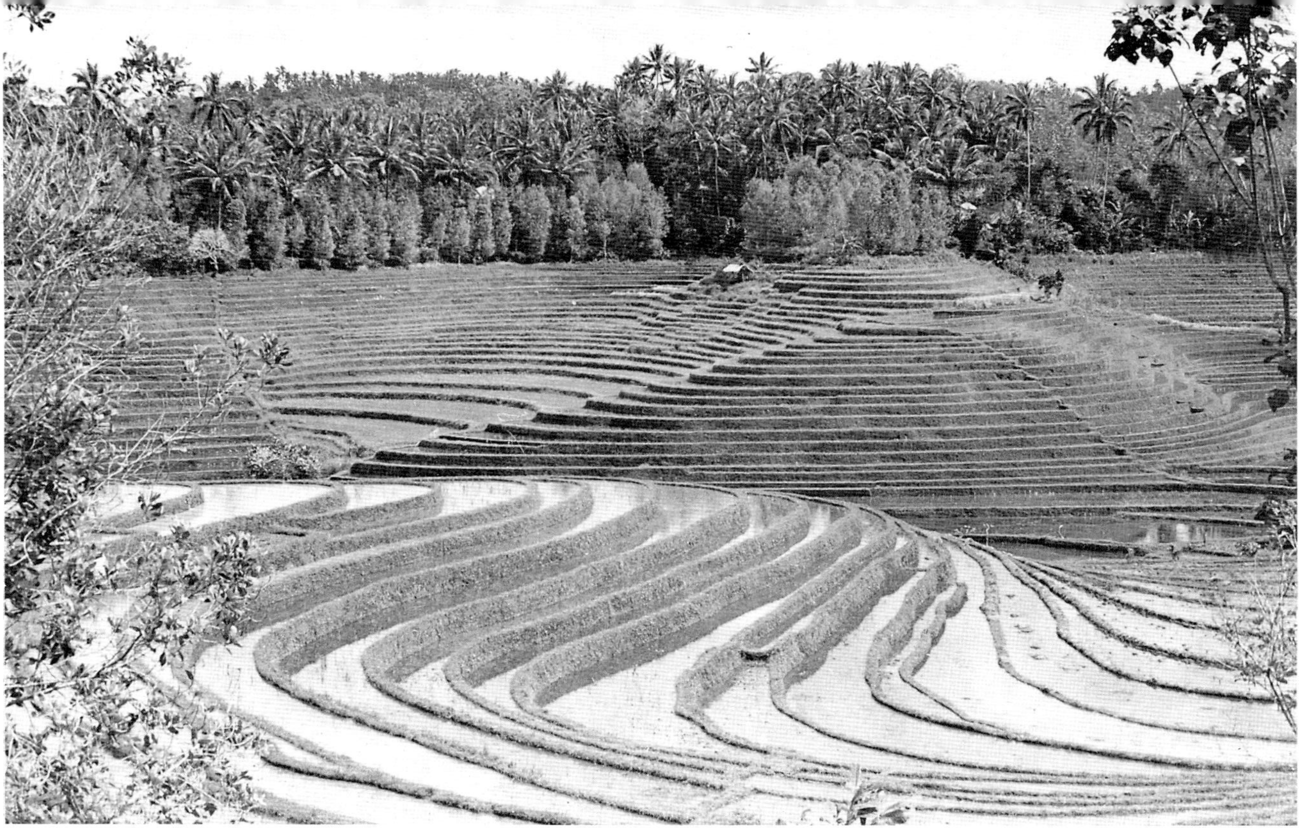

5 Rice, a dietary staple in Bali and a result of the gods' assistance, is grown on steep hillsides as well as on the plains. The goddess of rice presides over the irrigation system (*subak*), designed to deliver water to myriads of different levels of paddies.

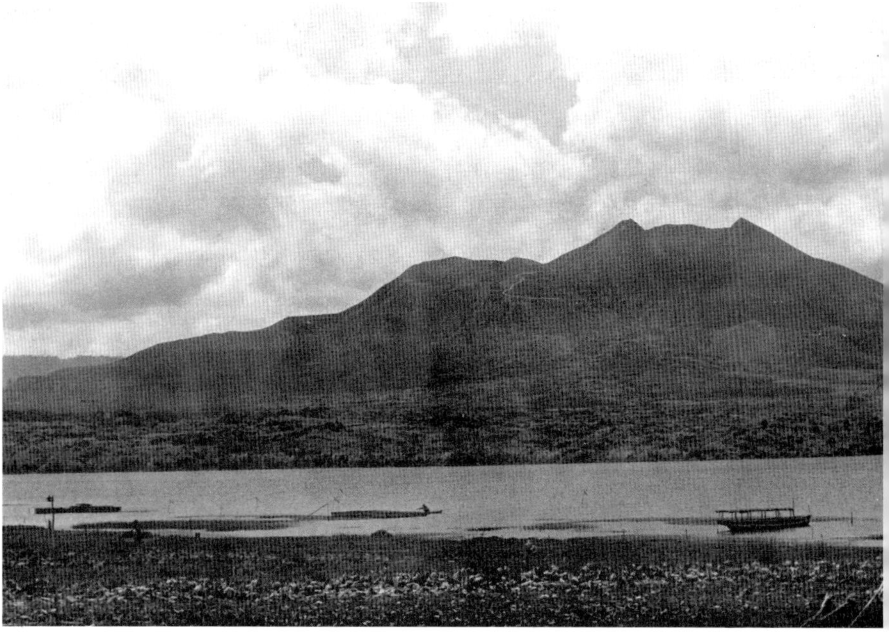

6 In the Kintamani area, Mt. Batur is regarded as the holy mountain and place of the gods. The crater lake below, believed to be the home of a goddess of the lake, is considered to be holy as well. These examples illustrate the Balinese Hindu belief in the religious aspect of nature.

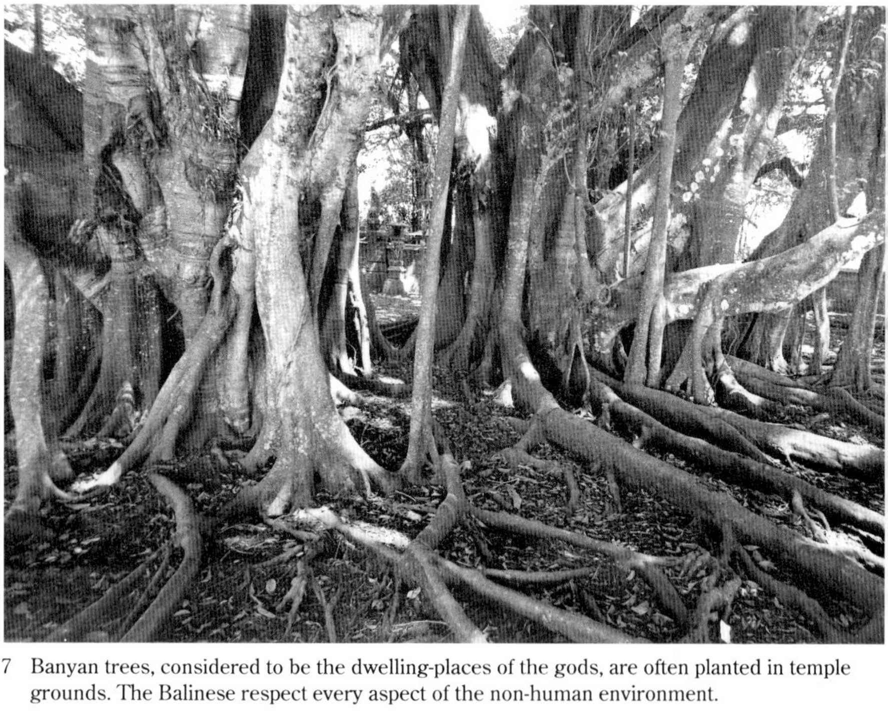

7 Banyan trees, considered to be the dwelling-places of the gods, are often planted in temple grounds. The Balinese respect every aspect of the non-human environment.

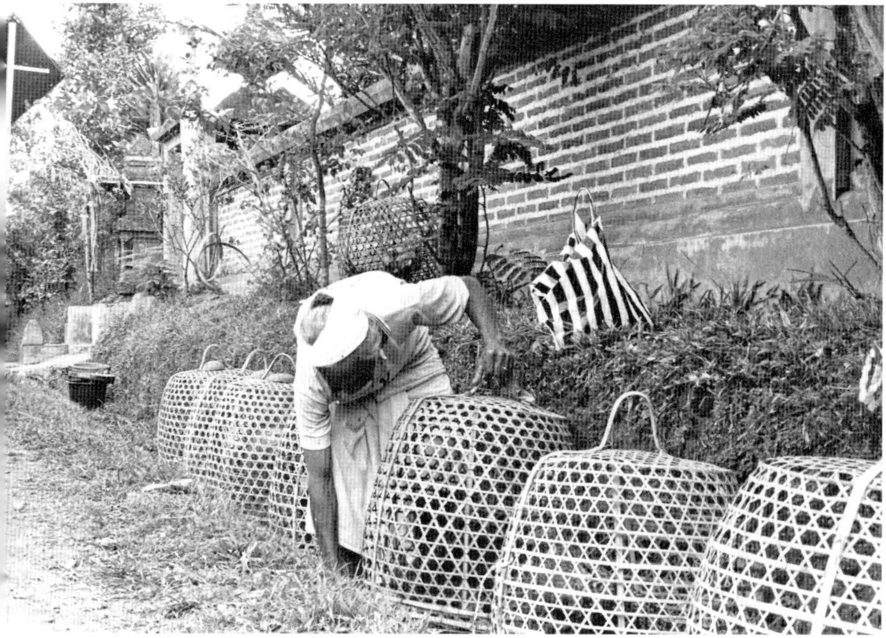

Cocks raised for fighting are seen in every village. This old man is tending to the daily feeding of rice and corn. Ceremonial cock-fights have religious significance: spilled blood from the fight appeases the evil spirits who live near the ground. Most cock-fights function primarily as arenas for betting and associated social interaction of men.

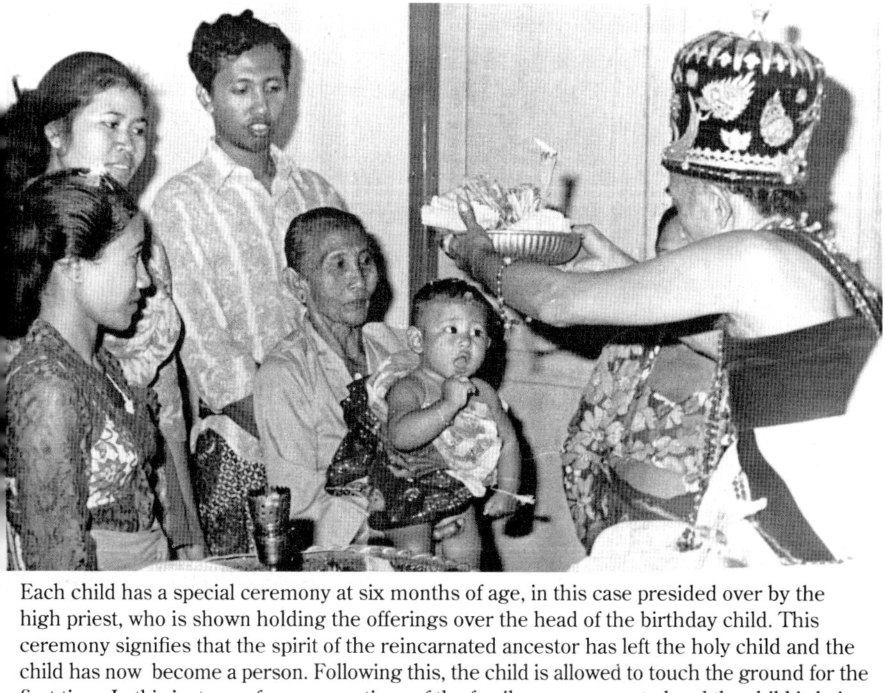

Each child has a special ceremony at six months of age, in this case presided over by the high priest, who is shown holding the offerings over the head of the birthday child. This ceremony signifies that the spirit of the reincarnated ancestor has left the holy child and the child has now become a person. Following this, the child is allowed to touch the ground for the first time. In this instance, four generations of the family are represented and the child is being carried by the great-grandmother.

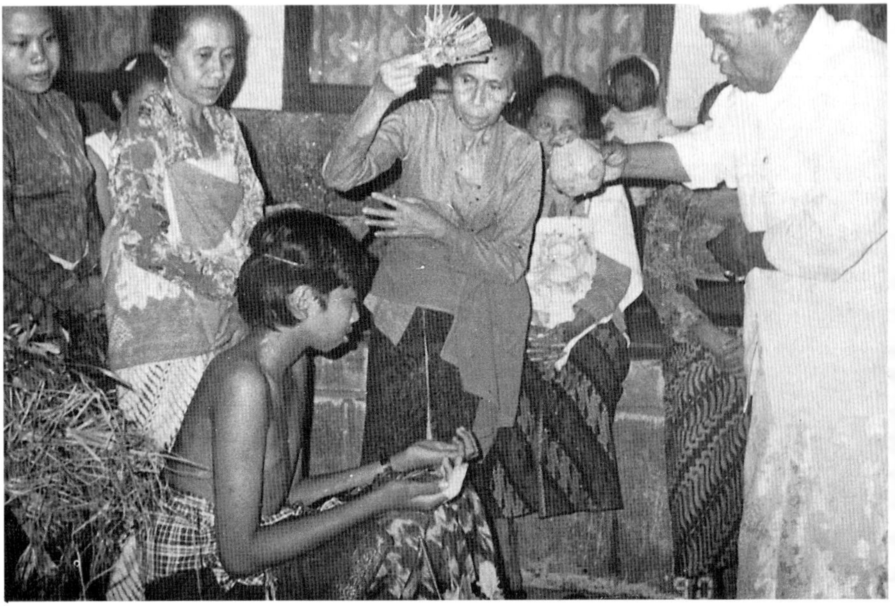

10 A child who was born on a bad day (*wuku wayang*) attends a special ceremony to promote a good personality in him. At midnight, after a shadow puppet performance (*wayang kulit*), he is purified by holy water from a sacred puppet.

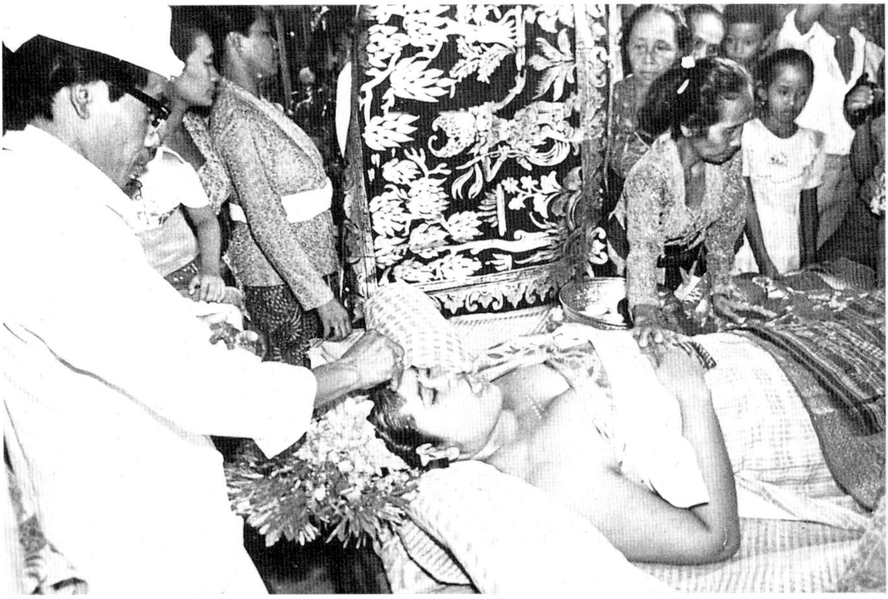

11 The tooth-filing ceremony, usually held in adolescence, is a very important rite of passage and signifies the expulsion of undesirable, naturally inborn feelings such as jealousy and anger. It is presided over by a priest (left) with the extended family in attendance. The filing of the canines to make them even with the incisors is now slight and symbolic rather than complete and painful as in years past.

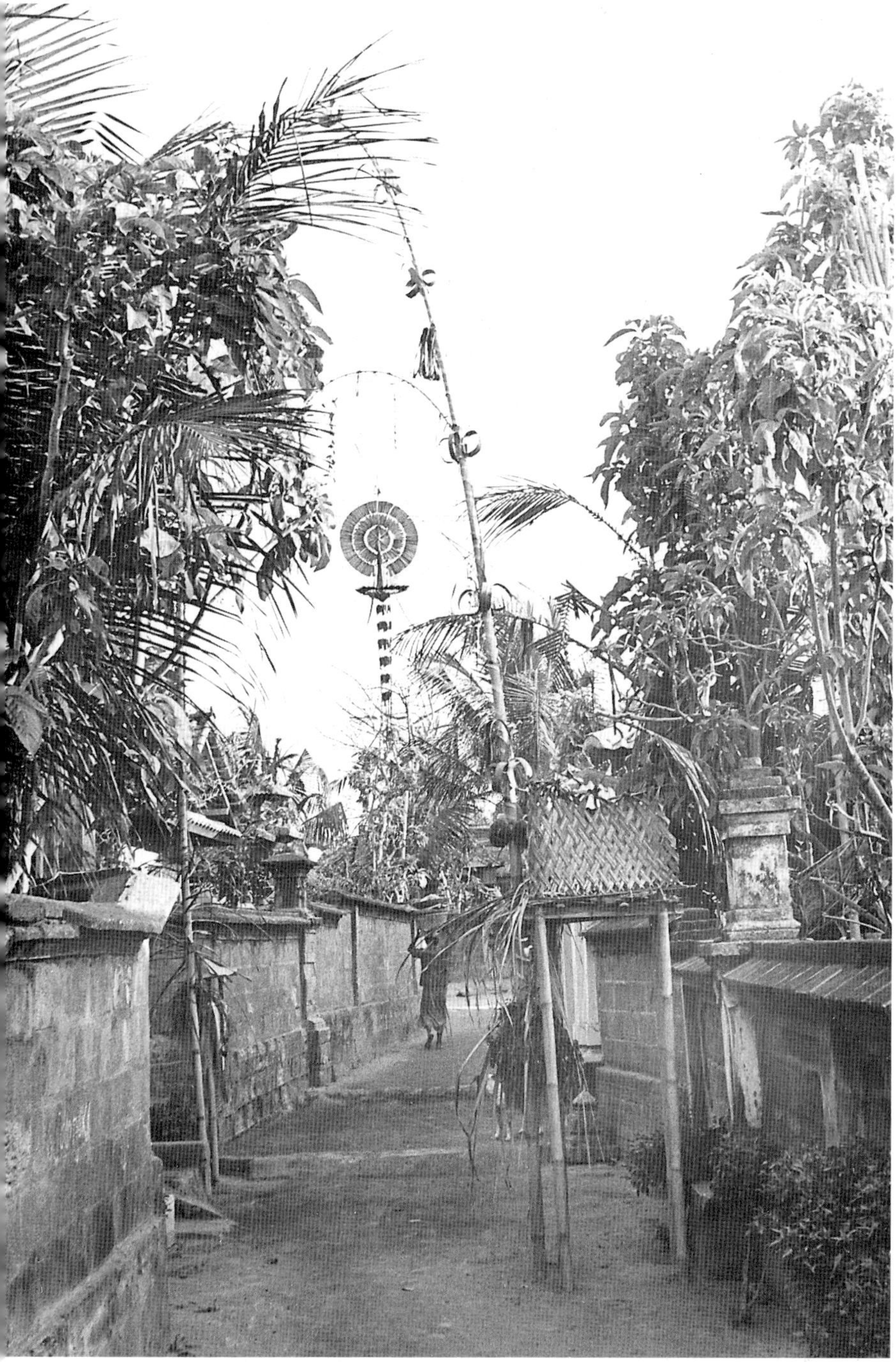

12 Every *galungun* (210 days by the Balinese calendar), each household places a *penjor* in front of its house. This is a bamboo pole decorated with symbols to give thanks to the gods for providing the household with products such as rice and coconut. A small bamboo shrine at the base is for offerings.

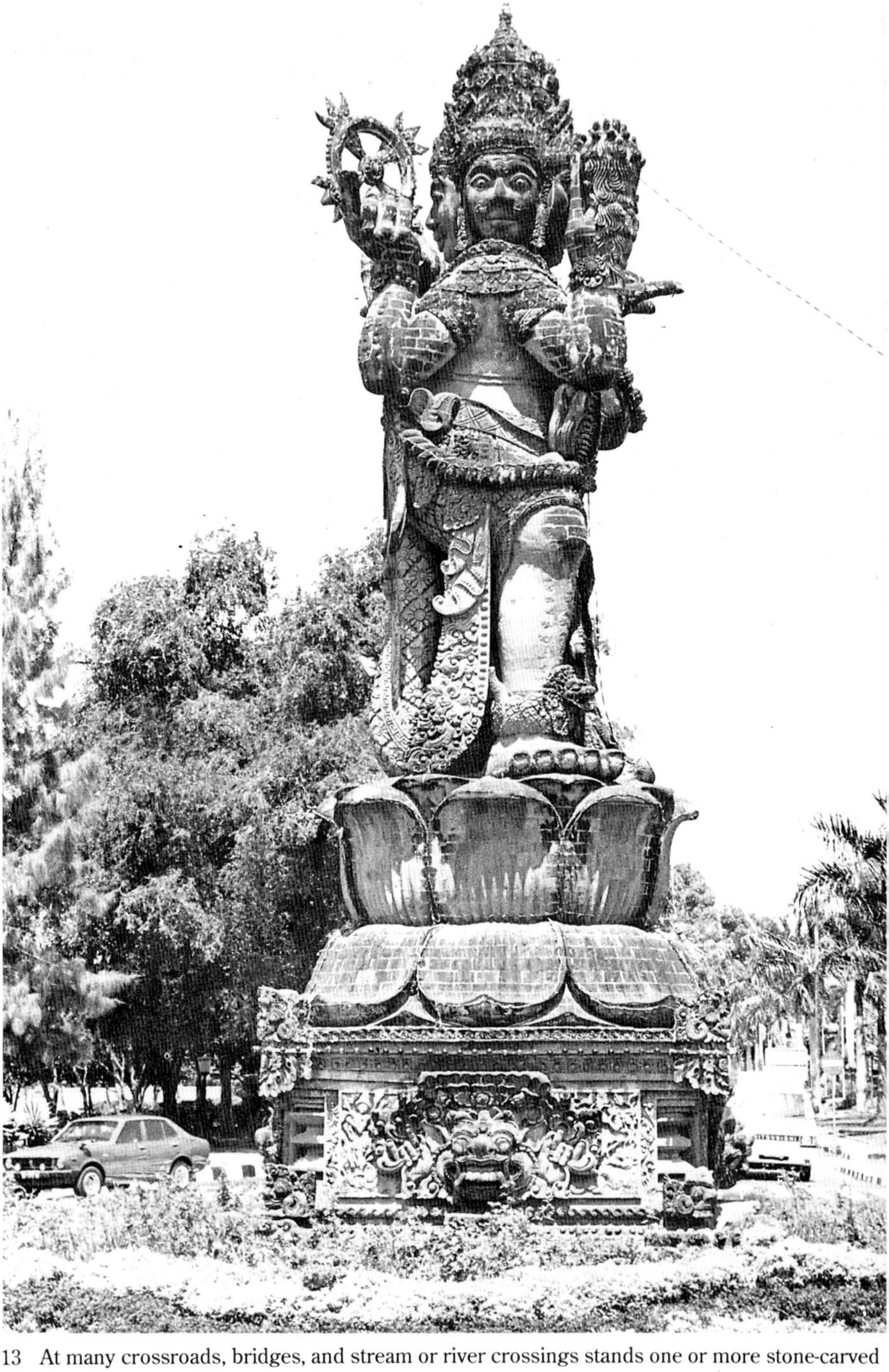

13 At many crossroads, bridges, and stream or river crossings stands one or more stone-carved gods whose purpose is to ensure safe travel. This four-sided monument in the centre of the capital city of Denpasar is huge with a body and face looking towards each of the four directions. It stands on a lotus blossom, the holy flower.

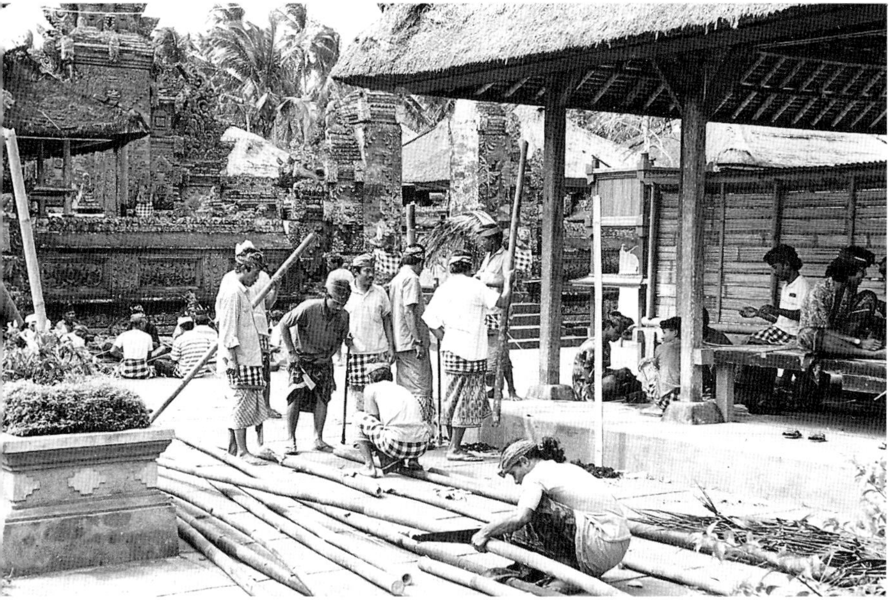

14 Men of a village in the plains working together to prepare decorations and furnishings for a village ceremony at their temple.

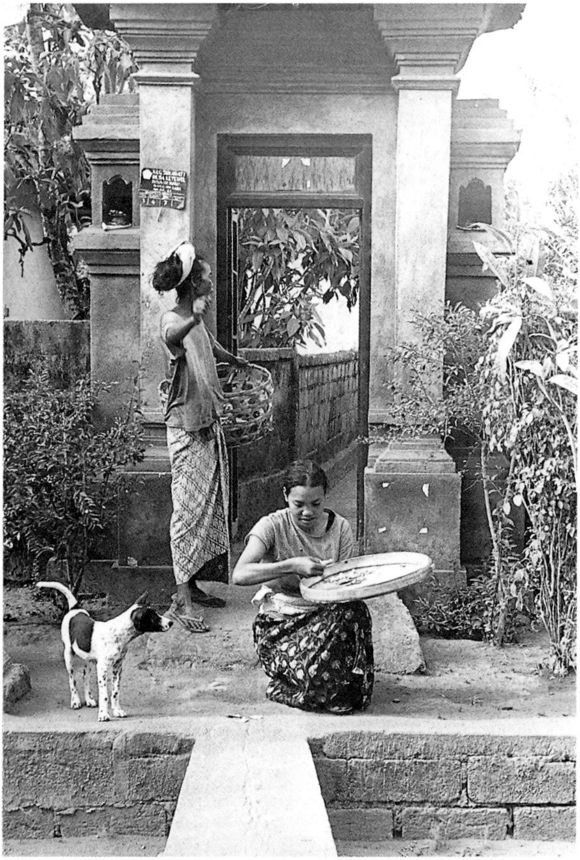

15 Daily offerings are given to the gods and spirits. This young woman is shown setting small offerings of rice, onion, and salt—prepared in the morning before the family has eaten any of these—on a banana leaf on the ground in front of her household gate. Such offerings are also placed at many locations in the household.

16 On ceremonial days, beautifully arranged offerings of fruits, rice, and chicken are prepared in special ways. One member of each family is chosen to bring the offering for the gods to the temple where it will be blessed by the priest and subsequently taken back home for consumption by the family.

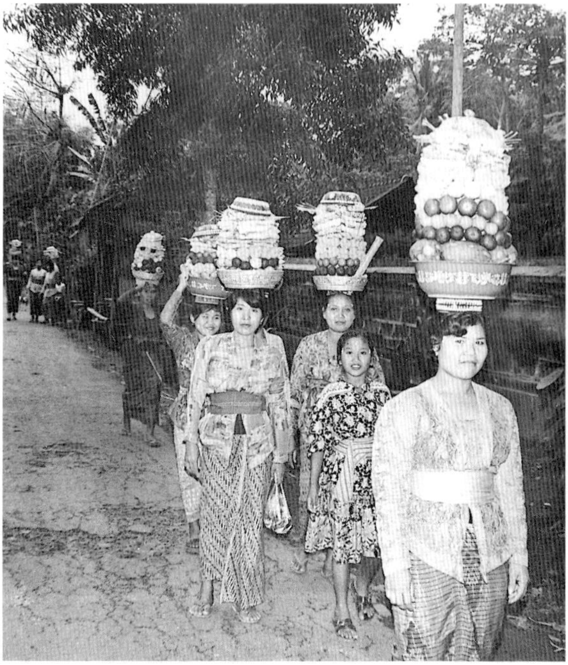

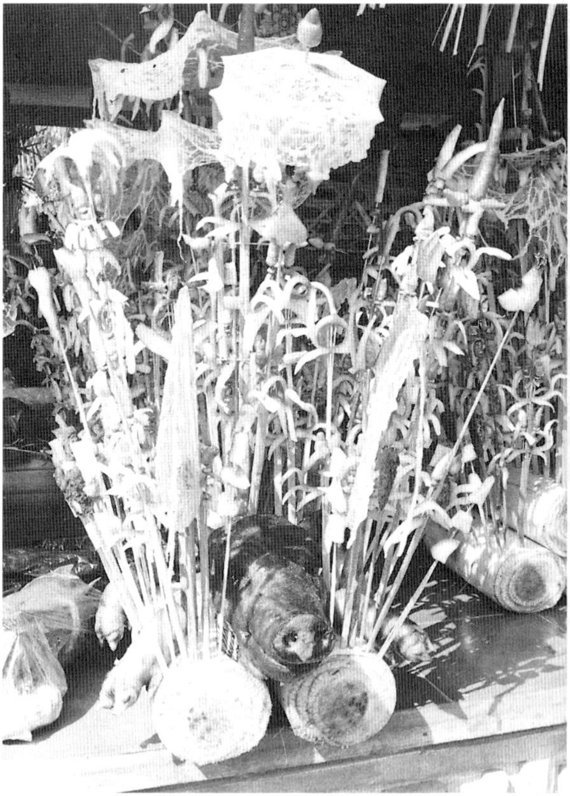

17 At a yearly ceremony, in this instance at the village of Jimbaran near Denpasar, an elaborate and artistic offering made of fried pigskin and the pig's head and feet is provided for the gods at the village temple.

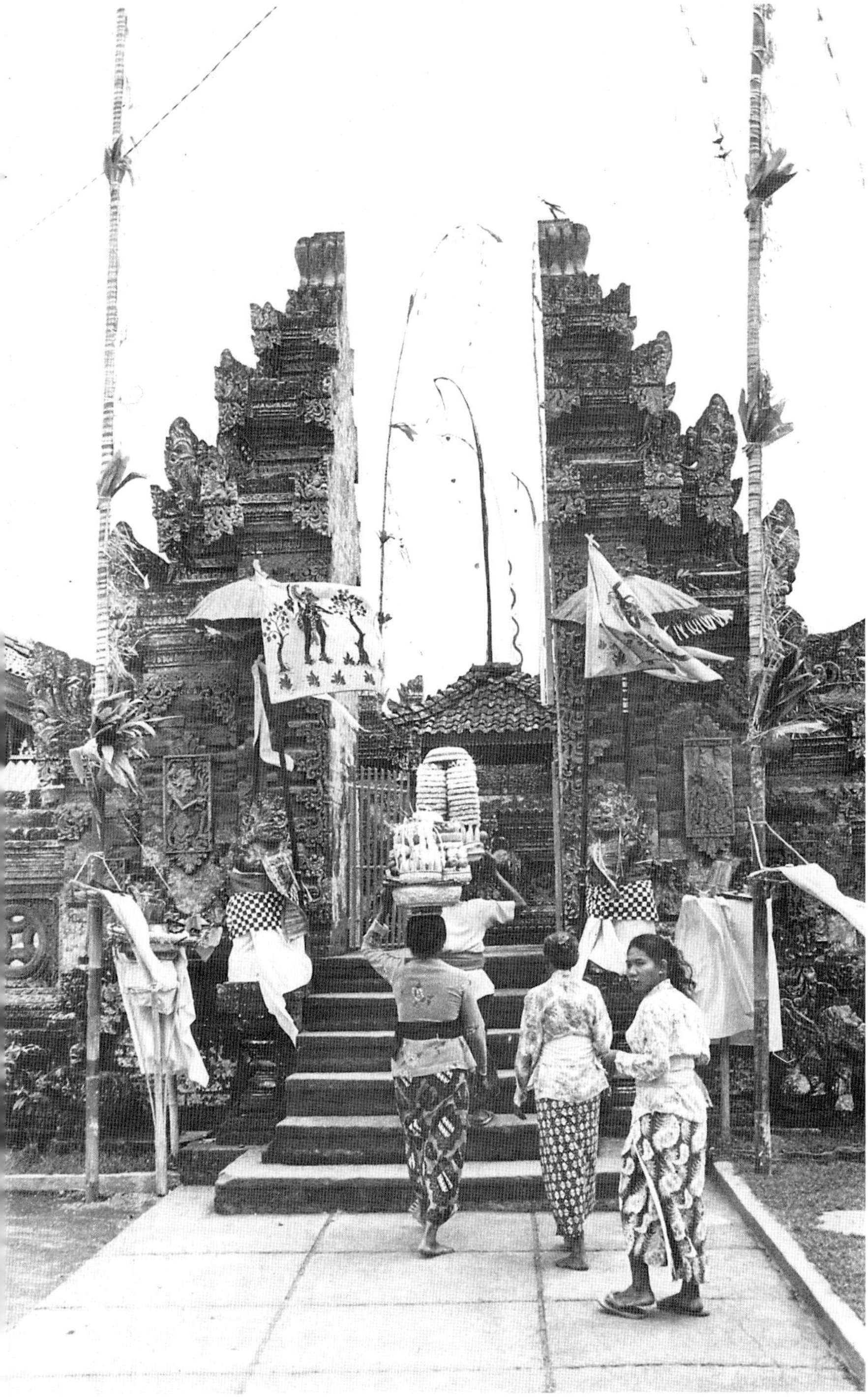

8 Women carrying offerings on their heads for a temple ceremony (*odalan*) through the split gate of a village temple in Bangli.

19 Carved stone statues adorn every temple. This statue in Pura Dalem, in the monkey forest at Ubud, depicts the queen of the witches, the evil Rangda. She is in the act of eating her food—a baby held in her arms.

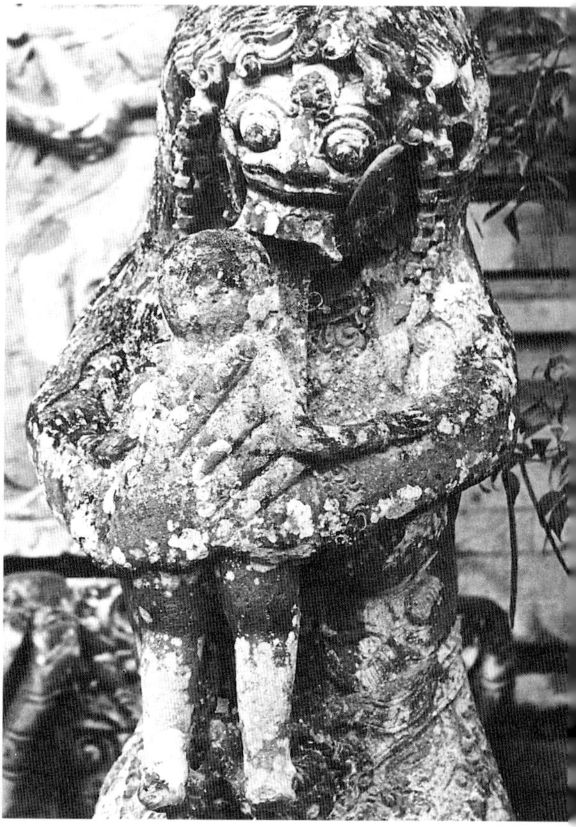

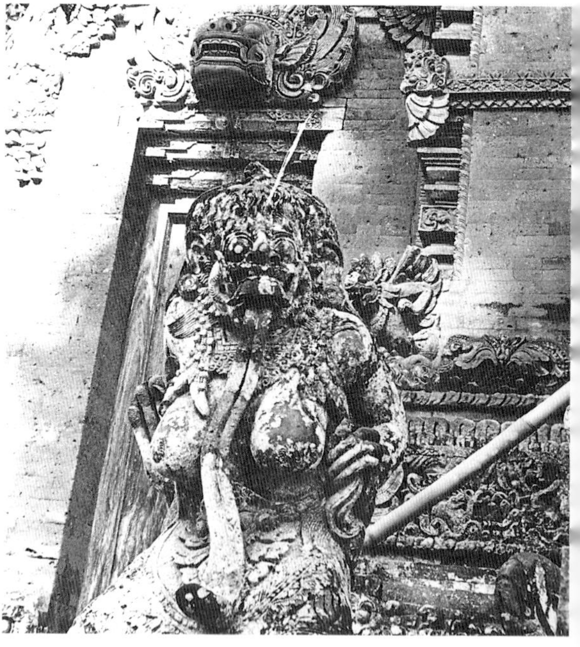

20 Stone carvings at Balinese temples are ornate and graphic. The temple at Ubud features the evil goddess Druga, with pendulous breasts and a 1-metre-long tongue. Behind her is a gate with a typical carved stone symbol of Boma above the doorway, which is believed to help ward off evil spirits.

21 The brightly coloured, mirror-glistening Barong at a ceremony at the mountain village of Kintamani. The holy Barong is a welcome part of many regular ceremonies.

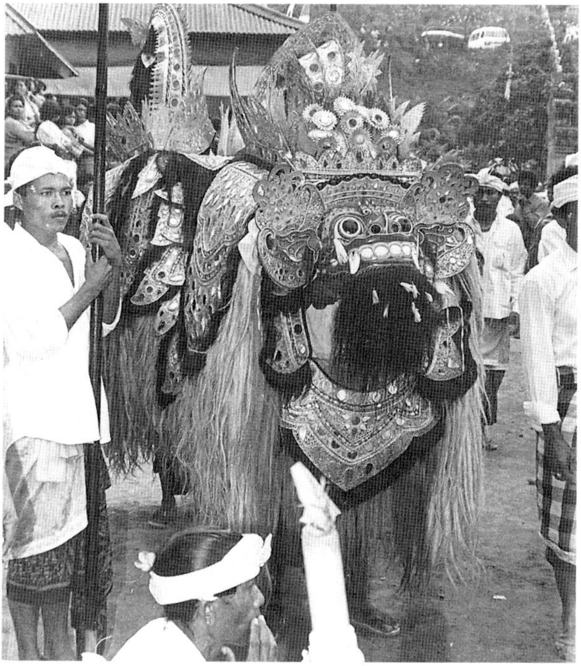

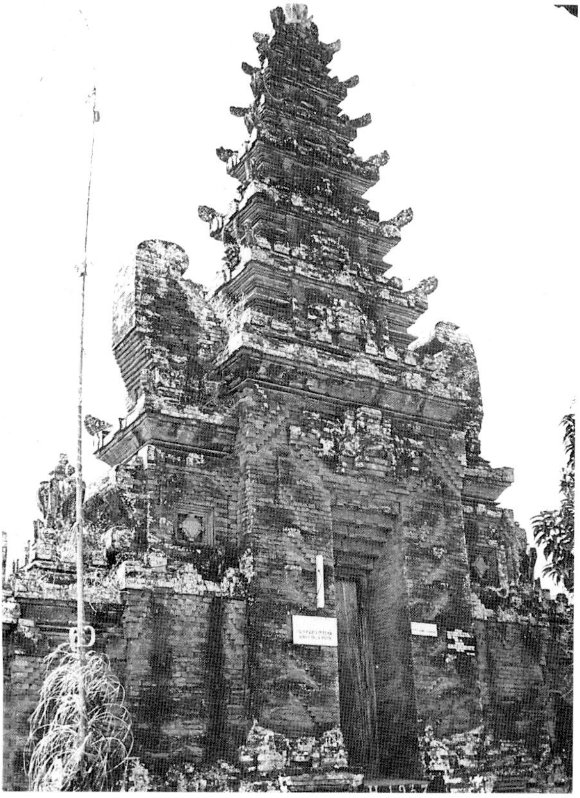

2 The closed temple gate at Kesiman on a non-ceremonial day.

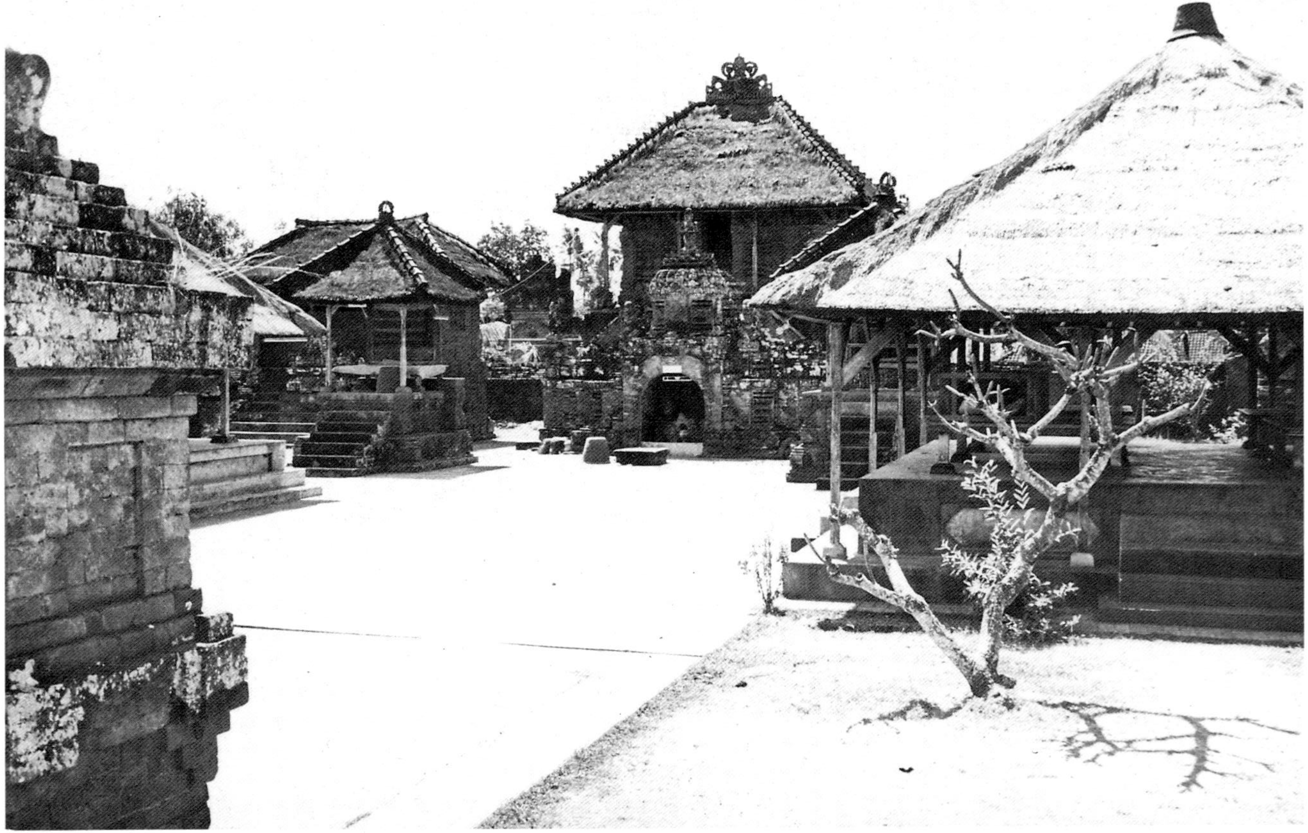

22 Inside the most sacred part of the temple at Kesiman on a non-ceremonial day

24 A woman with *latah* at the point of surprise stimulation by the person seated next to her (hand visible on the right).

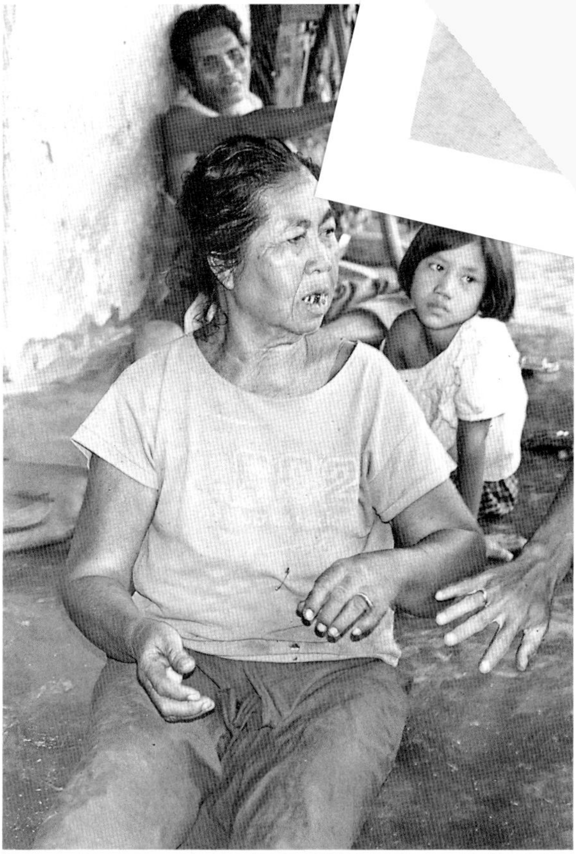

25 The woman in Plate 24, still in the *latah* state, performing a dance suggested by the person who startled her.

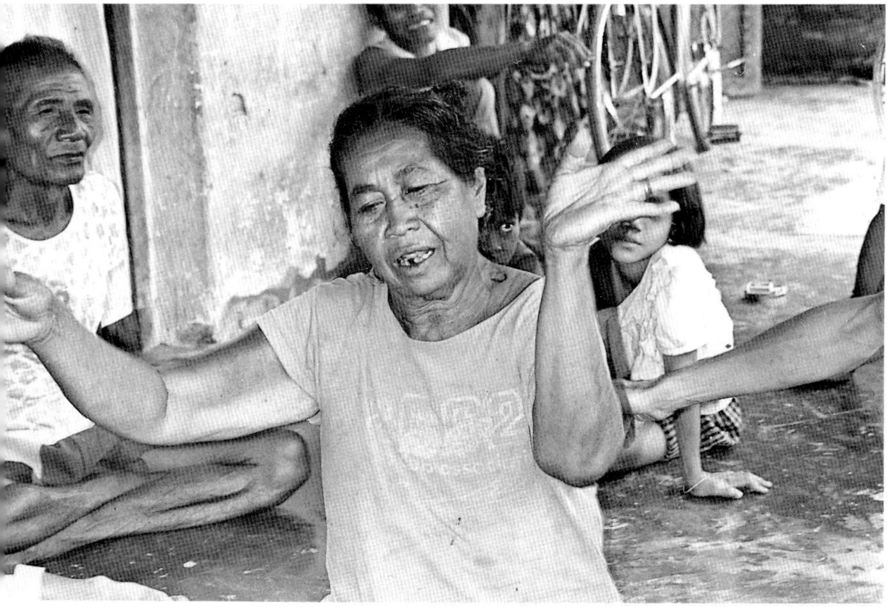

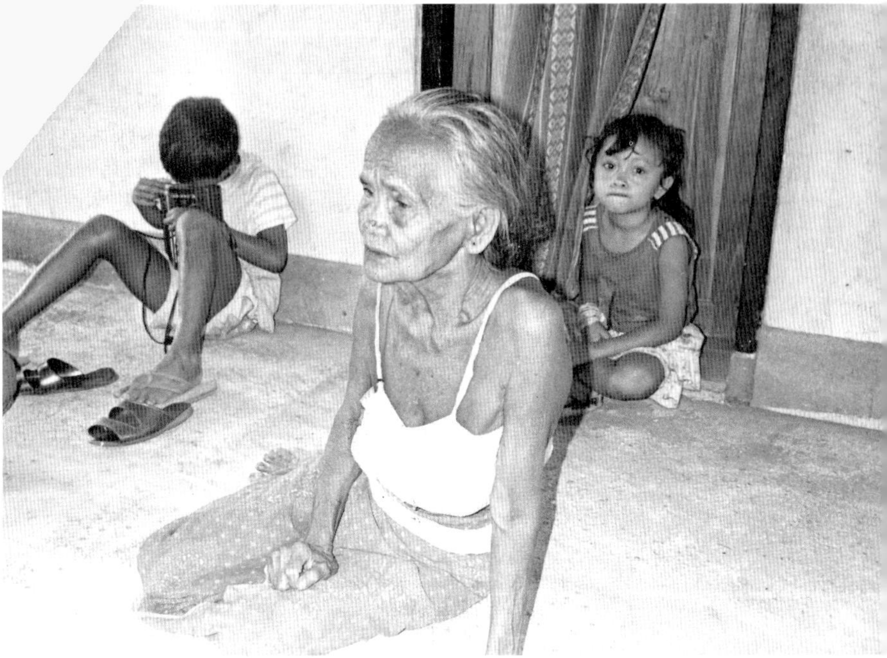

26 A 65-year-old woman who has had *latah* for many years sits quietly and calmly, responding t[illegible] Suryani's questions.

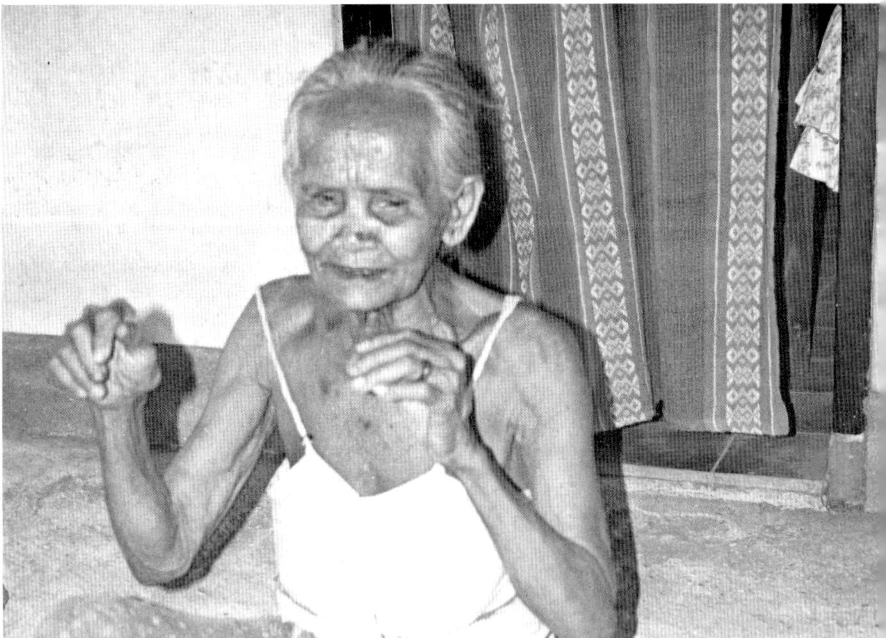

27 The woman in Plate 26 behaving mechanically in a state of *latah* after being startled by a family member.

Chapter 3

Trance and Trance-possession in Traditional Healers and Their Clients

THE traditional healers (*balian*) of Bali were chosen for detailed study because they are among the chief practitioners of trance and trance-possession and have much to reveal about the nature of possession itself, including the inherent special and unusual psychological and psychic abilities. This investigation did not focus on the rituals, psychophysiological mechanisms, or efficacy of the healing ministrations of traditional healers;[1] rather it concentrated on descriptions of the background of the healers, the objective and subjective changes that occur in the trance and trance-possession states, the physical, psychological, and psychic processes involved in the treatment of problems and illnesses, and their place within a Western psychological perspective.

The traditional healers in Bali are the primary source of care for all sorts of problems and ailments, both mental and physical.[2] It is estimated that there are more than 2,500 such healers in Bali. They use a number of methods and techniques for diagnosis and treatment. Some healers limit themselves to one technique, but most use a mixture or combination.[3] *Balian* may be identified by a name indicating their predominant method. For example, *balian usada* base their powers on reading the *lontar* (ancient Balinese sacred books inscribed on palm leaves). *Balian apun* use the technique of massage combined occasionally with supernatural manipulation of mystical forces through mantras and offerings. Such massage is employed particularly for setting bones, healing sprains, and correcting dislocations. *Balian taksu* are trance-mediums who contact gods or spirits or are possessed by these in order to cure sickness, treat bereavement, or advise on family problems associated with deceased relatives. Most *balian* who utilize trance prefer to be called *pengadeg dasaran* (a term meaning 'god uses the body') or *taksu*.[4] *Balian kebal* specialize in magical paraphernalia such as amulets and rings; they also dispense love potions and sometimes a drawing that the client is expected to wear to protect himself from spirits. Of more recent origin is a type of *balian* who uses massage but in the process removes—often ostensibly—pieces of bone from the client's head, abdomen, or other parts of the body that are believed to have been placed there through black magic practices and considered to be the cause of the problems or illnesses. Although no *balian* intentionally hypnotize their clients, the authors' observations indicate that some clients do experience altered states of consciousness, including trance or trance-possession, during treatment.

The Balinese seek help from *balian* in preference to physicians for several reasons. *Balian* spend more time with the family, with or without their clients, and discuss the problem with them; they also give intense attention to their clients and are more personal. Furthermore, clients and their families have great confidence in *balian* who are able to diagnose the problem without being given any prior information about it.

Most traditional healers do not ask their clients about their problems; rather, in a trance-possession state, they tell their clients what their problems are and why they have come to them. For example, a *balian* in trance-possession by a god told a client that she had come because her son was stabbed by a kris and that was in fact precisely the case. Trance-mediums usually begin treatment by asking the client and his or her family a few questions in order to set them at ease, such as 'How is your family?' and 'Where do you come from?', but they do not ask questions seeking clues to the diagnosis. Some *balian* may ask the client directly what complaints or problems they have for which they seek help, what they want advice about, or whether they want advice or treatment.

The style of treatment of a trance practitioner described by Belo (1960: 23) in the 1930s is similar, in many respects, to the trance-possession treatment employed by some *balian* today.

On one occasion when I was at her house a man came in with two followers bearing presents and the necessary offering. They came before her as she sat on the little porch of her house, made obeisance, and addressed her by her title as trance practitioner, Koelit. She accepted the gifts—rice, vegetables, dried fish, and fruit which was out of season. The offering contained a coconut, eggs, and money—Chinese cash. She asked what they wanted to consult her about and sat quietly chewing betel for a time. Then she rose and went to the bathing spout at the back of her house, washed her hands and face, and let the water spatter a bit on her torso. She combed back her hair and plucked a red hibiscus from the hedge, placing it on the top of her head.

Then she came back and seated herself on the raised platform on the porch of her house. She sat across-legged as a man does and rested her hands on her thighs. After only a few minutes, sitting quietly with her eyes closed, she suddenly raised her arms and clapped her thighs, her customary sign that the god has entered into her. She lifted her arms and performed a few movements of the dance. Her eyes, open now, were staring, and her entire attitude was usual to her in a trance. She uttered many unintelligible sounds and finally, becoming more articulate, referred to the question of the medicine. After this she was silent again, only making dance movements. Then she announced the prescription: a newly laid egg from a black hen, followed by drinking seven times water mixed with certain leaves. A few more dance movements, and she clapped her hands over her head, coming out of trance, and made three times the gesture of reference to the god. She continued talking then, in her normal personality, asking the visitors if they had understood. Then she began to chew betel again and sat chatting informally with them as the conversation became general.

Treatment of Grief or Bereavement by Trance-mediums

Trance-mediums or *balian taksu* practise a specialized form of trance-possession by the souls of deceased family members of their clients whereby they communicate with these souls for the purposes of counselling or assisting the family in dealing with unanswered questions and unresolved feelings about the deceased. This generally amounts to a treatment of bereavement.

A *balian taksu* whom the authors visited a number of times lives and practises near Sukawati, not far from Denpasar. To reach her house, one needs to travel several kilometres on a narrow dirt road through rice paddies. She is 50 years old, married with a child, and she has been practising as a *balian* since she was 7. Just prior to becoming a *balian*, she was chronically ill and almost near death, but she has been healthy ever since she became a *balian*. She practises daily, from morning to night, sometimes until midnight, and she always appears energetic. During one observation, she displayed a sustained level of energy as she attended to eight families in the morning. She took a few minutes' break between families and did not admit to feeling tired. People from all over Bali come to see her for many reasons, including to seek treatment for physical illness, to ask for help regarding relatives who have died, and to learn who is reincarnated in their baby. In the treatment of grief or bereavement, she acts as a trance-medium for the deceased soul to communicate with or to visit her client's family.

In practice, she prays to God and the souls of the deceased who may either appear visually to her and communicate with her or enter her and speak through her. In 1990, she claimed that she was possessed by her god, the god of the client, and the holy ancestor's soul. (The soul of a person not yet cremated is unholy and is not able to possess one.) At the interview in 1991, she contradicted this, saying that she could not be possessed by another god, only by her own god; she also said that the ancestor's spirits appeared and spoke as if on television, and as she saw them she imitated them in speaking to her clients and their families.

This *balian* likens falling into trance to 'sleeping—without feelings'. When she is controlled by her god, her voice is automatic, 'like electricity, television, or radio; . . . wire on which the current travels'. She is unable to recall most of what happens while she is in trance-possession. She cannot dispense advice without being in trance-possession: only if a god or spirit enters her can she give advice. Most *balian* say that they do not know what they do in trance-possession; they only know that their ability depends upon the deity (God or god) who enters them. They generally say, as she did, 'I'm sorry, don't ask me questions [when I'm] out of possession, ask me [when I'm] in possession.' Probably she would be able to recall some things if questioned appropriately, just like the Balinese dancers and others in ceremonial trance-possession who initially deny any ability to recall their possession experience but who nevertheless proceed to give some description of it if more detailed questions are posed.

At her treatment sessions, this *balian* dresses in a white coat and white sarong and sits on a slightly elevated, covered platform which has a large shelf with offerings brought by her clients; at her side are jars of herbs and concoctions that she dispenses to clients. The family, usually consisting of three to six members, sit cross-legged on a mat in front of her, looking intently up at her as she speaks.

She commences treatment by lighting incense followed by prayers and mantra. First, she asks the client and his family if they have obtained permission from their ancestors to come to the healer. They usually say 'yes'. If not, they have to pray for permission. Then the healer introduces them to the gods. After this introduction, she is possessed by her god which gives her a special ability to know the purpose of the client's visit. She sits back a little and then becomes possessed by the souls of dead persons (*inatuun*). Her voice and often her behavioural gestures change to take on the characteristics of the particular holy ancestor spirit. She asks the family very few questions but allows them to ask her questions. The family members are often enthralled and sometimes tearful, as the ancestor's spirit speaks through her. Her (the gods' and holy ancestors') verbalizations and messages to the family are often lengthy and they include a number of actions that could qualify as techniques of psychotherapy in the Western sense. For example, she acknowledges the concern of the family, relieves anger and guilt, assuages feelings of revenge, elicits feelings of loss or sadness, explains problems, offers advice and support to solve problems, interacts with the family, and accepts their grief abreaction. Each session with a family takes 30–90 minutes.

At the end of the session she abruptly comes out of trance and then acts her usual (non-possessed) self again. Finally, she asks the family if they have got the message (*polih baos*). If they answer affirmatively, she will receive their offering. If the family does not receive a message or if the god or soul of the dead person fails to 'come down' for the healer, she tells them to take their offering home. She gets up from her platform and walks off to her compound to smoke a clove cigarette, returning in a few minutes for the next session.

In the following case-studies of this *balian*'s patients (and in the other case-studies in this chapter), an attempt has been made to preserve the atmosphere of the treatment session and to keep as close to the original language as possible.

Case 1

The clients were six family members, including the widowed husband, offspring, and nieces. The *balian* went into trance-possession, and after God appeared, communicated as follows: 'You have come here because you are worried about one of your family members who had died,' although the family had not made any mention of the deceased. The *balian* then explained why the woman had died: 'She got black magic from people who did not like her. She was ill for a long time, suffering from headache, epigastric pain, and recently, vertigo.' The *balian* then said, 'Now the soul of the woman will talk to you.' The possessed soul started speaking, 'My son, uncle, grandson, [etc.], thank you for coming to see me. I was pretty and slender before and now after I'm old, I look bad, with no teeth and a wrinkled chin. Can you give me tobacco?' The family responded by handing the *balian* a tobacco leaf which she put into her mouth to chew. 'Don't call me aunt. Call me Mom.' On hearing this, the family was very attentive, with bright eyes, smiles, and laughter. (Later they said that the *balian* sounded, looked, and acted just like the deceased woman when she was alive.) She continued, 'All grandchildren should work hard to earn money for the house and to keep their health. *Kurenan tiang* (my husband), give me your hand. I want to touch your hand. It's been a long time since I've seen you.' The elderly man took the *balian's* hand, smiling and chuckling happily. She then went on to say, 'Don't think that I have died; I will protect, help, and care for you from my world. In my life you helped me, now I will help you. Don't think about who wanted to kill me. Don't do bad, because it is all finished. This is my future now, to be with God. Please help my husband because he is sick.' The mother's soul then proceeded to joke about their lives together which relieved the sadness of some family members. The grandchildren asked her to help them to get good results from hard work and to advise them on what to do in order to be a success in life. She answered, 'Don't worry, I will help you every time even though you don't ask me. This is my job.' After the 30-minute session, the *balian* abruptly came out of trance-possession and expressed thanks to God.

In the interview with the family members after the treatment, it was learned that the woman had died two months previously at the age of 65 from heart failure. The family believed that she had died because God ordained it. The children said that they had come to see the *balian* because they felt a deep sense of loss at their mother's death and they wanted to ask the *balian* what mistakes the family had made and why they always have family problems. They said that it was true that she was a slender woman and that her soul's voice, movements, and gestures were similar to those when she was alive. The family felt happy to be able to talk to her soul and said that all of their burdens had been lifted. They had come with the intention of finding out if they had made mistakes in any part of the death ceremony, including the cremation.[5] They were satisfied with the soul's reassurance and by the *balian*'s work.

Case 2

There were five clients in this family group. The *balian* fell into trance and asked politely, 'Where do you come from and what caste are you? I have never seen you before.' She went on to pass several other social remarks to make them feel comfortable and to establish rapport. She listened to their answers and then said, 'If what I say is true, you can agree by saying yes. If you're not in agreement, please tell me.' In a state of possession by a god, the family appeared to her and she said, 'I see that the family is quiet. There is no quarrelling and your income is good, but you feel uneasy, and for this you have come here to speak with the god (*nunas baos*). The [deceased] woman's illness was sudden. There was pain in her joints, caused by an amulet someone put in your house.' The god said they must make offerings to get rid of the power of this amulet since the power causes illness. 'The woman died because other people wanted to kill her. Don't think it was her mind. It was the power of the amulet which killed her.' Next, the *balian* was possessed by the souls of the holy ancestors—the grandparents—a man and a woman who then spoke and described why the woman had died. He reassured them that all their ancestors had a good place in heaven (*tongosne melah*) and would always help to care for their descendants. The *balian* then said abruptly, 'I want some coffee.' The family answered, 'We are sorry but we did not bring any.' The *balian* responded, 'It's okay. Give me some when you get home. Put it in the shrine.' The soul of the dead person then spoke, 'Don't be upset about me because I can handle myself. This is not your business. Don't try to take revenge. It's not good for you. Now my life here in this other world is good. I'm happy; I have no problems.' The *balian* then gave her clients some advice to prevent them from being disturbed again: they should prepare a mixture of leaves and oils and put this in the ground by the front gate of the house. Throughout this session, most of the family members looked sad and tearful, and appeared grieved.

At an interview after this treatment, the family revealed that what the *balian* said was true: their relative had died suddenly and she did suffer from pains in the joints. They had worried that their mother or grandmother did not have a good life in the other world. Now reassured, they no longer felt the need for retaliation or revenge. They believed that their problems had been solved.

Case 3

This case also involved a deceased woman. When the *balian* fell into trance-possession, the god appeared and explained to the family that the woman's death was not caused by God or by an ancestor punishing her but by two persons. One was a woman and the other was a man. These two people, who were not relatives but neighbours, had put something with magical power in their house gate. This had caused her to lose interest in things, feel pain in the epigastrium, develop vertigo, become irritable, and eventually die. The *balian* then said, 'Now the soul of the dead woman will come to see you and try to discover what is the matter with your family. Do you agree?' The family answered, 'Yes.' The soul speaking through the *balian* then said:

> I died because someone wanted to hurt me. I am still distressed about this. I want revenge, but don't do it by yourself. I will do it. This is my business. I am sorry I died so quickly. I only care about my children, not my grandchildren. After my cremation, I hope you have a good relationship with each other. Don't try to find out who killed me. You must try to have a good relationship with everyone. Don't worry about me; I still have a good chance to make a good life for myself. I will help you from my world.

Next, the soul of an ancestor spoke, 'We know you have approached many people—e.g. the doctor and the traditional healer—to help your mother, but to no avail.' The family at this point asked the *balian*, 'Who disturbed her?' The ancestor's soul replied, 'A power in a bone, nail, or stone disturbed her. They put it in one place. Don't try to discover the name of the person who did it because this would be bad for you. If you know the name, you'll want to retaliate and this is not good for your family. Try to maintain good relationships with others and believe that God will help you.'

In an interview following the treatment, the family said that it was true that they did want to get revenge because several family members had died recently and they wanted to know who had disturbed them or caused their deaths. Many family members also believed that they knew who had disturbed the deceased but after speaking with the souls of the ancestors and hearing what they said, they would change their attitude and no longer think about revenge. This case illustrates the degree of trust the Balinese have in their ancestors: if the ancestors ask them to do something, they will obey.

Another female *balian taksu* living in Ubud, and specializing in helping relatives of the deceased, demonstrated psychic ability during possession as she treated a Western client, who sought help in resolving grief over the death of her husband which had occurred 10 years earlier when she was in Bali on her honeymoon.

The client only informed the healer that she had been married. The healer, using some of the same techniques as the first *balian*, told the client certain things—e.g. the fact that her husband used to read Shakespeare to her when he was alive—which convinced her that she (the healer) was indeed possessed by the deceased husband's spirit. Speaking through the healer, the husband said that he now had a good life and hoped that she would go on with her life separate from him; that she was free to choose a boyfriend and lead a good life too. This was the kind of result she was seeking. His spirit also warned her not to walk alone through the rice paddies at night (which she had been doing) because he felt it was dangerous. This single session had a significant curative effect on the client's prolonged grief.

A third female *balian* studied by the authors lives in Denpasar. A 46-year-old woman with 4 children and a husband who works for the government, she has been practising since 1976, when she had a one-month illness with paralysis of both legs which rendered her unable to walk. Although she went to many physicians and traditional healers, none could help her. Finally, one healer told her that she should not go to doctors again because she could treat her illness herself and that she would become a healer. Soon after, she received a message from a god that she should treat her paralysis with her urine, mixed with the bark of a certain kind of tree at the cemetery. She applied this to the skin, felt better, and one week later, was able to walk again. At this point, she performed a special ceremony (*pawintenan*) to become a holy person. Since then, she has been practising as a *balian* from 8.00 a.m. to 3.00 p.m. daily.

Her method is to pray to a god from Nusa Penida, an island just off the coast of South Bali, who appears visually to her as a big man with very dark skin. The god appears as on a colour television screen and a voice relays messages (as over a telephone) explaining the reason the client has come to see her (e.g. an illness, a deceased relative, or a need to communicate with the ancestors). She then feels that her body is changed by the god. At this point, she recalls nothing further. At the end of each seance, she regains consciousness.

This *balian* was videotaped in entirety in a seance with a young couple and their 7-year-old daughter. The healer did not know the family nor the reason for their visit. (In the interview after the seance, the family revealed that they wanted to find out who was reincarnated in their newborn son, then 2 weeks old.)

The family sat on a bench about 8 feet behind the *balian*, who lit incense, prayed, and then spoke, 'Your great-grandfather has been reincarnated in your son. He wants to care for and help his descendants. All of you are poor because he did not leave any inheritance and your life has not taught you good habits, so that is why the baby is reincarnated by him.'

The family asked, 'Who are you? What is our relationship with you?'

The *balian* (addressing the baby's father) said, 'I am your great-grandfather. The baby is my great-great-grandson. I never gave advice to you before. Now I can advise you. Do you want to know the name of your great-grandfather?'

The father answered, 'Yes.'

The healer then said, 'It is Ida Bagus Anom. I lived a long time ago and I wanted to see my descendants. I hope they are not in a bad way. You are living from hand to mouth and I want you to learn a good way to live so that you will be a success and will not suffer from illness. That is why I am born into the world through this baby. You must meet your ancestor god. You must say goodbye to your mother (god). Before, you always lose your money and fall sick. You go to many doctors to get cured, but your father is still sick. Your father is a stupid person. You should say goodbye to your family at the original family temple. You went there but you forgot to say goodbye. The father now tries to influence you but he is stupid. You neglected to say goodbye to your ancestor at the clan temple (*kawitam*), and [that is why] you always have illness. Now you have to say goodbye to your ancestor at your clan temple, to Batara Guru (a special god) at the clan temple, and to the original human shrine (*sanggah kamulan*).'

The father interjected, 'I have done it.'

The healer said, 'You said goodbye to me maybe but not at the original family temple. You must say goodbye at both.'

The father said, 'No, I made two offerings.'

The healer asked, 'Where did you put them?'

He said, 'In one place.'

The healer said, 'That was wrong; you must put one in one place and the other in another place for the god.'

The father said, 'I didn't know I had to make two separate offerings in two different places. When can I do it?'

The wife now spoke up and said, 'Sorry, I can't do it now. Can I do it after one month?'

The healer replied, 'Yes, but tomorrow you must make a little offering.'

Then she continued 'Your ancestor needs holy water and an all-white dress. When he was young, he was a high priest and he knew the good days for ceremonies. This ancestor is born in your son, and he needs a *pejati* offering ceremony on his sixth-month birthday ceremony.'

This was the extent of the seance which lasted approximately 15 minutes. The healer prayed briefly and then abruptly came out of trance-possession; she opened her eyes and showed a different facial expression as she spoke with the authors.

At the interview after the seance, the father said that his parents lived in Negara in West Bali, but his family originally came from Denpasar, where he now lives. He said that it is true that they had come to this healer to get information about the reincarnation of their newborn child and that the healer's comment about their difficulty with money was correct.

The changes in perception reported by four other trance-mediums further illustrate their ASC experiences. Three were women, practising in villages in the city of Denpasar. Each related changed perceptions upon falling into their trance-possession state. The first *balian* feels big, heavy, and 'like the spirit', i.e. if the spirit feels sick, she feels sick; if the spirit cries, she cries. She said that she does not 'realize herself' nor can she recall what she talks about in the trance state.

The second *balian* reported that in trance she feels as if she is floating and her mind is controlled by a spirit. She sees and hears spirits, 'like they are on colour television', and is able to recall them. She said that the possession state is more intense than the spirit trance state (i.e. a trance in which spirits appear)., and she cannot remember what happens in possession. Whenever she is possessed by a god at temple festivals, she only knows that she screams loudly at the time.

The third female *balian* said that in trance she has the feeling her body is lightweight, 'like smoke', without any control. When spirits enter her, she does not know what they are saying, but her clients appear to understand these spirits. When the spirits leave her, her body weight returns to normal.

A 45-year-old male *balian*, who works as a traditional healer in the evenings and as a hotel service employee in Sanur during the day, sometimes consults Suryani about his puzzling cases. His subjective experiences of trance resemble those of the foregoing *balian* but are unique in some ways. He first became familiar with trance and possession during his personal possession experiences at temple ceremonies. Since then he has become very familiar with possession and is able to describe his sensations clearly. These include a feeling that he is bigger than his normal self and a sensation of his entire body shaking. He is nevertheless able to control himself in this trance state. For example, he said that in trance he is able to drive a car to the temple with his eyes closed. When he is in trance-possession, he often asks people to give him fire (a torch) which he puts into his mouth without sustaining any burns. On one occasion, he asked his ancestors for permission to visit the high priest, which he then did, and the priest asked him to take some incense in his hand. He said, 'No, give me fire', to which the high priest responded, 'You are not my student, you are on a higher level [of trance-possession].'

All the healers who practise trance-possession are self-trained; after a number of experiences, they find it easy to fall into trance-possession and may do so quickly. However, shifting into trance-possession each time depends upon the choice of the gods.

The subjective experiences of *balian* in possession states and the healing techniques used, as reported here, are illustrative and typical of other trance-mediums in Bali. The authors' interviews of *balian* verified that their trance states were genuine. Dr Denny Thong, former Director of the Bangli Mental Hospital in Bali, studied Balinese *balian* and believed that trance could be faked by some practitioners. However, the Balinese believe that if a traditional healer is not authentic, people will no longer go to him or her.

The *balian*'s work in healing is presented here in a Balinese context, but it can also be viewed from a Western psychological perspective. *Balian taksu* follow a standard procedure: first, they introduce the clients and their families to the gods, God, or their ancestors; then, they speak with the clients to establish rapport; next, they tell the clients why they have come and what their problems are; finally, they give advice on how to solve the problems. The information and advice given follow the Balinese Hindu beliefs of the clients and have common themes, e.g. problems, illnesses, or death due to offences against the gods or black magic from other sources. The explanations offered are readily understandable, and believable, to the Balinese. The advice given is generally consistent with Western psychotherapeutic techniques and concepts, including support, relief of feelings of guilt, suspicion, revenge, and anger, motivation to build better family and social relationships, and encouragement to form constructive, not destructive, interpersonal relationships. It appears that the clients' emotional experiences of contacting and interacting with the spirits are extremely effective in resolving bereavement. The closest Western parallel is transference to the psychotherapist.

A Trance-medium (*Balian Taksu*)

A female *balian taksu* in Denpasar was interviewed both before and after trance and observed during trance-medium sessions. Her daughter and several neighbours were also interviewed. She was 51 years of age at the time of the first observations in 1981. A Balinese Hindu who is unmarried, she lives in Denpasar and has three sisters, all of whom are married. Her parents, both deceased, were poor farmers when she was young. Their marriage was described as good with very few problems, and their relationships with their children were also good. Her grandfather was a *balian* and his father was appointed by the gods to become a *balian* but chose not to do so. A few months after he refused, he became ill and died, a consequence of having offended the gods. She left school after the fourth grade because her family was poor and went to work as a labourer in road and building construction. She was very energetic and helpful to her neighbours and whoever needed help. Interviews with her neighbours indicated that she was an obedient, quiet person who had good relationships with many friends and her behaviour was normal like that of her friends. Every day when she worked as a labourer, she was possessed by the gods. When possessed, she shouted loudly and the neighbours thought that she was mad. She said that suddenly, at one point, her hair train (i.e. long hair) fell off and her hair became very tight and difficult to separate into strands. Because of her 'possession', she had to stop work as a labourer and after that, she lived for 3 years in a very crude, dirty home, like a farmer's shed in the fields. She had no money to live a better life. During this 3-year period, she said that the gods tested her to see if she could do what they asked. She became a vegetarian. In her room, there were many kinds of snakes: green, yellow, white, and other coloured snakes, a cobra-like snake, and a snake with two heads. She said that the snakes did not bite and that she fed them every day by giving them offerings. She also described more than 100 black birds, similar to crows, who came daily to her room and to whom she gave offerings as well. The birds ate and then left. She also said her house was full of *tokek* (large lizards), which never bit or disturbed her and to these she also gave food and offerings. Caring for these animals kept her very busy. For 3 years, she did what the gods wanted and did not think about her neighbours. She felt that if she did not do it, the gods would punish her. Her neighbours were asked if they knew of the animals and they said they did not and that the only people able to see them were those who were possessed and had a 'special sense' of the gods. She said that once a god asked her to go to many temples and sleep in them. She meditated at Pura Besakih and other temples in the mountains. She said that she was at a mountain in Java (Mt Semeru) and also at the Himalayas in India. After this period of being tested by the gods, she was entered by Ratu Gde Dalem Peed (RGDP),[6] the god from Nusa Penida Island, near Bali. She said this possession by RGDP was not like a *balian*'s possession.

On 1 February 1961, she came home and obtained guidance from RGDP to make a shrine in her own house. RGDP gave her directions on the form and location of the shrine in her compound and also provided pictures of the statues for the shrine, which her family members were asked to make. People in her neighbourhood contributed money to build the shrine. When it was finished, there was a big ceremony with offerings; priests came to the ceremony, and a variety of forest animals were present (e.g. snakes and lizards). After the ceremony, many people came to ask her to treat their illnesses, to help to keep their families harmonious, and to consult her about religious ceremonies, for example, auspicious days to perform these. After receiving treatment by RGDP, grateful clients faithfully attended the *balian*'s ceremonies and gave money to build a new house for her.

In 1969, she became pregnant—still unmarried and, she claimed, without having had sexual intercourse—because the gods needed her to have progeny who could follow her heritage. All her neighbours knew that she was pregnant but no one criticized her. Many thought that this was what the god decreed. Some felt it was impossible to conceive without having intercourse. Her daughter, now 23 years of age, is married; she has a child 1½ years of age and lives with a neighbour beside her mother's house. She and her husband appear to honour her mother and to believe that she is controlled by RGDP.

At home, when she is not in trance-possession, this *balian* wears only a sarong or a sarong and a shirt. When she is possessed, she dresses formally in male clothes: a white shirt, a wide sarong with a yellow cuff around the bottom, and a sash. Her hair is tied up high on her head, similar to the way a high priest wears his hair, with a flower in it, and she has grains of rice stuck on her forehead as is usual for people who have returned from a temple after prayer and being blessed. She uses a walking staff. Her attitude in possession is like that of an old but energetic man with a long beard and moustache which she frequently 'twirls' with her fingers as if it were real.

According to the neighbours, this *balian* loves another woman with whom she has a good relationship, a woman who is a priest at another place in the city. She visits this priest daily and sometimes the priest comes to her home to pray and work together with her. Neighbours know of her relationship with the woman priest but they accept it by saying that the two gods love each other. When the people living in her house were asked what she does at home, they said that if no one comes to see her for treatment, she walks around without apparent purpose and then goes to sleep at 2.00 a.m., waking up around 9.00 or 10.00 a.m. After her bath, she returns to her room and closes the door. The people living at her house must prepare the offerings, the household shrines, and the altar to receive the god. She comes out of her room if the god asks her to see a client.

In daily life, she does not receive guests graciously. She is forgetful and does not remember people who have come to see her. Sometimes she asks her visitors why they have come. Then she says, 'I'm sorry, I do not know anything and I can't serve people well because I'm stupid.' She may ask her visitors whether they would like tea or a cigarette and repeat this a few times, in a persistent manner. In striking contrast when she is in trance-possession, she looks happy and optimistic, speaks fluently in a friendly manner, and treats her guests and clients very graciously; for example, she chats cordially, asking people where they have come from, or if she knows the people, with whom they have come. When new guests arrive, she invites them politely to sit down; she is very pleasant and friendly, and follows rules of etiquette, for example, by not asking people of higher status what their status is. Her eyes are bright and alert, and she moves about quickly. Sometimes she can also be very humorous, joking with the guests, but she is always respectful towards the gods.

She receives clients in the afternoon every day except market day (*pasah*; the third day of the Balinese week). Every person who comes seeking her help must bring a special offering, called a *pejati*, consisting of coconut, rice, money, or some other product. She goes into trance-possession when she sits in front of the altar praying, with incense smoke rising in front of her, and making an offering to God. Before she commences giving advice, she asks her clients where they have come from, how many of them are here, and how they have come. After establishing rapport, she turns her attention to their problems. She gleans her clients' situations from a large leaf, which she takes in her hands and studies, rather in the manner of some seers reading tea-leaves or looking into a crystal ball. From this she tells her clients and their families what has happened to them, why they have come to visit her, and what they must do to solve their problem. When she talks, her clients must simply listen; only after she has finished talking can they ask her questions if they do not understand or if they disagree with what has been said. Usually if the clients disagree with the *balian*, they seldom speak because they know they have come not only to receive advice but also to learn if the *balian* knows about their problem.

In the treatment session, the family members usually come without the patient, and they are free to discuss the problem and ask questions, which the *balian* answers patiently, talking like a parent to her children. If the family members feel sad or helpless, she makes them calm and optimistic. If they feel sick, she helps them combat their illness. She seldom says who has made the patient ill or that she knows someone's mistake has caused illness; in this way she does not imply a family member is 'bad' or guilty. She usually advises her clients against trying to find out who was responsible for their troubles and instead encourages them to become calmer, healthier, and happier. Only once in the observations did she identify a guilty person; her reason was that the client's ancestors asked her to do so because they were very sorry to see the client suffer. If her clients are of low education, she gives many examples to illustrate her explanations. Discussions with the family take about 20–30 minutes. Sometimes, she tells a story to help a client understand, and this may take up to 60 minutes. She is generally successful at managing her clients' problems.

At the end of a session, she takes holy water near her shrine, throws it out, and abruptly comes out of trance. She then goes to her room and changes back into her usual clothes. When she reappears, she resumes her non-*balian* personality: her vocalization is slow and dull in contrast to her fluent and witty speech during trance. She says she does not recall what she did or what happened during trance-possession, and she is reluctant to talk about it further.

This *balian*'s changes in personality and attitude bear out Gauld's

(1977: 580) statement that 'in the case of mediums who pass into trance, the ordinary personality may often, after a short interval, seem to be completely replaced by that of the deceased person or other discarnate being. The new personality may in some instances attain almost complete control of the medium's organism.' Out of trance, this *balian* appears abnormal but not psychotic; she merely withdraws to her room for long periods. She shows no evidence of delusions or hallucinations although the history of her 'illness' prior to becoming a *balian* indicates that she probably had delusions and hallucinations then. In normal circumstances, when she is not possessed, she acts as if she is demented or of borderline intelligence and finds it very difficult to focus on any type of conversation. She does not realize what she has said during trance or at least denies any knowledge of it; in trance, she claims to be God. These observations are consistent with those of trance-mediums in other cultures.

The following case-studies provide further examples of how this *balian* works.

Case 1

A 25-year-old, single, male labourer, with no past psychiatric history, and his family had apparently sought help to deal with his difficulty in forming relationships, his withdrawal, irritability, and anger if the family advised him, his anxiety about the future, his weakness and laziness, all of 1-month duration. The family came because they felt they had caused the problems by offending one of their ancestors and asked what they must do to make amends. In trance-possession, the *balian* said, 'You came here because you want to pray to God, because you want to make a big ceremony and request that all will be a success.' The family all agreed and said 'yes'. The healer then said, 'You are crying because your ancestor comes. Some of your ancestors stay at the temple (Dalem Puri).' She continued, 'The job is not finished. If you are sick, you go to the doctor but if you are sick because you have made a mistake with regard to your ancestors, you must find out how to erase your sin. You can do it in a big ceremony with the complete offerings.' The family said, 'We don't have enough money to hold a big ceremony. If it is a small ceremony, we can do it.' The healer said, 'The ceremony is the biggest one (*madudus agung*) but in practice, you can choose which size of ceremony you are able to afford. You did not conduct a ceremony to get permission from the god of

Dalem Puri for your family to leave the temple. The god is angry because you did not do it.' The healer followed this up with a long recitation of advice on how to prepare the ceremony.

Follow-up visits to the client at his home were made at 3 days, 20 days, and 30 days after the *balian*'s seance. At the initial visit following therapy, he was shy but spoke easily. His family said that at home, he fell calmer and seldom quarrelled; his relationships had improved, he seemed more peaceful, and he had become involved in more activities. The entire family were pleased and were grateful to the gods. The family had held a large ceremony which was quite costly (1.5 million rupiahs or about US$1,000.00 at that time), but the gods had helped them economize. At Suryani's next visit one month after treatment, many changes were evident in their home: they had new chairs, a television, and a Vespa motor scooter in the driveway. They attributed the improvement to their work and good family relationships. The client had returned to work and was energetic. He suffered from fewer headaches, and he was establishing more and better relationships with people. At the interview he was fluent, smiling, and self-confident. The family said that all the things they and he did had yielded good results and consequently their income had increased.

Case 2

This case involved a married woman, 42 years of age who had complained of physical and and mental problems for the past 3 years. She had an itchy skin and a repulsive, eczema-like rash which a dermatologist and a general practitioner had treated without success. Her facial appearance was another cause for concern: the skin looked blue, with dilated veins, and her eyes were perpetually averted, making her appear frightened and 'dangerous', at the same time. Other somatic complaints included back problems (e.g. she had difficulty standing) and stomach pains. In addition, the woman suffered from depression and she was talking less and less. Her case history indicated that her husband had taken a second wife approximately 10 years ago, and Suryani's initial clinical impression was anxiety disorder and psychological factors affecting physical condition.

This woman came to consult the *balian* with her mother and her daughter. The *balian* said, 'You are here because you want to know what is happening to yourself. You look pretty, but your heart is crying. You come here because you are sad and depressed. Your husband has another wife.' The woman answered, 'Yes.' The *balian* continued, 'You are the first wife. Don't be angry if I say the truth. You are sad and don't know why and you want to die. If you don't remember your children, you may kill yourself. You are always anxious and tense, and recently you failed to get help for what you wanted to do. Your livelihood is lost. Many people borrow from you and do not repay you, and all this makes you feel sad.' The *balian* spoke in a solemn and serious manner, like a father talking to a daughter. She continued, 'All your problems have arisen because of the second wife who wants to kill you by making you confused so that you will kill yourself. She makes you feel itchy all over your body. She makes your husband unable to think and is scared of her and your husband forgot about you and your children. You are a good person. The god of Dalem told you the truth.' As the *balian* said these words, the client looked down and her daughter looked sad and held on to her mother because she was afraid that she might lose her. The client asked the *balian* what she should do to avoid suffering. The mother of the client said that her granddaughter and all the other grandchildren depended upon their mother for school and so on. The mother of the client looked very scared and worried. The *balian* continued, 'Pretty woman, you come here to get peace' and proceeded to advise her on what she must do in order to achieve peace.

Suryani visited this client 10 days after her final treatment by the *balian*. Initially the woman did not believe that the *balian* could help her: it was her mother and daughter who had asked her to go. However, by this time, she already felt an improvement. On a second interview 2 months after her treatment, she looked happy and was able to talk but only in response to questions. She said that her thinking was calmer and less confused, she felt less sad, she cried less, and she was no longer suicidal. One month and 7 days after her treatment by the *balian*, she was able to work calmly. She seldom scratched her skin, the blueness of her face had disappeared, she was less shy, and she was able to establish good relationships. The Western clinical diagnosis in retrospect was moderate depression (dysthymia) and psychological factors affecting physical condition.

Case 3

The first clients of the evening, a mother and her daughter, presented themselves without saying why they had come, and were told by the *balian* in trance-possession that they had come because her son (and the daughter's brother) had been 'stabbed by a kris'. This was, in fact, their concern. He had suffered a wound in the chest while performing at a ceremony with a kris and was in the hospital recovering. The client wondered why it had happened. The *balian* explained that in a previous life, the young man had been asked by the gods to be a priest but he had declined on the grounds that it did not pay enough and the kris accident was a punishment from the gods. The *balian* assured the young man's mother that he would be all right.

Suryani interviewed eight other clients of this *balian*. All but one had satisfactory results from the treatment. One family had a problem of rats eating their rice crop. The *balian* advised them to place some rice at each corner of their field. As a consequence, they were no longer plagued by rats and their rice crop matured. In another case which involved a dying husband, the *balian* told the family that she could not help them as it was time for him to die. She advised them not to seek a cure because he would die the following day. Instead, she advised them to pray to God to help him achieve a good way to die. The husband died the next day.

This *balian*'s ability to foretell her clients' problems is typical. Westerners may be sceptical of her ability as it is difficult for them to believe that she could know the problems of her clients without being told by someone. However, in the case of this *balian*, it does not appear that she has gleaned information from common village knowledge since many of her clients come from other areas. A Western interpretation of this phenomenon is psychic ability akin to that demonstrated or claimed by Western clairvoyants. From observations of over 100 treatments by *balian*, Suryani estimates that about 50 per cent of clients' problems are correctly divined.

This *balian*'s initial 3-year experience of possession, with seclusion, delusions, and hallucinations, meets the criteria for a diagnosis of psychosis. This is a common pattern among *balian*: a severe illness and/or psychosis usually lasting one to several months prior to becoming a *balian*. Connor (1982) termed this 'divine madness'. Although this *balian* no longer has delusions or hallucinations in her non-possessed state, her personality can best be characterized as schizoid.

The differences in this *balian*'s appearance and personality between her trance-possession state and her non-possession state are striking. The change in behaviour is not readily explained in

Western terms. Behaviour characteristics of personality disorders do not usually disappear under hypnosis. Her shifts from one personality to another meet the diagnostic criteria for the clinical condition of multiple personality disorder. An incongruity peculiar to this *balian* is her masculine manner under possession, but perhaps this is understandable since she is possessed by a male god. Similarly, patients with multiple personalities may show such changes in gender behaviour as their alters of the opposite sex take over.

Annotated Translation of a *Balian Taksu*'s Treatment

The following is an account of the interaction between a female *balian taksu* in Denpasar and her first clients of the day, two women who presented themselves without saying anything about why they had come.

The *balian* prayed in a very loud, strong voice, different from her usual voice, and announced to the god that the clients had come with an offering to see him (the god). In trance she addressed the clients, 'You have come here because you need to know something about your baby (neither woman was the mother; they were relatives of the mother). The little child is newborn. You want to know which god or goddess [ancestor] is born in this child. [This was in fact the reason for their visit.] Your ancestor has come here, a man and a woman. The woman is unmarried. She has a child.' (The *balian* was visualizing and was being addressed by the ancestor but she was not yet possessed.) 'Now about this baby: the reincarnated ancestor had a family temple but did not have a baby in her past life.'

The first woman client then spoke, 'We don't know who it is who is not married.'

The *balian* replied, 'Yes, it was a long time ago. The great-grandmother of the baby is the woman [who is reincarnated]. She is not married. The baby is called by her.'

The first woman asked, 'What is her name?'

The *balian* replied, 'People call her Nyoman.'

The first woman asked, 'Please give me her full name.'

The *balian* said, 'I can't tell her full name because she is a god.'

The first woman asked, 'If I don't know her name, how can I know which ancestor is reincarnated?'

The *balian* replied, 'She is a god now, so she has no name. If you still want to know her name, I'll give you only her first initial: S.'

The second woman, trying to calm the first one, said, 'It's enough that we know the name is Nyoman.'

The first woman again asked, 'Who is Nyoman?'

The *balian* switched topics and advised them to perform a ceremony at 1, 3, and 6 months and said, 'When you conduct a ceremony at 3 months, bring white and yellow cloth, and at 6 months, when the baby's hair is cut, please bring me 30 pieces of Chinese money.' [The 6-month ceremony signifies that the infant has now become human; the ancestor then discontinues his life in the other world and assumes a real life in the baby.]

The *balian*, now speaking as the ancestor possessed, told the two women that when the baby becomes an adolescent, they should 'arrange a "marriage ceremony" (*masakapan*) to be held at the ocean'. [This means that the person will have a relationship with the mountains and the ocean.]

The women answered that they would do it if they had the money.

The *balian* replied, 'Yes, I know that you are short of money.' She then repeated the advice for the benefit of her clients.

Afterwards, when asked about her experience during the session, the *balian* said simply that she had fallen into trance-possession (*kalinggihan*) and would say no more about it.

Connor, Asch, and Asch (1986) published a detailed, verbatim account, and also produced an ethnographic film, of a trance-medium *balian* named Jero, who practises in South Bali. Jero is not able to recall the feelings or perceptions she experiences during a seance. However, she 'hears her own voice from afar coming from above her head, as if it belonged to someone else'. For example, this would tell her the spirit's wishes for a cremation or post-cremation ritual and let her know if the family had omitted certain offerings. Jero uses the word 'forgetting' (*engsap*) to refer to the change in herself when she is possessed. During the possession, the spirit may direct her to a particular potion for the patient to take home to treat his or her symptoms. 'In achieving a state of light trance, by praying and chanting, her personality is transformed. A supernatural being takes possession and converses with the practitioner.' According to Connor, Asch, and Asch, some Westerners believe that Jero is a fraud when she states that she is a medium for others. They note that Jero's voice changes entirely in character when she is possessed by the son of a petitioner in contrast to when she is possessed by a deity. It is also noted that much of the speech of the deities and spirits relayed through Jero is ambiguous. (See Connor, Asch, and Asch, 1986: 96, 102, 107, 116, 127.) All the above characteristics were present in the trance-medium *balian* observed by the authors, including depersonalization phenomena, possession by spirits, possession by relatives, and transformation of the voice to that of the possessed entity.

A *Balian* Who Treats by Physical Manipulation

This *balian* at Bangli refers to himself as a *balian usada*. In his view, a *balian* is a mediator in the process of restoring health to clients. He treats clients with all kinds of problems and ailments. He regards himself as a specialist in helping people rid themselves of evil spirits (*roh-jahat*) and in balancing the body energy. His technique involves knowing the energy centres, meridians, and pressure points of the body (*urat-saraf*). He uses his energy to cleanse clients of evil spirits, a special talent given to him by God, tempered by his study of the *lontar* (sacred palm leaf books) and by meditation. When he was 20 years old, he had an urge to become a healer and a strong desire to help others; this led him to make many offerings to his temple and to ask the gods if he should pursue such a path. He received an encouraging answer from the gods and was told how he should become a healer. In the tradition of the *usada* healer, he studied the *lontar* seriously for 5 years and through meditation he received answers to all his questions. It was during this time that he developed a special gift for healing people by using his spiritual energy. It is a method peculiar to himself, which he believes is given to him by God during meditation. He is of the opinion that everyone can learn to use his or her spiritual energy through meditation but unless one has a spiritual calling, one would not be able to do the type of healing that he does. He is quite well known and respected in his community. His son has chosen to go into the field of medicine so that he may heal others as well.

Patients, dressed semi-formally in sarong and sash, come to his office with offerings and donations of rupiah. This *balian* always dresses completely in white. He treats about 20 patients in a day, the typical treatment for one client lasting about 20 minutes. Clients are always accompanied by friends or family members.

He has regular methods for treating all clients. After his mantra, introduction of the client to the god, prayer, request to the god to cure the client, and a ritual sprinkling of himself with some holy water, he steps up to the client, who is seated in a chair in his treatment room. He begins by opening up a 'positive energy channel' on top of the client's head. This is done by parting the hair, putting two drops of coconut oil which has been blessed on the head, and rubbing the spot with the middle finger of his right hand as he chants a mantra. He then blows a breath of 'unseen white fire' down through the top of the head of the person, and quickly follows this up by touching the main pressure points on the patient's body. Then he applies light pressure to the neck, shoulders, arms, elbows, legs, and knees, pointing with his index fingers on each side of the chest at the heart, the solar plexus, and the stomach. He then begins to feel the spots where the evil spirit is residing in the client, beginning with the back of the neck, with the right hand pressing firmly on the muscles. Then he holds the patient's arm outstretched and blows into the palm in a straight line down the length of the arm. He will know where the evil spirit is when the white fire that is travelling through the person creates sparks at the point where they meet. Quite often, he senses spots of imbalance in the neck. He concentrates on the specific areas where the evil spirit is located by applying pressure with his fingers on the arm and upper body or with his heel on the leg, knee, or foot. This causes considerable pain as indicated by the patient's wincing and crying out. Only when the evil spirit has left the person will he no longer experience any pain. The treatment is completed when the *balian* touches those areas which were painful before but are no longer so, indicating that the evil spirit has left.

This *balian* was observed on a number of occasions treating more than a dozen clients for various complaints. One of his clients was a 34-year-old woman, a Western graduate student in psychology, who had come to him for treatment of an ovarian tumour. He asked the client if she wished to be treated or be given advice, and she said she wanted to be treated. He did not ask about her problem nor did she tell him. He prepared himself with a ritual mantra and holy water blessing for the client. He first opened up an energy channel on top of her head in order to establish a free flow of energy. He explained that this was to open the fontanelle so that he could see what was happening in her body. He was able to visualize coloured smoke which told him where the problem was and what it was—an evil spirit. He then blew on her head and started touching the pressure points, according to his ritual. Palpation of her neck and shoulders elicited excruciating pain. As the recipient of the possessed god, he blew power on to his left elbow, then on to his right hand, and after that he felt her elbow. He then stepped on the dorsum of his client's foot with his heel and said, 'She has a weakness, not an illness or a pain.' He added that the client 'always complains about her weakness [fatigue and lack of energy]'. Suryani asked him what the problem was and he replied that it was 'caused by the supernatural', possibly because the patient had made a mistake in another place which was manifest by the evil spirit entering her. He continued, 'For example, she might have gone to a temple during her menstruation and that is the reason she is tired. It is caused by the evil spirit.' Addressing the client, he said, 'Fortunately you came here. If you were to go home to America, no one could handle this there.' He explained further that 'Bali is magic. Sometimes visitors who come to Bali get sick. Bali is different from the rest of Indonesia: it has more magic.'

He felt the client's neck again, causing her a great deal of pain. He claimed that he did not touch her very hard. He then touched both her arms and commented, 'Now you don't feel any pain, although I touched your arms in the same way as before.'

He then applied pressure on her knee with his bare foot, which elicited severe pain. He said to Suryani, 'I touched her very lightly. After the evil spirit is thrown out, she will feel no pain.' He explained that if she had no disorder from an evil spirit, she would not feel any pain. He then stood on her knee again with his foot and this time it was not at all painful.

Suryani then asked him about the tumour. 'It will take a long time.' He said, 'Its cause is not supernatural but natural. It is better and more quickly treated by doctors. Why not do it?' The client responded that she was scared of surgery. Suryani explained to him that her surgeon in America was planning to operate on this tumour. He agreed to try to treat it and proceeded to blow on his arm while touching the patient, felt her back again, blew on his hand, felt her arm, blew breath on her head, then palpated her abdomen and her head, none of which was painful. He asked the client how it felt and she replied that it tickled. Holding her waist, he blew again on his arm to drive out the evil spirits and asked her if she felt any pain. She replied, 'No.' He appeared to have finished his treatment and said that he thought he could treat her problem. He asked her if she could come again for two more treatments.

After the *balian* came out of trance, he verbalized aspects of his treatment. As the smoke from the incense entered his body, he felt warm; he sensed his body getting bigger, and then he was imbued with the power of the god to treat illness and other problems. During treatment, he was possessed by the god Saraswati, a manifestation of the supreme God. He explained that each part of the client's body which was painful at his touch was an encounter between the god's power and the evil spirit; he believed that god's power effected the cure by extruding the black magic.

After the treatment, the client admitted that she did in fact have a physical problem of weakness and severe malaise brought on by ingesting sugar in any form, such as soft drinks, candy, or doughnuts. This condition, which had affected her for about 10 years, began around the time she lived for several months in Indonesia. All sorts of medical tests and examinations in America failed to yield a diagnosis and nothing had helped. The following day, when she tested the *balian*'s 'cure' by taking a soft drink and eating cake, she did not experience any negative symptoms. Follow-up on this client 6, 12, and 18 months later in the United States revealed that the sugar/tiredness problem did not recur. However, because of her brief stay in Bali, this client was not able to return to the *balian* for further treatment of her tumour. It was subsequently surgically removed and proved to be endometriosis.

A *Balian* Who Uses Trance, Chinese Coins, and *Lontar*

This *balian*, a Balinese who practises in Denpasar, utilizes trance and old Chinese coins in his treatment. According to him, the god Saraswati (the goddess of knowledge) appears during his trance and conveys to him the advice he delivers. When the authors visited him, he had no clients, so Suryani presented herself as a patient. First he prayed to request the god Saraswati to help him because a client had come to see him. After this brief ceremony, he asked Suryani to take some Chinese coins from each of two stacks on a plate. She took several from each stack and handed them to him. He quickly arranged the coins around the plate and after looking at this arrangement for several seconds, he picked up a *lontar* to determine her reason for coming to see him. He stated:

> You want to know about a man who has a problem with his job. His income has decreased; his livelihood has decreased; his effort has decreased. He must avoid the 'friends' who want to destroy his work if he wants to succeed in his job because he has a good livelihood and he gets good results from his usual work. He has two wives but he does not have any big problems from them. He does not need drugs or treatment, but he must take a holiday, a break, to become calm and relaxed, so that he can make good decisions.

Halfway into his 'reading' of the *lontar*, Suryani observed that, although he looked intently at the *lontar* and appeared to be following the words with his index finger, the *lontar* was blank and without inscriptions at all. On several subsequent occasions, he repeated his performance: he appeared to be reading without hesitation, as if the words were written. This phenomenon is comparable to automatic writing in a state of hypnosis.

After this seance, Suryani contacted her brother and learned that what the *balian* had said was true. She had not previously known the extent of his problems at work and she had wrongly suspected that he had problems with one of his wives.

A *Balian* Who Extracts Bones from Clients

This *balian* was observed on a number of different occasions treating more than 20 different clients, ranging in age from 3 months to 65 years. There were about equal numbers of males and females. From about one-third of these, the *balian* extracted bones during his very painful massage of the client. On each occasion, 1–6 bones were extracted—some long and sharp, others shaped like kernels or small pebbles. These usually came from the umbilicus but there were some from the abdomen, behind the knee and from the back of the head. During this procedure, all these patients experienced or evidenced behaviour indicating excruciating pain. Often there were signs of trauma to the skin with some redness and swelling at the site of the bone extraction. Although the authors and several colleagues watched this *balian* closely during all his manipulations, it was not possible to establish that he might have concealed these bones in his hand prior to their removal from the clients. The *balian* explained that these pieces of bone and the associated pain of removal were manifestations of evil spirits; the removal of such evil spirits would lead to a cure. Following treatment, clients were frequently given a prescription or remedy that they could take home, usually an organic substance. For example, the *balian*'s wife would ask the client to name something they could use to help themselves, to keep them in balance. The client would usually choose the *balian*'s medication, usually a certain leaf or flower to ingest or anoint. Clients interviewed immediately after treatment generally indicated feelings of relief and satisfaction.

A young physician from America presented himself as a client to this *balian* because he wished to be treated for high blood pressure. Suryani accompanied him and brought the appropriate special offering to the temple at the *balian*'s house. The *balian*'s wife, who usually prayed and ministered to the clients upon their arrival, appeared to fall into trance immediately, as was evident by the closing of her eyes, fluttering of her eyelids, flattening of her facial expression, and changes in her voice, manner of speaking, and gestures. She asked, 'What do you need?' Suryani answered, 'We want to know what the problem is that he has', referring to her colleague and phrasing her statement so as to 'test' the *balian* to see if he would know. She responded, 'I know that you are here to test me.' At that point Suryani denied it. The woman continued, 'He has a problem in the mind; he has difficulty concentrating, he is losing his memory, and he is confused. His main problem lies in the food he eats. It makes him that way. Sometimes his thoughts are empty. To treat his problem, he must eat more vegetables.' The young physician told Suryani that what she had said was true to some extent. He said that his hypertension was reduced when he ate more vegetables. He proceeded with his treatment by this *balian*, who massaged his abdomen forcefully and then 'removed' a small sliver of bone from his umbilicus, a very painful experience indeed because of the deep, sustained pressure applied by the *balian* to this spot. Three days later, the umbilical soreness had subsided and he reported feeling calmer and less confused. Suryani advised him to stop taking his anti-hypertensive medication because she felt that his hypertension was primarily a psychological problem and at this point, his blood pressure was normal. Daily repeat blood pressure measurements over 20 subsequent days were also normal. While he attributed this change mainly to the *balian*'s treatment, another factor could have played a role: every day he also performed Suryani's technique of 'healing meditation' (see Chapter 8).

The *balian*'s wife, who was not a *balian*, also went into trance and behaved in some respects like a *balian*. In trance, she appeared to demonstrate psychic abilities; for example, she could discern the client's motivation and problems. According to the client, she was fairly accurate. This was the first time that the authors have observed a *balian* working with his wife as a team.

Jensen and one of his Western colleagues submitted themselves for treatment by this *balian* in order to experience his work at first hand. Although he had not been briefed by either client, the body parts he worked on proved to be the areas for which each had sought help. His physical treatments included hard pressure with the stone of a ring on the terminal bone of the client's fingers and toes; hard, deep massage on the abdomen; and intense pressure on body parts (i.e. back of the head or the umbilicus) to 'remove' the bone, all of which produced excruciating pain. Afterwards, both Jensen and his colleague were convinced that he did not remove a piece of bone from either of them; he surreptitiously made it appear as if he did. He showed all observers the sharply pointed piece of bone that he had ostensibly removed, about 2.5 centimetres long by 1 centimetre wide, but he would not allow them to handle or keep it, and he quickly concealed it. The effects of the treatment were both painful and traumatic (physically and emotionally) and were not at all therapeutic. While Jensen was convinced that the 'bone work' was trickery,[7] two Balinese medical colleagues did not view it this way. On the contrary, several aspects indicated to them that he was genuine in what he did: they actually saw the piece of bone being removed; this healer had a long-standing reputation of more than 25 years for successful healing; clients came from far and wide to see him; and they believed that his treatments had different effects on individuals. This evidence, combined with belief, was so strong that it overrode their Western logic and scientific knowledge.

Even if this traditional healer's bone removal technique was 'charlatanism' in the Western sense, this would not necessarily detract from the healing power of the entire procedure for some clients. The procedure could be therapeutically significant overall because of elements other than the bone removal *per se*, such as the ventilation of emotions, the palpable and painful awareness by the client that something definite was being done, the emotional exhortation associated with the pain, the belief in the supernatural aspects of the problem or illness, and faith in the healing procedures.

A *Balian* Who Uses Massage

This small, slender, wiry, 60-year-old man had been a farmer all his life at Batubulan near Denpasar when one day, 6 years ago, he was spontaneously possessed at a religious ceremony and was told by a god to become a *balian*. He declined and in the following year, his crops failed, his cows and pigs died, and he feared that he himself would die unless he became a *balian*. At the time, his sister-in-law who had always had a difficult time with delayed deliveries, and now was pregnant for the fifth time, was in her ninth month of pregnancy. He vowed then that if she delivered now, he would become a *balian*, and she promptly delivered without any problems.

Subsequently, many people with illnesses came to consult him and he has practised steadily since. A number of Suryani's psychiatric patients had been successfully treated by him.

His method of therapy involved massage, for which, he explained, he did not need to be trained, having been given the skill by the gods. The authors had a massage by him, observed him treating each other, and questioned him about what happened as he massaged. He said that his hands and fingers moved by themselves as if they were under 'another power', and that he did not have to think about how to massage, even when he set fractures or replaced dislocated joints. It was evident that he used up a lot of energy and muscular strength while he was massaging, but he said he did not feel tired even when he treated up to five clients in a morning. During the interview before massage, he was rather distant and socially awkward. In contrast during massage, he was friendly and spoke fluently, and he was able to converse on a variety of social topics. He reported experiences of possession at temple ceremonies. These data indicate that this *balian* was in trance and probably possessed while carrying out his massage treatment.

Clients of *Balian* Who Fall into Trance-possession

At a small village north of Klungkung, a *balian usada* (who uses *lontar*) specializes in treating clients possessed by an evil spirit or black magic which causes *bebainan* (see Chapter 7). Many of his clients fall into trance-possession during treatment. He is a widower with nine children, a very jovial, animated, and talkative man who was happy to discuss his work, particularly when he learned that Suryani is from the royal family in Klungkung. He wore two large rings inset with big stones on each hand. A ring with a very large, carved evil spirit's head on it—the head of Boma, which looks somewhat like Rangda—was placed on a shelf above his head in view of his clients. This was one of his two 'test' (*penued*) objects. If a client sees this ring and it appears bigger than it is in reality, it indicates that the client is possessed by an evil spirit. Another test object is a metal cylinder which appears to be a pewter salt shaker about 2 centimetres in diameter and 4 centimetres long. Testing with this involves placing it on the forehead of the client and holding it there firmly for several minutes. Patients who are diagnosed by him to be possessed by an evil spirit or black magic, which is the cause of the complaint or illness which they present, fall into trance with eyes closed, shaking their body, sometimes screaming and crying, and stiffening their extremities, as if they are experiencing considerable pain. The metal cylinder is pressed against the client's forehead for about 3–5 minutes more, and the client then comes out of trance if the black magic has been caused by an evil spirit from the island of Lombok or from East Java. If the evil spirit originates from West Java, the trance lasts about 10 minutes. If the evil spirit is from Bali, the trance may last up to 3 hours, which, according to him, indicates that the Balinese black magic is exceptionally strong. During the time that the client is in trance, the family may witness concrete evidence of the black magic in the form of hair or a large beetle extruded from the client. During the trance, the client's verbalizations, crying, and yelling are regarded as those of the evil spirit who possesses them. Following the trance, the client may have complete amnesia regarding the episode, and experiences feelings of relief or calm, presumably from relief of the problems or symptoms.

An 18-year-old Balinese college student who accompanied the authors submitted himself for a 'check-up'. Suryani held the metal cylinder firmly to his forehead for several minutes and then the *balian* placed a wooden peg, about 1 millimetre in diameter, with small knobs on the surface, between the fingers of his left hand. This had no effect until it was placed between the third and fourth fingers, at which point it immediately evoked excruciating pain, causing the young man to wince, writhe, and cry out. The pain lasted for about 2 minutes and then completely disappeared. The *balian* explained that black magic had been placed in him at his school by a girl who loved him and wanted to cast a spell on him and that the pain was due to the exit of the black magic from his body. When the pain disappeared, he was declared free of the black magic. The authors' Western explanation of the phenomenon was that the young man experienced pain as a manifestation of trance.

Half of the clients who experienced trance-possession with this *balian* were men and half were women; they ranged from adolescents to old people but most of them were young adults. One elderly woman did not appear to the authors to be in trance but, according to the *balian*, she was, as indicated by the paleness of her face, a change in her breathing, and sleepiness while the metal cylinder was placed on her forehead. The total time that the cylinder was placed on the forehead was approximately 5 minutes. This indicated to him that she had black magic from a Muslim and whatever problem she had did not need further curative work because the black magic had been removed. Not all of the clients who came to him fell into trance-possession and manifested *bebainan*; with these clients he used the *lontar* to give advice.

The clients come to him from all over South Bali and are aware that he is a specialist in treating *bebainan* caused by the possession of evil spirit or black magic. Perhaps this is the reason that his clients are prone to enter trance-possession during his ritualistic treatment procedure. Whereas it is quite common to see clients enter a trance state during treatment by a *balian*, this is only one of two *balian* observed whose patients enter trance-possession in this rather ritualistic pattern and apparently under some control by the *balian*. This represents a parallel to Western hypnotherapy.

Observations of another *balian* in Klungkung further illustrate trance in clients. This middle-aged *balian*, also a junior high schoolteacher, treats patients in his home. He explained that most of what he knows as well as his healing powers was given to him by God during meditation. He believes that anyone can learn methods of healing through meditation. This *balian* has an air of bravado and arrogance, often telling everyone how powerful he is. He enjoys relating specific instances of his cures and stories about people from around the world who have come to observe him and study with him. He is very eager to teach what he knows and to discuss his work with anyone. In so doing, he is generous and patient.

The first client was a 70-year-old man who complained of headache and stomach fullness of 10 years' duration for which he had seen many doctors and traditional healers without success. He said his head felt like it was frozen, that it did not work right, and he still had a headache. Three days previously, he had had his first treatment by this healer. After his prayer and mantra, the *balian* lit a handful of incense and passed the smoke over the back and upper body of the client. He then placed stick-like instruments ('wands'), one on the forehead and one on the back in different areas, which caused the client to experience warmth and pain, and to cry out uncontrollably and scream, writhing with an extraordinary grimace on his face, as if in severe pain. This behaviour lasted about 3 minutes and then gradually subsided, at which point the *balian* said that he was pressing just as hard with the wands but they were no longer painful because the black magic had left. After the first treatment, the client said that his headache was somewhat better and after this treatment, he felt even better. He stated that he felt happier and more comfortable and that he could now relax in contrast to feeling tense before the treatment. He appeared very much at ease after the treatment and was happy to talk about the treatment and his improvement.

The next client observed was a 28-year-old married woman, accompanied by her husband, who complained of pain all over her body, including her head and her abdomen; this pain had been going on for 5 years and she had also sought help from a number of doctors, again without any sign of relief. This was her eighth visit to this healer. Under observation two weeks previously, she responded much like the patient described above, with extreme pain and emotional and uncontrollable crying as he placed the wands on her chest and forehead. On this visit, she experienced relatively little pain from the same treatment, although she cried a bit. She looked much healthier and more at ease than she had on the earlier visit. She reported that her pains were not completely gone but were about 75 per cent cured, and she was able to eat better.

Both of these patients appeared to be in a state of trance during the treatment, as indicated by a change in sensation resulting in pain at one point and release of it at another, under similar conditions. They also appeared to express themselves in a very primitive, uncontrolled manner, comparable to the way an infant cries without being able to say what is wrong with himself. This kind of emotional expression is not seen in ordinary Balinese life, except under special conditions, such as trance. In terms of Western diagnosis, it seemed likely that both the above clients had a somatoform disorder which in the West is generally treated with psychotherapy and medication, although it may also be treated with hypnotherapy.

A third client who complained of discomfort in her abdomen was treated by this *balian* in the same manner as the first two clients above but experienced no pain from the touch of his wands. The *balian* pronounced that she did not suffer from black magic, but rather had a physical problem.

A possession disorder was observed in a client treated by the *balian usada* in Bangli who specialized in problems caused by evil spirits. This was a 55-year-old woman who had a variety of somatic symptoms. The *balian* first went through his ritual of prayer and mantra and the patient also prayed. The *balian* began with his standard massage technique to the client's neck which caused her suddenly to twitch and shake violently. As he applied more pressure to her neck with his hand, she began to shout and a spirit began to speak through her. It said it did not want to leave her and it told how it had been living in her body, moving around inside it. Her voice at this time was noticeably different from her usual and she began to move differently too. The *balian* put more pressure on her neck and he stated that the spirit was now moving from her hips to her throat and that he was going to force it out of her mouth.

The spirit then began speaking in a high voice, sounding very agitated. After the patient gave a final shudder of her body, the *balian* said that the evil spirit had left and the patient felt immediate relief. The *balian* explained that the evil spirit had been inside her for 15 days and that she was now cured because it had left her.

Part of the foregoing report represents the *balian*'s interpretation but part of it is also consistent with a state of possession, as indicated by the changed quality of the woman's voice as an entity spoke through her. Her closed eyes and loss of usual facial expression are also indicative of a trance state. The treatment in this case consisted essentially of an exorcism of the evil spirit. A similar instance of possession disorder was observed in a case treated with hypnotherapy by Suryani (see Chapter 8).

A Balinese Physician's Personal Experience with *Balian*

A practising Balinese physician trained in Western medicine was interviewed about his experiences with and attitudes towards traditional healers. He related detailed personal experiences similar to those of the trance-mediums' sessions reported above which he considered as valid, meaningful, and helpful contacts and messages from the gods or spirits of his ancestors. Although he had no formal education regarding traditional healers and no professional contacts with any, he knew them through his own childhood and family experiences and he respected them.

He related his personal experiences with traditional healing as follows (J. Isherwood, personal communication). After his younger sister was killed in a motor vehicle accident, he and the dead woman's husband and daughter went to a *balian*. The healer went into trance-possession, and without being told the reason for their visit, suddenly cried out and, smacking herself hard on the head, said that she was dead. In this manner the healer acted out the pain and fatal blow to the deceased sister's head in the motor vehicle accident. The sister's spirit then spoke through the healer to her daughter, calling her by name and also mentioning an incident known only to the husband: namely, that the dead woman had been seen at home staring into space and thinking about death just a few days before the accident.

This physician related two other experiences with traditional healers. After his mother's death, the family visited a healer and upon entering into trance-possession, the healer changed posture and sat just as his mother often did and spoke with phrases that sounded very much like hers. The physician recounted an even more remarkable event that occurred at a visit to a *balian* by his family after he had been seriously injured in a motor vehicle accident. Without being told anything about the accident, the *balian* told the family that their son was seriously hurt, 'not in Bali but in Sulawesi (an island in Indonesia), that he would not die but would take a long time to recover, and that the accident was sent to remind the family of an important ancestor, one of the sons of a king from Klungkung'. When the family asked why it had been necessary to call attention to their ancestor in this way, the healer said that there had been a previous attempt to draw their attention to this matter when a boy in the extended family had been injured by a needle in his eye. After learning this, the family made enquiries at Klungkung, located the ancestor's temple, and made appropriate offerings and ceremonies. The injured doctor recovered as predicted. This physician regarded traditional healing as a positive mental health resource for the Balinese. His grandfather was a traditional healer. In spite of his Western medical education, he maintained a firm belief in consultation with *balian* and would seek help from them if he had similar problems in the future.

Balian and Shamans: A Comparison

The phenomenology and methodology of the trance-mediums in Bali are comparable in many respects to the practices of shamans in China and in central India, both of which have an ancient history (Tseng, 1976). They enter into trance-possession and explain the supernatural causes of the patient's problems or illness and give advice consistent with cultural beliefs in supernatural causes of illness and religiously based concepts of restoring interpersonal harmony. A variation of the practice of these trance-medium shaman is a self-mutilation component (Fuchs, 1964; Li, 1976), which does not occur in Bali.

While the process and techniques of *balian* can be compared with Western psychotherapy and with Eastern shamanism, in a number of aspects it is additionally illuminating to compare the work of *balian* with that of American Indian shaman healers. Halifax (1992) identified what she referred to as eight 'modes' of treatments used by shamans, all of which relate to the 'practical process of healing the rift between the self and other'. All of the modes of the shamans, except one, are strikingly similar to those observed in the *balian*; this is especially astonishing when one considers that not only are the two cultures separated by half a world but they are unrelated and have no contact with each other. The eight modes are given below:

1. The aspect of enchantment is revealed in the process of ceremony: the physical aspects of creating a sacred ground or place, songs or mantras, herbs, and the psychic aspect of concentration. Ceremony is further structured to create a 'field' where everything is seen as magic; through concentration, the magic is brought out. The power spot refers to the sacred place where 'minding', or concentration, allows the evocation of the power.
2. The shaman is awake and lucid, functioning as if in a dream, and he may become part of the patient's state of consciousness. It is essential that the shaman should be able to retain or restore control of himself and return to a state of reality after his seances.
3. The shaman reconciles and counsels. He reconciles opposing realms of thought and counsels his clients on relationships, such as the relationship with God.
4. The shaman is able to see into the future, and can understand the causes and effects of life's experiences. He may be able to predict how one lives and how one needs to live.
5. The shaman is a pathfinder or guide. Metaphorically speaking, he is able to see the path in the darkest territory, just as a wolf is able to find the trackless way. In this mode, the shaman helps the patient explore 'territory' (experiences) not previously interpreted or described.
6. The use of the 'plants' intelligence' refers to the natural botanical medicinals, of which there are many.
7. The shaman experiences an ecstatic state or state of trance or possession in which he makes magical flights which involve his spirit leaving this world to join other spirits.
8. The shaman is also an 'ordinary' person.

All of the above aspects of shamans' work are similarly characteristic of the work of *balian* except for the shaman's magic flights. Another mode of the shaman not seen in the *balian* is that in which the shaman goes on a journey in which he dies and is reborn. *Balian* may go on a journey through the client's body and extract malevolent spirits that have intruded. An ability of some *balian* which is similar to shaman journeying, and which is learned from the *lontar*, is to travel to another town to visit a person whom he usually threatens to harm or kill. Such a *balian* is then regarded as a *leak*. The Balinese people caution against learning this ability.

Western Channellers

Channelling is a relatively new term for a process described as the transmission of information which appears to come from a personality source outside of the conscious mind and which is purposely directed towards an audience (Hastings, 1991). The phenomenon of modern-day American channellers is similar to that of Balinese trance-mediums in several ways. In one form of channelling a person goes into trance and another 'being' speaks through him/her, in a manner similar to possession states (Hastings, 1991: 11, 12). Hastings (1991: 2, 71) considered the possibility that channelling may be a non-pathological form of multiple personality or 'dissociated subpersonalities', secondary personalties, and he elaborated on the theory that channelling is a process of the unconscious mind communicating with the conscious mind in the form of a voice or entity. Channellers experience entities near themselves or entering into their bodies, a process many refer to as 'blending' (by which they mean a harmonious merging), a term they prefer in contrast to the concept of 'domination by possession' (Hughes, 1989). They exhibit varying degrees of amnesia concerning their experiences (Hughes, 1989). Some channellers' entities have characteristics of modern Western culture (e.g. they may come from outer space) and differ from other cultures in that they do not represent familiar embodied persons who have lived on earth before. This difference illustrates how the experience of trance in channelling is culturally determined: beliefs and ideas about trance states determine their content. Hughes (1989) interviewed channellers before and after trance and he also interviewed the channelled entities themselves. The latter report using the channeller's 'tool kit vocabulary and symbol system' to give expression to their ideas. Both channellers and their entities speak of 'signatory sensations' which enable them to identify each other. The channellers describe their motivation as 'personal growth' and as, being of service to others'. Channelling can be viewed as an inherently religious activity (Hughes, 1989).

Western Psychiatric Treatment of Balinese Patients

Psychotic Balinese patients, those who manifest delusions, hallucinations, thought disorganization, and changed affect (e.g. mania), such as is typical for schizophrenia, bipolar affective disorder, and certain acute psychoses, who are brought to traditional healers and not cured, are often referred by the healers or brought by their family for treatment by psychiatrists and are likely to be hospitalized at either Udayana General Hospital in Denpasar or at the mental hospital at Bangli, Bali. There they are treated with conventional Western pharmacotherapy, especially major tranquillizers such as Thorazine, chlopromazine, and haloperidol. Most of them respond to such therapy, by becoming asymptomatic but not completely well, and are returned to their homes after a 1–2-week hospitalization. Their families again take them for treatment by traditional healers and carry out ritual ceremonies that are recommended. It is clear from the authors' clinical experience that the major psychoses are more effectively treated and managed with the adjunctive modern pharmacotherapy. However, some psychotically ill patients are resistant to pharmacotherapy; they become chronically ill and require long-term hospitalization, as has occurred in the West.

In the following case treated by Suryani, a 31-year-old traditional healer who lived near Besakih suffered from daily attacks of panic (with palpitations) lasting 1–2 hours, which made him feel as if he was going to fall down and die. Although he was reputed to be a very clever man (reportedly able to bring dead chickens back to life), he was unable to cure himself and had been suffering for four years. He worried incessantly about the possibility of a repeat attack. He came to Suryani as a private patient and she treated him with the medications Amineptine and Clobasam. After three months' treatment, he returned to normal, relatively symptom-free. Since then, he has had only one mild attack but he continues to worry that the attacks may recur.

If trance-mediums and other types of traditional healers of Bali have implications for Western medicine and mental health, it would appear to be in their demonstration of the effectiveness of ASC, therapists' intuition, and the powerful healing effects of belief by the therapist, the client or patient, and the respective families. These elements offered by Balinese culture support and may broaden the views and skills of Western medical practitioners.

* * *

Some of the thousands of traditional healers (*balian*) in Bali utilize trance and trance-possession in their work with clients and families. Most are referred to as *balian taksu* or trance-mediums. They are given their skills by the gods and in therapy sessions become possessed by God, gods, holy spirits, or souls, enabling clients and family members to communicate with them and receive their advice. Some *balian* demonstrate psychic ability in diagnosing the problems of their clients without asking for such information from the clients themselves. *Balian* give advice and treat many types of problems—physical, behavioural, and emotional, particularly bereavement. Many of their techniques have much in common with Western psychotherapy, including establishing rapport, furnishing explanations of causes, allowing ventilation of feelings, relieving guilt, providing support, giving hope for the future, assuaging anger, discouraging revenge, and dispensing advice for pursuing concrete, positive restorative goals and behaviour. Some *balian* who go into trance use physical techniques such as massage. Tricks or 'sleight of hand' are rarely used. Treatment by an individual *balian* often, but not always, helps with problems and cures illness, even in a single session. The personalities of some highly functional *balian taksu* resemble the Western condition of multiple personality. The work of Chinese shamans, Western modern-day channellers, and American Indian shamans shares many similarities with Balinese trance-mediums; their differences are culturally based. Occasionally, some *balian* seek Western psychiatric help for their personal problems and disorders.

The work done by most *balian*, carried out in states of trance-possession, is tied in with their cultural beliefs of the cause and cure of illness; it is always framed in spiritual or religious terms. Traditional healers are quite effective in dealing with problems, especially those concerning bereavement and the family. Their success in resolving problems, healing clients, and curing diseases attest to the power of Balinese spirituality. Their techniques appear to be no less effective when used in other cultures, including Western cultures, in which spiritual or religious elements prevail.

1. Connor, Asch, and Asch (1986) provided a detailed account and produced a film of one traditional healer at Bangli in South Bali, which illustrates the ritual and observed process.

2. The shaman or 'medicine man' is a parallel in other cultures. Their origins may have been similar and could possibly be traced to the rock paintings of the Lascaux Cave in France from the Old Stone Age (Goodman, 1990).

3. See Leimena and Thong (1983) and Connor, Asch, and Asch (1986: 24–6) for more details on types of techniques used by the healers.

4. The word *taksu* has several meanings. First, it means possession of a body by a god. Secondly, it refers to an inner power—a spiritual power conferred by the gods—which gives an artist intelligence and genuine creativity (Bandem, 1990) and

helps him to excel beyond what is customary by the normal performance or execution of his art. Every dancer strives to obtain *taksu* of this sort. Thirdly, *taksu* means the place where a *balian* receives a special power from the gods for the paraphernalia (e.g. ring and cylinder) used in treating his clients, as is the case with a traditional healer at Klungkung.

5. It is believed that if the family makes a mistake in the death ceremony, the ancestor god may be angry and fail to bring good fortune or help to the living family. Because the death ceremony is elaborate, it is easy to make a 'mistake' in some aspect of it.

6. According to Balinese legend, Ratu Gde Dalem Peed was descended from God Siwa and his wife who had intercourse when they flew above the sea and whose sperm and ovum dropped into the sea between Bali and the island of Nusa Panida. The god (RGDP) is believed to have the ability to harm or kill people who have been bad and also to help people by protecting them and curing diseases.

7. Tricks are recognized as part of the practice of shamanism (Walsh, 1990: 101). The remarkable cures and hoaxes of psychic surgery in the Philippines have been well described (Elaide, 1966; Leff, 1981: 109; Valentine, 1973).

Chapter 4
Mass Trance-possession in Ceremonies

TRANCERS involved in mass or communal trance-possession ceremonies offer another window on the trance-possession phenomena. They are not characterized by the self-control of the traditional trance-medium but require the assistance of helpers in the immediate environment, particularly for guidance and control of their behaviour and for termination of the trance-possession state. These trance-possession states are contagious. The trancers demonstrate unusual physiological abilities during the trance-possession state, such as forceful 'self-stabbing' by a kris (*keris*) and contacting fire without injury, and they often experience the positive emotional after-effects of possession.

Mass Trance-possession at Timbrah

At the time of *kuningan*, which occurs at intervals of 210 days by the Balinese calendar, a small village in East Bali has an 11-day celebration, one day of which involves a trance of 80 or more of the villagers at once.[1] This trance ceremony is one of the most riveting and emotionally climactic events a Westerner can witness. It has been performed every 210 days for as long as the people can remember.[2] Several village residents said that the present ceremony is on a smaller scale than the ones staged during their childhood because families today wish to spend their money on other things such as education for their children. However, there is no less devotion and no change in their beliefs or values.

Preparations leading up to the event include decorating the temple with banners and hanging colourful cloth around the pavilions, preparing the receptacles for six gods to be carried on bamboo frames (*joli*), preparing food for all the youngsters in the village and for many of the adult men, making elaborate food offerings for the gods, and practising the gamelan and gong. The day's event lasts all day, ending about 1.00 a.m.

The temple is approached on foot, up narrow dirt paths with river stone steps and inclines at intervals. Upon arrival at the temple, one can hear the gong orchestra playing in a pavilion at the corner of the outer temple grounds about 50 metres square, the least sacred area of the temple. Just beyond this is the second temple area and next to it is the most sacred part of the temple. Its high gate in classic Balinese style has six high steps going up and six going down into the grounds.

At a mass trance-possession ceremony in this village witnessed by the authors in 1991, about 100 people had gathered outside the main temple by 4.00 p.m. Women were walking into the temple with tall stacks of food offerings on their heads, and about 40 young boys and girls from 4 to 12 years of age were sitting on the ground in a long row, stretching from the steps of the temple gate to the outer temple grounds. Between the two rows of children was a long 'table' of green banana leaves on the ground. Inside the temple walls, all was quiet except for the sounds of the orchestra and the shouting of the children outside. Pavilions in the temple were stacked with hundreds of colourful food offerings. At one side of the temple, arranged all in a row, lay the six receptacles for the gods, each looking like a small grass house on two long bamboo poles by which they would be carried. Just inside the temple gates were many offerings of food and rice laid out for the gods, who would soon descend. In another pavilion of the temple was a huge pile of cooked rice, presented as an offering to the gods, which would ultimately be eaten by the children and the adults.[3]

About 5.00 p.m., the temple priest, a woman in her sixties wearing a white coat, came to the inner temple to bless the offerings and the rice; the rice was then carried on palm leaves by five men to the long palm leaf 'table' on the ground where the small children were waiting to eat. They ate the rice along with roast pork (*sate*) and vegetables (*lawar*) in traditional Balinese style, with their fingers. After the children had eaten, about six or eight groups of 7–8 men each ate rice, *sate*, and *lawar* served on palm leaves on the ground. The gamelan played off and on, while villagers and a sprinkling of tourists with cameras gathered around the edge of the outer temple expectantly awaiting the trance ceremony. After eating, the men gathered up the uneaten rice and cleaned up the palm leaves. The slit gong in the corner pavilion was struck about 30 times to call the participants. After a few minutes, about 20 women with offerings and effigies of the gods on their heads and the *joli* of the six gods, each on bamboo poles carried by two young men (who felt they had been specially chosen by a god to carry it), passed carefully out of the temple through the narrow temple gate. The men moved out of the outer temple grounds, joined by about 80 young men dressed in sarongs with bare torsos, by rows of women villagers dressed in fine traditional clothing, by the young girls, dressed in beautiful costumes with fresh yellow marigold flower head-dresses, who would be the singers, and by boys carrying flags and spears. This stream of several hundred people wound its way through the narrow streets of the village, down the steep path to the river, as the women chanted in monotonous tones. At the edge of the river, the *joli* were set down, the men bathed briefly in the river, and the villagers sat down in a large semicircle. The journey to the river is symbolic of bathing the gods prior to entering the temple. The gong, drum, and cymbal orchestra played intermittently, while the group chanted and sang. This type of singing facilitates trance induction. The people prayed and holy water was sprinkled on everyone. Soon, all the people at the river's edge rose and began the climb back up the cliff trail to the temple.

When the group reached a clearing some 30 metres before the temple, several men with long spears started performing dance steps which involved balancing on one leg, and the pairs of men carrying the six *joli* charged about jostling and narrowly missing each other in increasingly swift dance-like movements. It appeared that these men were in trance as they covered the short distance to the temple where the many young men joined them and the young women standing in a group next to the temple gate chanted, in a continuous monotone, the words *suryak* (shout jubilantly) and *sare* (sleep).

At dusk, that brief period before dark, the groups of men holding the six *joli* circled the outer temple grounds three times, and the atmosphere became more exciting, each group careering wildly, often unexpectedly lurching into the surrounding crowd. Several men in trance held long pole-like spears while others stood balanced on one leg. The gong orchestra played constantly with an accelerating tempo. At this point, increasing numbers of men went into trance-possession as they formed groups of about 10 men with each *joli*. There was a contagion-like spread of the trance as one man followed another in proximity. The men shouted noisily as each *joli* was carried abruptly, unpredictably, and swiftly from one side of the temple grounds to the other; in the process, some of the men fell and were trampled by the others but they picked themselves up and grabbed the bamboo poles again to carry the *joli* further. As groups of men with each *joli* approached the steps, their violent movements raised a lot of dust which filled the air and everyone's nostrils. The darkness was broken only by a lantern on each side of the temple steps and by tourists' camera flashes. Each group of men, most of whom were in trance-possession, struggled vigorously to get their *joli* through the gate. Whereas carrying a *joli* held by two men out of the temple gate was a relatively smooth and easy task, carrying it back in surrounded by many men acting in a largely uncoordinated fashion was a struggle. This part of the ceremony took about 30 minutes. As the men and gods went through, so did a stream of women and children, many moving silently in trance.

The crowd gathered inside the temple and some trancers became subdued as they came out of trance-possession after the priest had sprinkled holy water on them. The *joli* were set to rest, where they had been placed originally. Some men in trance were given krises and they self-stabbed themselves until restrained by the persons surrounding them. In the crowd there were older priests and other village men trying to stay out of trance so that they could physically help to control the trancers. A number of men who fell unconscious were picked up and carried into the temple. Some of them moved violently in a convulsive-like manner and required firm and strong physical restraint by about six men, who struggled to carry the unconscious men up the temple steps and into the sacred temple. Villagers reported that there had never been any serious injuries from this rather dangerous-looking behaviour of the men carrying the *joli* in trance. One man in trance stood on one leg with a live, small chicken in his mouth, the neck held firmly between his teeth. Later, he would bite off the head of the chicken and suck the blood from it as a ritual symbol of drawing animal blood as an offering to the evil spirits. In Bali, cock-fights are the most common ritual to spill blood as an offering to the evil spirits (*buta-kala*) in the *mecaru* ceremony.

Inside the temple, a tall, slender, young man—shouting and gesticulating vigorously as if performing a long dramatic monologue—walked among the crowd, none of whom were now in trance-possession. The crowd crouched or sat down and all looked towards him with quiet, respectful attention appropriate for the divine because he was possessed, speaking as the god of the temple. He said that he was very disappointed and angry that the villagers had placed the gong beside the offerings of rice. Someone responded with 'Where shall we put it?' and he answered angrily, 'You know where it goes.' He berated the villagers for several things, one of which was that not all had come with offerings even though some were poor. He said that they should bring something from their heart and not only the 'rich' people should make offerings. 'I don't think you are a good person only because you offer expensive things; the important thing is how you feel in your heart.' The villagers listened to him with rapt and respectful attention as he stomped up and down a clear strip of ground in the temple not covered by sitting people, sometimes pounding his chest and sometimes bending a banner on a long bamboo pole to the ground in a violent gesture. He proceeded in this manner for about 20 minutes, all the while holding the rapt attention of the villagers. Several villagers, commenting on this man's personality, claimed that he was usually quiet and not talkative.

At a similar ceremony 210 days earlier, the authors had observed almost identical events with the exception of the man possessed who had addressed the villagers towards the end. The priest helped the trancers to regain consciousness by sprinkling holy water on them. After all had come out of trance-possession, the crowd moved slowly, patiently, and silently up the steps, through the gate, and into the outer temple grounds. At this point, no one appeared to be possessed. Many of the trancers were dripping wet with sweat and the bodies of some were covered with dirt from having fallen on the ground. By this time, the music had stopped; so had the chanting and singing. The villagers prayed to God and were blessed by the priests, and all was quiet except for the shuffling of bare feet on the dirt as they walked out of the temple. On the conclusion of this part of the ceremony, the people moved down the dark paths towards their homes to bath. They would then return to the temple to pray again. Afterwards they would feel a sense of 'peace' because they had properly shown devotion to the gods.

Seven days after the ceremony, the authors returned to this village to interview 10 male participants who had fallen into trance at the above ceremony. They were selected at random from a group of many men who were preparing a stage at the temple for a religious drama to be presented as part of the 11-day celebration.

Five of the subjects described their experiences as follows: at the sound of the slit gong or the processional music and singing, they abruptly experienced changed perceptions, e.g. they felt that 'darkness' was coming and they could no longer see, although they knew there were people around them. They could hear the women singing which dominated their perception. They felt cheerful and full of energy. They felt the god coming into them. Their behaviour seemed automatic. Suddenly, they felt driven to carry the *joli*. They recalled being tossed around by the men struggling to carry the *joli*, falling down, and being trampled but they felt no discomfort or pain. This state continued until they were sprinkled with holy water. At that point, they felt they were back in the real world, with a sense of peace and happiness that was unusual and not experienced at other times in their lives. This state generally lasted 1–3 days. The day after the ceremony, they became aware of bruises and abrasions and felt some muscular soreness. Two men said that they felt different for 10 days, until the end of all the celebrations and, during this time, they had no motivation to work—they only felt drawn to return to the temple and felt happy at the temple with their friends. At the end of the entire ceremonial, they returned to their usual state. These men regarded those men who were in trance-possession (*kapangluh*) as having been chosen by the gods.

Five men interviewed experienced a period of complete amnesia and apparent unconsciousness during the ceremony. Their trance state began like the five described above, usually with the sound of the slit gong as they entered the temple. Some recalled circling around the temple. At the point when the *joli* were being carried up the steps into the temple, they became unconscious. When they awakened (from trance-possession), after being sprinkled with holy water, they realized there was a lapsed period for which they had no memory.

All 10 subjects interviewed had participated in this ceremony in previous years and had undergone the same experience each time. They felt very positive about these ceremonies and several said they looked forward to each new year's ceremony. None felt any negative social ramifications, and they minimized the pain and abrasions sustained in the mêlée.

Sometimes it was difficult to be sure from a single observation whether or not a person was in trance. Those in trance had closed eyes and a flattened facial expression. Two different states described by the 10 men were both consistent with the criteria for trance. One is an altered state with changes in perception, cognition, and physiological changes, and the other is an unconscious state with generalized convulsive-like movements. This suggests the need for differentiating trance-possession into two kinds: (1) trance-possession with loss of consciousness and inability to perform purposeful actions; and (2) trance-possession with sufficient consciousness to perform purposeful actions.

Suryani has observed this mass trance-possession ceremony at Timbrah every *kuningan* since 1973 and has noted only one change: the men who entered trance formerly wore shirts, but since 1984 they have stopped wearing them because an ancestor (through one of the possessed) informed them that they should carry out the ceremony in the same way as did their ancestors, wearing only a sarong.

Bateson and Mead (1942) and Belo (1960) believed that trance for the Balinese was therapeutic, i.e. it allowed the expression of culturally unacceptable emotions, which, lacking an outlet in normal life, might trouble the individual. Following this train of thought, the communal or mass trance should also be therapeutic and result in a better state of mental health and fewer mental disorders in villages which hold mass trance ceremonies compared with villages lacking in such ceremonies. To test this hypothesis is not feasible because it is not possible to control the many variables involved. A rough indication of the prevalence of mental disorder in the villages was obtained from village headmen. There had been no known cases of psychosis, *amok*, or other problems for which villagers sought help from any of the psychiatric services provided by the island or from *balian*. Two suicides have occurred between 1989 and 1991, but none in the 10 years preceding 1989. These data need to be compared with data from a control village for a more definitive interpretation.

Mass Trance-possession at Kesiman

The village of Kesiman lies at the edge of Denpasar, along the main road that leads to the south side of the island of Bali and towards the popular tourist town of Ubud. Eight days after *kuningan*, a ceremony with mass trance takes place. The ceremony witnessed by the authors began in the morning at the outer temple with a cock-fight as hundreds of men crowded together around the central area to watch and bet. Although cock-fights are outlawed by the Indonesian government, they still occur frequently, and this one at Kesiman is legal because it is accepted as a part of the traditional ceremony; the blood is used for offerings on the ground to evil spirits in the *mecaru* ceremony at midday so that they will not disturb the members of the community.

In the afternoon, processions of people, several hundred men and women dressed in traditional costumes, came from surrounding villages to meet at the common large temple. Each woman carried offerings for the gods or effigies (symbols of the gods), accompanied by a gong orchestra of drums and cymbals. Groups from some villages split off to go to their local temples to bring out their Barong[4] which would become part of the ceremony. Hundreds of people in a steady stream then entered through the narrow central gate of the temple to pray and give offerings. They returned through smaller doorways located on each side of the central gate.

At about 5.00 p.m., the men and Rangda[5] entered trance-possession while they were inside the sacred temple and they began filing through the temple gate: each trancer was assisted by a man on either side, both of whom had a firm and confident manner and a respectful and gentle demeanour. As the trancers passed through the gate, they began to thrash about violently with their arms, legs, and heads, shouting with eyes closed, as the helpers or assistants struggled to keep them from charging wildly and dangerously into the crowds of people watching outside the sacred temple. A total of about 50 trancers came through the gate, interspersed with about 10 Rangdas also in trance-possession (*karauhan*), each assisted by a man on either side. Occasionally, the men assisting the trancers went spontaneously into trance-possession and men in the group rushed in to restrain and assist them. Only two women were in trance-possession at this ceremony. Two Barongs also came through the gate. After descending the temple steps, the entire group of trancers, their helpers who were not in trance, the Barongs, the Rangdas, the priests, and the gong orchestra paraded around the outer temple building. As they did so, many of the trancers periodically became violent as if in convulsions, arching their bodies, shaking their hands, and shouting 'Kris, kris, give me kris'. A man standing nearby holding a kris up in the air would hand it to a trancer, who proceeded to direct the point to his chest, lean back, and press the kris with such force that at times the steel blade bowed or bent. (Each kris consisted of a rigid blade, about 35 centimetres long, with a sharp tip and a handle.) As the men self-stabbed, they often fell to the ground and were then surrounded by about six men. After 10–30 seconds of self-stabbing, these men took the kris forcibly away and gave it to another man who held it up, ready for the next self-stabber, perhaps two or three trancers further along in the parade. The crowd was tense, expectant, and pleased. The gong orchestra with loud, rapid, vibrating tones was part of the parade. When a trancer became violent and difficult to restrain, a priest splashed his face with holy water to decrease his violence, or to bring him out of trance. The parade wound its way three times around the temple, passing through the gauntlet of spectators.

After this, the entire retinue came back through the sacred temple gate. The men and women were still in trance-possession at this point, many unconscious, some limp, and some still lurching violently or moving convulsively. Not all of the trancers were unconscious; nor did all fall or feel convulsed or require assistance to walk or stand at the point of passing through the temple gate. None showed signs of blood from kris stabbing though one had a punctured and torn shirt. Inside the sacred temple, the trancers, participants, and spectators gathered for the final part of the ceremony which included many men self-stabbing, a group of women dancers (some in trance-possession), individual men dancing in trance-possession, priests sprinkling holy water on trancers seated in front of an altar with offerings, and smoking braziers to bring them out of trance-possession. The Rangda head-dresses were removed from the Rangdas and placed in their containers for the journey back to their temples of residence.

Belo's (1960) description of self-stabbing (*ngurek*), during communal trance in 1937, is still valid today:

> With a sudden yell, a young man, I Rapoeg, tears across the upper end of the court, dashes up the steps of the same pavilion, and stands there doing *ngurek* before the Barong and the Rangdas. The music begins again. More people rush up to take hold of Rapoeg. Both he and Goesti Gedjir are lifted down to the ground, where they *ngurek*. A woman shrieks, and begins to hurl her body about, seizing one of the priests who is near her around the waist. Immediately another woman goes in trance; she has a *keris* and begins to *ngurek*. Simultaneously, the music changes to the loud clanging rhythm called *bat'el*, which has no melody but beats and beats upon the ears with hypnotic insistence. All over the court the women now break into trance, screaming and thrashing their bodies till their hair comes down, making leaps from side to side. If they have a keris, they *ngurek*; if not, they cling to the priests' hands or seize them round the waist till they are given one. The scene, now at its climax, is wild and lurid. The women's screams, shrill and high, have a quality of intense excitement, akin to a sexual excitement which can reach no appeasement.

Two men who had participated in this ceremony described experiences similar to those of the trancers at the mass trance ceremony at Timbrah. They perceived a darkness, although it was daylight, and then they became unconscious. One recalled all of the kris stabbing (*ngurek*) episode while, the other recalled nothing. The one who recalled it had suffered a skin laceration from the kris because he was not fully in trance. It is generally believed that a person in trance will not be injured by the self-stabbing.

This ceremony represents a welcoming of the gods back to the temple, which is very important to the village because the gods are the protectors of the village and all its inhabitants. The ceremonies which honour the gods ensure their continued goodwill to the village. The men in trance are believed to be possessed by the gods and the self-stabbing (*ngurek*) demonstrates the power of the gods. This recalls the kris stabbers of the Barong dance, who attempt to attack Rangda. However, the Rangdas of the Kesiman ceremonies are good and not evil, unlike Rangda in the Barong dance. This is not inconsistent but rather is in keeping with the cultural beliefs that all things have two sides, good and bad. What one should strive for is balance.

Mass Trance-possession at Jimbaran

This unique ceremony, peculiar to this village, lasts for 6 months by the Balinese calendar and takes place at yearly intervals if the 'gods need it' and the villagers have enough money to support it. The purpose of the ceremony is for the gods of the Barong and Rangda to be among the people of the village. It begins 50 days before the ceremonial day, *galungan*, when the priest gets a message from the gods about whether they will perform the ceremony or not. On the day before *galungan*, a ceremony is held to connect the head of the Barong and Rangda. The gods of the Barong and Rangda are then present among the people from the first day after *galungan* until 10 days before the next *galungan*, which occurs at intervals of 210 days. Between these two times, ceremonies are conducted at every *kajeng kliwon* (intervals of 15 days).

At the particular ceremony witnessed by the authors, the process of connecting the head of the Barong to the Barong body and, later, placing the Rangda mask on the man possessed by the god of Rangda took up almost the whole of the first day. The ceremony began at 4.00 p.m. and ended at 2.00 a.m. It took place both in the sacred part of the temple, which is adjacent to the cemetery, and in the cemetery. First, the Barong and many of the villagers dressed in white traditional clothes paraded from the temple (where the Barong and Rangda are stored) down the street to the cemetery. There was a great deal of offerings, praying, blessings performed by the priests, both for the Barong and for the village participants. The villagers believe that at this ceremony, many of the chief ministers to the gods (*patih*) come to see them. Every *patih* has a special name and trait. One man was possessed by a monkey god and, in a state of trance-possession, abruptly climbed a coconut tree on the grounds of the temple, plucked a coconut, carried it down, tore the husk off with his teeth, stabbed a hole in it with a kris, and drank the coconut milk. Then Rangda and her two daughters received a message from the god of Rangda that he was coming and they danced to the temple and then to the cemetery to receive their masks. When the mask was placed on Rangda, she screamed loudly and invited the Barong to come and fight, saying, 'If you are brave, come here.' At the temple, many men began to cry and moan as they bent over in a sitting position and rocked, muscles tensing and jerking. At the sound of Rangda's voice in the cemetery, about 20 men who had entered trance-possession (*bebutan*) suddenly jumped up and raced towards the seven-foot high concrete wall that surrounds the temple. Many were restrained by the villagers; others broke loose and managed to run to the wall and climb it abruptly and swiftly as if it were a small hurdle, and then ran to the cemetery where Rangda was. When they reached Rangda, they fell down because they felt frightened at the sight of her eyes. There, they were brought out of trance-possession by holy water from the priests. Men who remained in the temple grounds began to stab themselves with krises and perform self-stabbing (*ngurek*) ceremonies for some time. Meanwhile, the Barong had returned to the temple and many of the men who were still in trance-possession and were considered to be his followers went up to the head of the Barong, grasped the beard, and put it on their faces. Many of these men were brought out of trance-possession at this time by holy water from the priests as well. After an hour or two of these activities, all the people walked slowly and quietly out of the temple and went home.

On the following day, the ceremony began at 3.00 p.m. inside the grounds of another temple located directly on the main road that passes through Jimbaran. This road had been decorated with many banana trees stuck in the ground at intervals along the road and with the traditional long, bamboo ornaments specially hung over the streets for this festive occasion. Inside the temple, six young men were being dressed in the elaborate costumes of women dancers. Some women sat around, preparing offerings made of woven palm leaves. A ceremonial cock-fight was held to signify the spilling of blood on the ground, an offering to the evil spirits. The Barong and the six adolescent male dancers (Sandar) with their white masks and fan held in one hand, all in identical costumes, paraded out of the temple and walked a short distance down the street. The gamelan played continuously. They stood near the gate of another temple for about an hour and then performed a dance, as helpers of the Barong. The young male dancers in their female costumes and masks appeared very feminine in their movements. The leader of this group of dancers (Telek Sandar) performed a dance following the dance by the Sandar, who then stood near the Barong. Four more dancers, called Omang, who wore masks with long black hair, tried to disturb the Barong and the six men while they were dancing. This performance lasted about an hour; when it ended, all the male dancers left and two 'daughter Rangdas' entered the temple. It is believed that they cause bad things to happen to the people. Rangda herself then appeared at the temple door with her magic white cloth draped over her head. She asked her daughters to find her a baby and if that was not possible, to give her the inner organs of the baby's body because she needed to eat them. After they had found the baby (a doll), they faced the Barong who said, 'Don't do it,' and took the baby from them. The two daughters then fought with the Barong but the Barong won. Angry, they went home and told their mother (Rangda) what had happened. One daughter said, 'You must beat him (the Barong). I cannot do it.' Rangda again asked her two daughters to bring food. This time, they brought the Barong, and so Rangda was forced to fight, saying, 'Now I will kill you.' Suddenly, about 10 men with krises appeared at the other end of the short part of the street and approached Rangda with menacing gestures, as if threatening to destroy her. Rangda moved towards them. At intervals, one of the men would suddenly charge towards Rangda but as he reached her and she waved her magic cloth, he fell unconscious at her feet and remained unconscious for the rest of the ceremony. Each of these men had to be carried off the street by villagers and laid down at the side of the road. There they lay, eyes closed, motionless, and completely unconscious in a trance-possession state. Many of the men advancing towards Rangda with krises turned the krises on themselves and self-stabbed themselves in front of Rangda.

This behaviour is apparently a show of devotion to the Barong standing behind Rangda, as the Barong is believed to have the ability of giving power to the men.

Finally, Rangda, no longer imbued with power, walked slowly back to her temple. Inside the temple, she spoke for about 5 minutes to the throng of villagers seated around her on the ground. She then sat down and her mask was removed and placed back in its container, where it would remain in the temple. The man possessed by Rangda was then splashed with a great deal of holy water—particularly over his head—by the priests, after which he slowly came out of trance. He was able to walk slowly on his own accord and in a normal manner to a pavilion in the temple. The spectators went back into the other temple to witness an hour of kris stabbing by *bebutan*. This ceremony concluded at about 6.30 p.m.

In these ceremonies, the individuals who are possessed are regarded as special since not all individuals can be possessed. Certain families are regarded as having inherited the ability of being possessed. The trancers report that the lower god says to them, 'I will possess (*ngayah*) you. I am the god so-and-so,' giving one of several names. Each trancer has a different type of experience depending on which god possesses him. People standing around give a kris to the possessed individual to execute his self-stabbing behaviour. When the god gives his name as Kobar Api, the individual feels that he needs fire to complete the trance. In this case, assistants surrounding the ceremony light large torches of straw and bring them to him and he stamps them out with his bare feet. If the god identifies himself as I Belatuk Tanah, the trancer needs a chick to complete the trance. He will twist off the head of the chick and suck the blood from its body; after this he needs *arak berem* to drink, followed by application of holy water, which brings him out of trance. The same god may possess another person after the possessed person comes out of trance. Later, these individuals usually claim that they acted automatically and were out of self-control.

At one of the previous ceremonies, a man who was self-stabbing himself with a kris injured himself when the kris entered his chest to a depth of about 3 centimetres. The priest handled this case by asking the man to sleep at the temple, and treated the wound by rubbing a red flower (*pucuk bang*) and sandalwood-treated water over it. The man recovered after 3 days.

In this ceremony, unlike the ones at Kesiman and Timbrah, the gamelan music was slow and soothing, a music eminently suitable for welcoming the gods, which did not appear to stimulate trance induction. Rather, trance-possession occurred at the sight and/or voice of Rangda.

This ceremony is performed in order to bring the gods back to the people. Offerings are given every day and the gods are believed to stay in the village for a matter of months. Every *kajeng kliwon*, the villagers may repeat some part of the ceremony, such as making offerings or placing the head back on the Barong and the Rangda.

A 35-year-old man, a *bebutan*, was interviewed. He is married with two children and has had five experiences with this ceremony. His parents were also *bebutan*. At the temple, he felt the hair on his body stand up and then he became amnesic, and he felt that something possessed him but he forgot what it was. After he was given holy water and *arak berem*, he felt normal again. During another experience, he described his body feeling as if it was on fire, and he was not aware of the situation around him. He felt very happy when he saw the kris. He felt an itching above his eyes and then on his neck and everywhere on his body. He stabbed the itchy spots with the kris. He recalled the kris stabbing and felt he could not control it. Although he felt he did it, yet at the same time he believed it was some other force or energy—a power of the god—that made him do it. His thoughts were focused only on the kris, but he felt as though some other person or agency held the kris rather than himself. When he was possessed, everything appeared shadowy to him. The priest looked like a referee at a football game, one which he automatically followed. When someone brought him a chicken or a flower, his feet turned cold and he asked for fire. Then he felt he wanted a chick; his body became hot and he needed the blood to suck. He did not perceive the blood as offensive. After he had sucked the blood, he drank *arak berem* and regained consciousness. The heat of his body disappeared as he became conscious.

When the man was possessed at the Uluwatu temple, he felt his head was heavy and all his body was hot; he felt as if people were tugging at his body and that they were moving like smoke. After his possession was over, he felt very tired, as if he had carried an extremely heavy load. Every time he fell into possession, the experience was approximately the same, but the name of the god who possessed him was different and his feelings differed depending on the god who possessed him. For example, the god who wants fire (I Kobar Api) makes his body feel cold. When the white monkey god (Bojog Putih) possesses him, he needs fruit and Balinese cake.

When the god Ulu Siwi possesses him, he needs coconut and then climbs a tree to eat the coconut like a monkey. Sometimes the god needs holy water and he then drinks more than a litre of water.

Relating his experience at the cemetery, he said that after hearing the voice of Rangda, he felt angry, so he ran away to find her with the aim of killing her. He felt a power or some energy pushing him as he ran to climb the 2-metre temple wall. When he saw the face of Rangda, he suddenly felt fear and wanted to retreat. He believed he was not responsible for his actions. When he fell to the ground, he knew he was himself and in control again, so he proceeded to find Rangda. He did not feel horrified by the decaying smell of flesh and rotting offerings in the cemetery and passed these without thinking. When he was near the big tree, he felt drugged, as if suffering from a hangover, and his body became hot; then he felt weak and fell down to the ground. As many people carried him, he experienced pain in his body and he sensed some people were bringing string to bind him up (a hallucination). He said that other people did not see this process and that people could not release his hands or his legs from the bands because they knew he was bound up by the god. People carried him to the Barong, and the priest gave him holy water. He saw Rangda and she turned her face away. He again felt brave and wanted to kill her. When he regained consciousness, he felt tired and experienced some soreness in his muscles.

He described his experience during a second ceremonial day. When he fell unconscious on the road, he said he did not feel any pain. After awakening from trance and possession, he felt shy because his clothes were dirty and tattered, unlike the other people around him who were neatly dressed. If he were to go home while he was possessed, he might destroy the furniture of the house, so he only went home when he was completely conscious. After awakening from trance, he felt clear-headed, calm, and at peace. These feelings lasted about a month and during this time, it was very easy to get a job and to complete it.

The priest at the Jimbaran ceremony was interviewed several days after the ceremony. In his daily life, he regards himself as a humble and quiet man. But in temple activities, his attitude and personality change; he becomes more like a leader and the people follow what he says. He said, 'I cannot do it without the god.' He prepares himself by fasting for a day. On the day of the ceremony, he suddenly feels unsteady, swaying with his body bent over; he experiences a floating sensation, he does not see or hear the people around him and everything to him looks 'empty' (i.e. there is nothing around him); and he perceives he has a 'new power', which makes him feel strong and self-confident. This contrasts with his feeling immediately after he comes out of trance when he feels tired, and sleepy, but mentally normal.

The above description pertained to his experience when he was carrying out the ritual performance of placing the head of the Barong and the head of Rangda on to the heads of the men possessed by the gods of these figures. He had the same experience at the time he severed the heads from the Barong and Rangda, which had rested in the temple for 7 months after the connecting ceremony. At this head-severing ceremony where the Rangda mask rested on a skull in a box at the temple, he described how he suddenly took out a kris which he felt he would throw at Rangda. At that time he perceived the environment to be very quiet and was apparently in trance. He also described the feeling of another power possessing him and inciting him to cut off Rangda's head. When he slashed at her head three times, he suddenly felt weak, without any energy; he fell down and afterwards was given holy water by another priest. At this point, he still did not feel normal; he experienced a cold sweat, and some people directed him to the temple so that he could make an offering to the gods. After receiving the holy water, he recalled everything that he had done and felt tired. Afterwards he slept for a few days and then he felt normal again.

The experiences of most trancers at Kesiman, Timbrah, and Jimbaran who fell down unconscious appeared to be similar. All expressed violent emotions, and the aspect of devotion to the gods, the social expectation, control, and approval seemed to be the same.

C. Muller (personal communication) described a ceremonial trance in a group of *balian* gathered in 1989 for the annual *kuningan* celebration on Turtle Island, near the capital city of Denpasar. Thousands of Balinese come here annually for temple ceremonies (*odalan*). The day before, effigies of the gods were brought to the island late at night and about 10 *balian*, both men and women dressed in white coats with hair piled up on their heads, assembled at the temple. They talked about current problems and the rituals to be performed in order to bring about harmony and balance into life. Abruptly, all the *balian* went into trance-possession and began to talk in strange-toned voices in an ancient Javanese language called Kawi, which is very little understood. At one point, one *balian* executed an astounding feat:

he suddenly sprang from a sitting position up into the air, his body outstretched and rigid, only to be caught in mid-air by the others. It appeared like an acrobatic circus stunt. The trancers did not act surprised and quietly resumed talking among themselves.

Mass Trance-possession at Family Ceremonies

At periodic intervals, sometimes yearly, some extended families hold ceremonies at the temples of the extended family for the purpose of honouring the gods and ancestor spirits. Two attended by the authors in 1991, one in Denpasar and one in the south peninsula, were similar in form. At Denpasar the family invited 28 male priests and 14 female priests. At the peninsula, 7 male priests came. At each ceremony there were offerings to the gods, including food, *banten*, and *arak berem* (an alcoholic drink not drunk by the participants), and the offerings were blessed. Groups of women sang in monotonous tones. A Rangda went into trance-possession and danced. After he had finished, he sat down; his mask-cum-head-dress was removed and he was slowly brought out of trance-possession by a priest's holy water ministrations. Some family members in trance-possession, mostly elderly, danced individually or in groups. The priests sat on an elevated platform of a pavilion, the gong orchestra at one end. As the gamelan played, the women sang and the priests entered into trance-possession. Most began to shake, with their arms extended in front of them, trembling, and with their faces contorted, while some lurched backwards to be caught and assisted back into the sitting posture by surrounding family members. The body spasms and trembling lasted about a minute and then the trancers sat quietly, eyes closed, face impassive.

Sometimes, some of the possessed gods spoke. At Denpasar two priests sat quietly, head bowed, with heavy strands of mucus, about 20 centimetres long, streaming down from their noses, the symbol of being entered by a certain high god. The highest god did not come down but the second highest did. The priests (now gods) were handed coats and head-dresses to put on. All accepted except one who said sharply, 'This is not my dress.' The people asked politely, 'Which dress do you need?' and he responded, 'You know.' He was then handed a coat and hat of the second god and he accepted it and put it on. Finally the spokesman for the family politely asked the gods if their offerings and ceremonies were acceptable to them and if they had done everything right. The priests (gods) assented in each case and the family spokesman politely said that they were free to leave now at which point each priest slowly came out of trance-possession. Following this ceremony a number of the male priests and all the female priests danced in trance-possession as a group. Then a number of priests and family members in trance-possession self-stabbed themselves with krises. The ceremony, which began at about 9.00 p.m., continued until about 2.00 a.m.

It is striking that the behaviour at a ceremony of this type described over 50 years ago by Belo (1960) is similar to that seen today. At a village she observed, Belo claimed that all of the members, including the smallest children, could enter and had entered trance:

> The very youngest of the children's bodies as they were gripped by convulsions, rigidity, tautness, or fell limp in collapse, produced an impression stronger than any I had experienced in witnessing such a scene. The Balinese say the children are 'nearer to the gods, having just come from there,' and perhaps it was the conception of this nearness which made their trance so fantastically unreal and at the same time a terrifyingly present actuality.

Mass trance-possession still occurs in a number of villages in Bali. The various types of trance described by Belo exist today in similar forms. This is understandable since they are integral parts of fundamental religious ceremonies.

The behaviour of these trancers is unlike that of Westerners in trance, even those in deep trance. Under hypnosis Westerners may express profound emotions, particularly crying, but they do not become violent; they seldom have convulsive-like behaviours, and they do not become possessed. It must be concluded that social expectation is critical in determining spontaneous behaviour in trance states of Westerners and Balinese. The possession accompanying trance in Bali is both a function of beliefs[6] and a representation of a structured type of biopsychosocial phenomena. It is different from the type of psychotic thought and behaviour that asserts that something or someone outside them has entered into them: that is a delusion (a fixed, unrealistic belief) which is not considered appropriate, and is not subject to control by the society and the group around them (see Chapter 9).

* * *

Trance with possession by God and gods occurs in participants at various private and public religious ceremonies in many parts of Bali. Communal or mass trance-possession in religious ceremonies continues to occur in the same villages and in much the same way as described over 50 years ago. Approximately 80–100 men and a few women enter a trance-possession state at yearly ceremonies to welcome the gods back to the village temple. When entering into trance, the subjects experience changed perceptions such as a 'darkness', a constriction of awareness of surrounding stimuli, happiness, and increased energy. With possession they sense that a god is coming into them, taking over their body-mind and their behaviour becomes automatic. The eyes close, the facial expression becomes flattened, and the mouth turns pale. After trance-possession, there is partial or complete amnesia regarding the trance-possession state. These trances with possession are expected, controlled, and highly valued by the society because they help maintain the prosperity, security, peace, and health of the community. Trance-possession enables the persons possessed to carry out exceptional muscular feats, to come into contact with fire without sustaining burns, and to perform self-stabbing behaviour without hurting themselves. In trance-possession, individuals express behaviour and emotions not socially permitted or acceptable in their usual state of consciousness, a catharsis that may be positive for mental health; in this way, trance-possession may be considered a form of self-therapy. Following trance-possession, individuals usually experience pleasurable feelings of peace and calm lasting several days.

1. This particular ceremony is held to give thanks to heroes who succeed in achieving good over bad (*darma* over *adarma*).

2. The ceremony in this village was described over 50 years ago by De Zoete and Spies (1970: 280–4) and appears to have been virtually the same as that observed in 1991.

3. The large mound of rice is placed in a pavilion as an offering to God. After the priest blesses the rice, it is given to the children to eat. This ceremony signifies that God provides food to the villagers.

4. A legendary mythical animal; the term is also used to denote the Barong costume worn by two men.

5. A classic witch in dramas and ceremonies, as well as a symbol of a goddess.

6. To the people in some areas of Bali, trance-possession in ceremonies is an indication that the gods or God has come down and participated in the ceremony. They will know that the offerings they have brought to the ceremony are complete and well received by God and the gods and perhaps they will receive a message from the gods about this coming into their life. For example, if there is an epidemic in the village, they may be told to make a white cross with stones on the house gate and put a leaf of the *pandan* tree on it.

Chapter 5
Trance-possession in Dance and Drama and Individual Trance-possession

DANCES and dramas, which are traditional and widespread in Bali, provide the most common examples of trance-possession on the island. They are also a rich source of information about the trance-possession state. This chapter analysed descriptive data from Balinese dance and drama for characteristics and consistencies in the trance-possession process in individuals, pairs, and groups.

Dance has been associated with trance in a number of diverse cultures, including those of ancient Greece, Africa, and Morocco. In Africa there are legends about actors being possessed by the spirits of the characters they impersonate (Yap, 1960). Balinese dancers, actors, and persons wearing the Rangda or the Barong mask in ceremonies often go into trance-possession (*katakson* or *kalinggihan*), usually at the point when the large, sacred mask is placed on their head.

Belo's (1960: 57) description of Rangda at a village temple ceremony in 1935 is similar to that seen in villages today:

The man placed in the Rangda mask was very violent in his trance. Though the mask is heavy, and it is difficult to see through it, he danced a great deal with a mincing step, waving his magical white cloth. . . . Rangda continued calling upon the spirits of evil to come to her. 'Leak, leak Men Gobleh, come here!' she shouted at the night sky with upraised arms and guttural noises interspersing the words. As she stomped out towards the gate, *Rekun* was close behind her, shouting 'Who is brave enough to invite Men Gobleh to come here?' Everyone remained absolutely quiet while the eeriness of the whole scene made people crowd close together and huddle at the back. Her arms were flung high over her head, the white cloth was waved to and fro, and she laughed the witches' laugh defiantly into the graying sky.

The Rangda dancers at the communal trance-possession ceremonies at Kesiman, at Jimbaran, and at the family clan ceremonies described in Chapter 4 were observed as they were coming out of trance-possession at the conclusion of their performances when the masks were removed. Each time, the Rangda dancer would sit down in the temple, with his legs extended or crossed, eyes closed, face expressionless, and body still, and a priest or his assistants would then carefully lift the mask off him. One to several minutes after the priest had sprinkled or splashed holy water over his head, the dancer's eyes slowly opened, his head moved slowly, and he gradually regained consciousness. Minutes later, he arose of his own volition and stood quietly subdued among the many people. The Rangda dancers reported being 'taken over' during the trance and they experienced partial amnesia.

The Little Girl Trance-possession Dance (*Sang Hyang Dedari*)

This dance, dating back to the pre-Hindu period, is performed to stop evil spirits from causing disease and death in the community and to drive them out. It is performed by two girls of pre-pubertal age to the accompaniment of separate choruses of men and women seated on each side of the stage. Belo described this dance as she observed it in 1935, and Bateson and Mead took movies of it in 1937. The performances they reported and photographed were those in mountain villages. *Sang Hyang Dedari* is still performed occasionally in some village ceremonies.

The following trance-possession induction described by Belo (1960) is typical of a *Sang Hyang Dedari* performance:

> The putting into trance took place in the outer court of one of the holiest temples of the village. In a thatched shelter, lit by one dim light, sat an old man, continuously uttering a discordant, wailing chant. A few girls, one of whom was the Sang Hyang, were busy with offerings beside an altar. The Sang Hyang wore only a long white *kain*, wrapped several times round waist and tied with strings attached to one end. She knelt down before an incense bowl, from which rose thick smoke, and sat with folded legs, her hands lightly resting on the ground in front. For over an hour she leaned above the smoke, occasionally swaying a little from side to side, or raising herself languidly she would fall back into the arms of the attendants, who sat beside her. Her face remained entirely passive, her eyes shut. Gradually, one by one, children and older boys and men assembled, and sang hymn after hymn with her attendants, against the background of the old

man's monotonous, cracked chant. A certain amount of laughter and conversation also mingled with the song. Now and then a woman would lean over the incense bowl to speak to her, and she would shake her head or lazily nod. At last her flower-covered crown was brought and placed before her on the opposite side of the incense bowl. The song changed as she passed into the different stages of her trance (possession) with sudden variations of tempo. During her moments of respite from the smoke her body hung in a lovely pose in the supporting arms of the women behind her. Sometimes she would rest her hands actually on the embers. At last she was judged to be sufficiently in trance (possession), though there were none of the usual convulsions or sudden cries. Her clothes were brought in baskets; she put on the head-dress herself, her languid fingers seeming to move intelligently. Then she was stood up and dressed, her arms supported on each side by a woman. She kept her white skirt, but was bound round and round from breast to hips with the cloth-of-gold belting of the Legong dancer, till she looked like some lovely golden idol. At last she was seated in her carved and painted litter, sprinkling the people who crowded round her with holy water, and the singing procession set out into the starry night. Her flower-covered crown waved above the crowd, her arms moved already in dance.

Today, performances are given regularly near Denpasar, specifically for tourists. When the authors first observed this dance at the village of Bona in South Bali, they questioned if the little girls, who danced in nearly perfect synchrony with eyes closed, were truly in trance, but subsequent observations and interviews convinced them that the trance was real.

One dancer whom the authors interviewed was an 11-year-old Balinese Hindu in the sixth grade. Although she had had two years' experience, like other *Sang Hyang Dedari* dancers, she had not been trained in the dance. This is in sharp contrast to other Balinese dancers, such as those performing the *legong*, who need years of intensive training. She said that she danced because she liked it. She came to the performance fully dressed in her costume, but worried (*nyeh*) about whether she would be possessed during the dance. This was evident from her facial expression and her verbalizations. During the interview just before the dance, she appeared tense and had difficulty answering questions, her stock response being 'no problem'.

At the interview after the dance, she presented a very different mood and countenance. She smiled, answered questions easily and quickly, and appeared graceful and charming in her movements in contrast to her tense, strained appearance before the dance. She said that at the beginning of her performance, the world became dark (*dunia tampak gelap*), she heard only the women's chorus singing, and then she lost consciousness. She recalled a change in perception during the dance: a hallucination of a beautiful woman in front of her and sometimes beside her. She paid no attention to the audience and did not see it. She heard the singers whose vocalizations encouraged her to dance and she danced automatically, as if controlled and moved by some other power, not her own. When she fell down (falling is a regular part of the dance itself), she felt that others, not herself, had caused that to happen.

The other dancer was a 12½-year-old Balinese Hindu, pre-pubertal, in her second year of secondary school. She had been dancing for one year. The interview before her dance was difficult because she appeared to be extremely shy, a trait confirmed by other people backstage. She had visible sweat on her face and neck and had difficulty answering questions.

In sharp contrast, after the dance, she was smiling and appeared happy, and she answered questions directly. She said that after she heard the women singing she had a headache, her vision became dark, and, after that, she had only patchy recall. She reported seeing an old woman with white clothes, and recalled that when she fell down in the dance, it was as if another person had fallen. She felt that she danced automatically, with eyes closed, and she found it very difficult to open them. Like the first dancer, she believed that some other person had given her the 'power' to dance. She remembered being brought out of trance-possession by the sprinkling of holy water from the priest.

It is significant that the religious aspect of *Sang Hyang Dedari* is retained, even though the performance is for tourists: the dancers always pray beforehand and the priest is conspicuous. It can be assumed that if the religious context is not present, the little girls will not experience trance-possession.

The Fire/Hobby-horse Dance (*Sang Hyang Jaran*)

This ancient dance, which is performed for tourists 5 days a week at Bona, near Denpasar, remains much the same as described by Belo (1960). First, two men will prepare a fire made of coconut husks, raking them into a mound of flaming embers just prior to the performance. Behind the stage the dancer prays to the gods to obtain permission for the dance. A hobby-horse with a wooden head and dried grass on a pole for a body is then placed on his shoulders, and he grasps it firmly with both hands. As he enters the arena in trance-possession, a women's chorus, sitting on the low stage, starts chanting. The words, sung in a monotonous and repetitious way, go something like this: 'Please don't worry, there is fire, it will not hurt you. Please jump into the fire.' He runs and skips quickly about the arena through the fire, scattering the embers, which the fire builders periodically rake back into a central pile. He dashes to the sides of the arena where the embers are scattered as if seeking to stamp them out. His face is blank and expressionless, his eyes closed. After running around for about 5 minutes, sweat covers his face and body. At the completion of the dance when most of the embers are out, he sits down on the ground and two attendants pry the horse from his fingers. Up to this point, his body and the horse are a single unit, not separate entities. As he sits on the ground with legs outstretched, his arms jerk convulsively. After the priest sprinkles holy water on him, he relaxes, opens his eyes, and slowly awakens. He then thanks the gods in prayer. The soles of his feet are coated with ashes but show no signs of burns.

A *Sang Hyang Jaran* dancer was interviewed by the authors after a performance. A 50-year-old married man with elementary school education, he has performed this dance since 1972. He became a *Sang Hyang Jaran* dancer because he was asked to do so by a god who possessed him when he fell into trance during a temple ceremony. Relating his experience, he said that after praying, he saw the coconut husk fire being prepared. When he heard the female chorus, he had no fear of the fire. He felt happy when they put the straw horse on his shoulders. Then the world turned dark, and his eyes closed automatically and he joyously followed the singers' invitation to come to the fire. When he saw the fire, he felt that 'a power' had entered his body. He was happy to see the fire and he felt physically big and energetic. As the fire got bigger, he became happier and more eager to begin his performance. While dancing, his body felt light, his movements fluid, and he enjoyed touching the fire. His attention was focused on the singing and the god, who was acting through him. Immediately after coming out of trance-possession, he was afraid to touch the fire and he no longer experienced the happiness he felt when he saw the fire during his trance.

The exposure to fire without sustaining burns is readily understandable when conceptualized in Western psychophysiological terms: trance/hypnosis phenomena offer sufficient explanation. The mechanisms include dissociation of the parts of the nervous system that register heat and pain, resulting in non-perception of pain and awareness in the brain, and therefore non-elicitation of responses to the heat of the fire, such as reflex motor withdrawal or inflammatory reactions of the tissues. Thus the skin may be charred by the heat of the fire, but there is no redness (vasodilation) and no blistering or consequential peeling of the skin. The heavy plantar calluses and dirt on the soles add further protection.

Interviews with other dancers confirmed the similarities between their trance-possession and communal trance: a religious context, singing, changed perceptions, the sense of a power taking over, and termination of the trance by holy water.

The *Kecak* Dance

This popular dance—in its present form created specifically for tourists in the 1930s—has its origin in an ancient *Sang Hyang* or trance dance in which the dancers are possessed by deities. The story derives in part from the old Indian *Ramayana* epic. It is a unique dance accompanied not by a gamelan but by a chorus of about 80 men, who sit in three concentric circles surrounding the actors.

At a *kecak* performance observed by the authors, interviews were conducted half an hour before the performance with some members of the chorus, a priest, the dancer who played the prince's wife (Sita), the leader of the chorus (who also danced), and several other actors, all farmers who work in the rice fields during the day. Prior to the dance, the priest in attendance prayed to God and the gods for permission to stage the performance and to request a good performance by all dancers. During the dance, the men of the chorus directed their attention towards the leader of the group. While singing, the leader periodically emitted an unusual sound, something like a blast from an antique car horn, as he suddenly popped up from a sitting position as if on a spring, a most unusual muscular action. The men interviewed claimed that their movements were automatic and required no concentration. The chorus performed in unison, swaying their bodies and emitting monkey-like chattering sounds. Most of the time, their eyes were open. Some of these men were in trance as evidenced by their changed perceptions, passive countenances, unusual motor feats, and automatism. They said that after coming out of trance at the completion of the performance, they felt tired, slept well at home, and awakened the next morning, feeling happy, revitalized, and ready to work.

Generally, the performers receive very little monetary payment, only 75,000 rupiah (approximately US$40) every three months for their work. Some of the money derived from the performance goes to the welfare of the community (e.g. for the upkeep of the *banjar* and the temple). Pay does not concern them because they enjoy dancing and feel it is not only for themselves but for the good of the community. Furthermore, they are pleased to make the audience happy. They are glad to have the attention of the audience and they desire to perform well so that the dance will provide good memories for the audience and will continue its run.

A Combination of Modern Western and Balinese Dances

In 1990, in Denpasar, an international troupe of both American and Balinese dancers performed a repertoire consisting of a combination of Western and Balinese dances which they had presented on tour in America and finally in Bali, primarily for a local audience. The only part of the repertoire that was clearly recognizable as Balinese in type was that derived from the *kecak* dance.

Following the performance, four of the American dancers, three women and one male chosen at random, were interviewed. None felt they had entered trance while dancing but they often felt a high or what they called an 'adrenaline rush' depending upon the audience's reaction and this good feeling lasted several hours. One recalled that she had entered into trance on two previous occasions while performing Brazilian dances. She described these episodes as sudden and unexpected feelings of energy that came over her and made her dancing seem automatic. She said the sounds became more intense and described the sensation as a wonderful feeling, nothing like her usual performance. The feeling lasted for several hours, and she felt no fatigue. During the Balinese performances, none of the American dancers experienced this.

Five Balinese dancers, four males and one female, were interviewed separately following the performance. Each described feeling nervousness before the performance, enjoyment during the performance, and emotions during the *kecak* dance which were entirely different from these during other parts of the performance. Special energy engulfed them and their 'concentration and thinking did not work'; they 'just followed the leader' and tended to hear only the voice of the leader; and they danced and acted almost automatically as if their bodies were controlled by 'another power'. By contrast, in the other dances they had to think about what they were doing or what they were going to do. During the *kecak* dance, their facial musculature flattened, a typical feature of trance; this was not evident in the other dances.

The dancers said that when they performed the dance involving fighting, a mixture of Eastern and Western dance forms, they enjoyed it but felt no special emotion as 'they played what the story and the rhythm called for'. They consciously tried to suppress all emotions and felt lucky to be able to do so.

Although *kecak* is not recognized as a 'trance dance', the interview data indicated that the Balinese dancers in this performance went into a trance state, possibly with possession, during the *kecak* dance, the only part which is characteristic of traditional Bali. Those dances which contained a mixture of both cultures or appeared more Western than Balinese were not associated with an ASC.

Individual Trance-possession

Individuals frequently fall into trance-possession during ordinary and special religious ceremonies in which trance is not part of the ritual. There may be accompanying music from a gamelan in a procession of which the trancer is a part or music may not be involved. This is illustrated by an interview with a physician who had vivid memories of his two trance-possession experiences. A faculty member at Udayana University, he had spent several years studying medicine abroad. The interview was conducted mostly in English in which he was fluent. He was cautious and careful about the interpretation and translation of Indonesian words into English.

This physician had inherited the role of temple helper from his grandfather, and the group of priests (*pemangku*) of the temple expected him to become a priest. He had no difficulty accepting this role because it would allow him to go to medical school and at the same time continue to function as a part-time priest or temple helper.

He recalled most clearly his second trance-possession experience at the age of 26 in 1973, when he was a medical student. On this occasion he had gone with his family, which included his father, aunts, and uncles, to the temple of their clan for the purpose of communicating with and honouring their ancestors. They had taken a tape recorder to record any messages that any one of them might receive from the gods or the spirits. Before the temple keeper could begin his prayers, the young man, without premonition or conscious intent, abruptly sat down, apparently without control of his movements. His eyes closed and he was unable to open them. He tried to think but could not: 'I couldn't think what I wanted to say.' However, he could hear people talking around him. He saw 'a darkness closing in without images, just black'. He felt his body was light and out of his control, which was an entirely novel sensation for him. While he was sitting, he felt he could not walk. However, he recalled feeling that he was moved by another power and forced to sit on the temple platform (*bale*) where he grabbed burning incense with his bare hands; this was not painful and did not result in any injury. His eyes continued to remain closed and he called his family by their nicknames, something he had not done before. He had no image of the power at this time and reported no hallucinations. He did not feel he had encountered a god or a spirit; rather he felt 'a superpower that could control a human'. He spoke automatically but his words did not seem to make sense to him. During the trance-possession, he believed that he told his family some messages that he had obtained from the ancestors. In trance, he was able to ponder on his situation and remembered thinking, 'Why do I do this? Why is this happening to me?' However, he was unable to express himself. He recalled that the trance-possession state was terminated by someone sprinkling holy water on him. Prior to the trance, he had not experienced any change in his thoughts or feelings and he was not expecting it when it happened. After the trance-possession, he was rather embarrassed about his rudeness in calling his relatives by their nicknames. However, he also reported feeling a sense of peace or 'emptiness', tiredness, quietness, and calmness, which lasted several days. Following the experience, his family explained to him that he had been possessed. No other family members had reported such a trance-possession experience.

This physician's first trance experience occurred a few years before the second and was similar. He was with his family clan in the family temple. He had sat down at the back of the family group when much to his surprise he went abruptly into trance and touched the burning incense without feeling any pain or receiving any burns. At the beginning of this trance, he moved to the front of the family group and sat down facing the pagoda tower (*meru*). He talked to his family in a kind of automatic speech which he was unable to control. The trance was terminated by someone sprinkling holy water on him. After the trance, he had the same terrible feeling of having been rude because he had talked improperly to his family; he felt he had exhibited some gross lack of respect. However, his family accepted his behaviour without comment. As in his second trance-possession experience, feelings of peace and calm following his awakening remained for several days.

This individual's episodes of trance-possession occurred during his youth, which is the common pattern. His possession experience was similar to that of many others. He did not feel a spirit or a god entering him but an outside power controlling his body and his mind. To the Balinese, this experience is equivalent to possession by a spirit or a god. Furthermore, he did not have a mental image of the power or any hallucinations, as may be expected with possession. Four aspects of the experience are consistent with what is known as the depersonalization phenomenon: (1) feelings of detachment, observing the self, and feeling unreal; (2) feeling of being an automaton; (3) feeling of the body being light; and (4) retention of reality testing. However, in several respects the trance experience differed from depersonalization: (1) the sensation of another power outside of himself controlling him; (2) changes in external behaviour; (3) a change in physiological response (no pain or burn from fire); (4) a subsequent emotional change; and (5) amnesia.

These data on individual trance with possession are particularly illuminating because they are provided by a man who is highly educated, articulate, psychologically minded, and who is intent on giving accurate information because of his sincere motivation to provide useful data about possession in the Balinese. He expressed the hope that the results would be translated into Indonesian so as to benefit his countrymen who he felt would have much to gain by learning more about their own behaviour and culture.

Suryani herself has had possession experiences which have helped to shape her personality. She began at the age of 14, when she was possessed by God and, at times, by a goddess who, over a 3-month period, taught her many things, including a philosophy of life, what it feels like to be sick, what one experiences when one dies, and how to heal people. Her experiences are more fully described in Chapter 8.

Trance-possession also occurs in pre-pubertal children and in the elderly (Belo, 1960). The physical 'afterglow' or special feelings of calmness which follow individual trance are similar to those reported by the traditional gamelan players in trance without possession (Chapter 6) and in the trancers who are possessed at mass ceremonies, some of whom are unconscious and amnesic for most of the experience (Chapter 4).

These data on trance-possession in individuals are consistent with data obtained from the trancers in mass trance-possession. They indicate a process at work in trance-possession that has not yet been defined or described in Western psychological terms. The trancer feels that the possession is not part of his body or himself, although he is aware that it enters him, and acts through or utilizes his body. Western psychology and psychiatry have no term for the concept of an outside power or entity acting through or controlling a normal person as in trance-possession.

* * *

Trance-possession in Balinese dancers at tourist performances and in the individuals studied helps to explain spectacular feats such as synchronous automatic dancing, and handling fire and walking on hot coals without suffering burns. These performances attest to the critical role of spiritualism/religion in the trance-possession process. The Westerner frequently poses such questions as 'Does a spirit or god or some power of the universe really come into the trancers? Is possession a demonstration of the reality of spirits?' The answers are unquestionably 'yes' for the Balinese. Analysis in Western terms and psychological concepts reduce possession to dissociation, a process by which certain areas of the brain/mind are accessed and made to express conscious and unconscious material. In taking this point of view, however, it is not possible to rule out the as yet scientifically unprovable spirit world as a factor in the process.

Chapter 6
Self-hypnosis in Gamelan Musicians

GAMELAN music is an ancient art which originated in Java and developed its own distinctive style in Bali. The sounds from a five-note scale played on xylophone-like instruments, with cymbals, flutes, drums, and gongs, are haunting and ethereal. The music is familiar to almost all Balinese and captivating to many Westerners. McPhee (1970: 276), who studied the music of Bali over 50 years ago, described gamelan thus:

The swift, aerial music of the Balinese orchestra, or gamelan, fills the open air with chiming resonance. Innumerable little gongs, large and small xylophone-like instruments with ringing bronze keys blend in an intricate polyphony that floats above the throbbing drums and periodic accents of deep and vibrant gongs. The air is shattered with a continuous shower of bright, percussive sound as the difficult music is performed by thirty or forty carefully rehearsed musicians. The music itself is based on a five-tone scale; beneath the complex ornamental patterns lies melody of unique grace and charm, constructed according to metric forms that have mathematically balanced proportions.

The tone colour and instrumentation of the gamelan varies with the nature of the performance. Small flutes, a pair of drums, cymbals, and a bamboo gong are enough to accompany the dancing and light, delicate singing of the *arja* operetta. The popular *joged* street dance takes place to the gay, staccato sound of an orchestra of xylophones. The large gamelan that accompanies historical mask plays and the heroic *baris*, or warrior-drill dance, has a brilliant, heavily metallic sound and an almost barbaric splendor, while the music for the swift, humming-bird movements of the little *legong* dancers is filled with an indescribable, sensuous iridescence. In and out of the glittering figuration the melody weaves, stressed softly from time to time by gongs of different pitches, while from beneath, the restless, agitated drums rise and fall, their syncopations intensified by the thin clash of tiny cymbals.

Many villages have their own gamelan orchestras made up of 30–40 village musicians who work as farmers, labourers, merchants, hotel workers, or artists during the day. The traditional music of Bali, gamelan was originally restricted to ceremonial dance and religious ceremonies. In recent decades, it is not uncommon to come across gamelan in non-religious ceremonies or to hear it being played simply for pleasure. The music itself is believed to be close to the gods. Gamelan has undergone numerous modifications in the course of its development. However, the traditional music remains unchanged. It is possible to distinguish three types of gamelan music: (1) the ceremonial or traditional; (2) the new creation (*kreasi baru*); and (3) the contemporary (*musik kontemporer*). Contemporary gamelan is 'currently new' music. *Kreasi baru* refers to 'previously new' arrangements of the older or traditional gamelan music. *Kreasi baru* melodies and arrangements, which were new at one time, may have been performed over many years or decades.[1]

Some background information on Balinese character and emotional expression is necessary to understand the significance of this chapter and its hypotheses. The Balinese believe that it is essential to maintain good relationships in all aspects of life, including relationships with the family, the clan (*dadia*), the community (*banjar*), animals, trees, ancestors, evil spirits, the gods, and God (Jensen and Suryani, 1992). Communication should be carried out in a manner that makes one accepted by others. This entails suppressing nearly all emotions that could disrupt a good relationship, especially anger. However, there are outlets for the expression of various emotions in daily life such as youth clubs (*seka truna-truni*), dance clubs (*seka ngigel*), and music clubs (*seka magambel*). In religious ceremonies, emotions can be expressed in offerings to the gods, in feelings of devotion, and sometimes in trance-possession (*kasurupan*), either individually or in groups.

The aim of the study reported in this chapter was to explore the effects of playing gamelan (instruments and music) on the expression of emotions and trance. It was hypothesized that gamelan is a vehicle for emotional expression, the contemporary more than the ceremonial, and that it is a positive influence on mental health. Prior to the study, it was not known if trance played a role in gamelan.

Selection and Interviews

In August 1990, 20 male subjects were studied: 3 composers and 17 players or instrumentalists. They were associated with STSI

(Sekolah Tinggi Seni Indonesia, the State Institution of the Arts), and they regularly performed all three types of gamelan music. These subjects were either professional musicians or conservatory students, and their lives revolved around music.[2] All the subjects were Balinese Hindus. The players, chosen at random from the larger groups working with each composer, were either students or lecturers at STSI. In addition to questions about routine information (e.g. age, sex, occupation, and gamelan experience), subjects were given two checklists to complete: one concerning personal problems in the past three months and the other, symptoms in the past one month. Suryani then clinically evaluated each player in order to determine if he had any mental disorders. All 20 subjects were subsequently interviewed on three occasions: at the conclusion of training; after recording; and after a performance of the musical works. The aim of the semi-structured interviews, lasting about 30 minutes each, was to learn about the experiences and feelings of musicians while playing and after playing the three different types of gamelan—traditional, *kreasi baru*, and contemporary—and to establish whether a particular type of music effects a trance state.

The composers were asked about the meanings of *kreasi baru* and contemporary gamelan music with regard to: (1) how they create the music; and (2) how they transmit it to the players. They were asked if they experienced different feelings when playing in a public performance as contrasted with playing in a religious ceremony and what feelings they experienced. In addition, the composers' training activities with the players were observed.

Results of the Study

The 17 Players

The players were first evaluated based on their answers to the questionnaires concerning personal problems and symptoms. The personal problems they indicated over the previous 3 months are: financial, $n = 16$; pessimism about the future; $n = 9$; not pleased with their physique (e.g. too thin, too fat), $n = 7$; and physical illness, $n = 6$. Their main complaints over the previous one month are: difficulty in sleeping, especially after a performance, $n = 6$; decreased interest in activities, $n = 6$; decreased memory, $n = 6$; nausea or stomach symptoms, $n = 6$; decreased self-esteem or inferiority, $n = 10$; palpitations, $n = 7$; difficulty in concentrating,

$n = 11$; tiredness, weakness, or low energy, $n = 10$; and tingling of feet while sitting, $n = 6$. On a psychiatric clinical evaluation, dysthymic disorder was noted in one subject and generalized anxiety disorder in one other.

In the interviews all subjects expressed dissatisfaction that they did not have an exact time for playing and that sometimes they had to train for a few hours at a time or long into the night. As a result of waiting and training they always felt tired. They believed they needed to sleep and eat more regularly in order to feel better. They felt different from their peers; they seldom exercised and they spent much of their time sitting. Most were from the lower socio-economic group, and they felt there was a conflict between enjoying gamelan and needing to earn more money for a better life.

All players gave similar answers to questions regarding recording and performance. At recordings they felt tense, not relaxed, and they focused only on playing perfectly so that they would not have to repeat. Not a single mistake is allowed in recording; otherwise the whole piece has to be repeated. When playing, they must remember all the instructions of the composer and they cannot express emotion; they see only the quiet room and the cameraman.

In public performances they were more relaxed and not so tense, because even when they made mistakes, the audience usually would not realize it and they could cover up by adjusting their playing. A performance is continuous without repeats. They felt that the audience provided an environment which favoured the expression of emotion and encouraged improvisation, activities which did not disturb the harmony of the group.

All players were unable to differentiate their feelings (e.g. mood) with regard to *kreasi baru* and contemporary gamelan. The two kinds allow freedom of emotional expression and improvisation, but there is a difference in concentration. *Kreasi baru* has been known to them since childhood and does not require effort to remember; it is 'automatic'. Contemporary gamelan is entirely new, so they must remember the composition and concentrate. Contemporary gamelan is only temporary, performed only a few times and then forgotten. *Kreasi baru* is longer lasting; it remains 'in the heart', and it is accepted by the public for repeat performances.

Interview data regarding what they felt when playing contemporary and ceremonial music are as follows. With regard to contemporary music, the players must use discipline and remember all the notes; furthermore, they cannot relax, as the time to play is limited. (In a ceremonial performance, they play for an hour or more.) When playing contemporary music, they can experience a full range of emotions while still keeping the 'harmony' or balance of the group. They may feel more relaxed, energetic, or happy, depending upon the music. After playing, they lose these emotions and return to their mood prior to playing, often physically tired.

Ceremonial gamelan music is for religious ceremony. It has a basic relatively simple unchangeable pattern. When playing ceremonial music, the players feel no tension, are relaxed, and seldom express any emotion except at special times, particularly during emotionally laden ceremonies such as mass trance or carrying the corpse at cremation. The playing is repetitious, and the rhythm is the same; it tends to be monotonous in volume and intensity. All subjects reported experiencing the sensation that their body is 'not here'; they feel as if they are floating above the ground, 'nearer to the gods' and 'in another world' amidst peace and quiet. They feel a sense of devotion to the gods while playing it.[3] This feeling is especially strong in players of *gender*, a xylophone-like instrument used for shadow puppet plays. They feel like they are 'following the gods who are coming to them'. This feeling continues throughout playing, persists at home, and sometimes lasts for 1–2 days. They do not feel tired or experience backache although they may play for hours sitting cross-legged on the hard floor with very little body movement and no back support. Any feelings of anger and disappointment are lost after playing. All of them like to play the three forms of gamelan but feel happiest when playing ceremonial gamelan. Playing the newer forms helps to increase their creativity, emotional range, and improvisational skills while playing ceremonial gamelan provides them with the peace that they need.

The Composers

The three composers selected had had experience playing and studying outside Bali and Indonesia and had established relationships with foreign musicians. They were male[4] lecturers at STSI, and their ages ranged from 18 to 35 years. Their responses are recorded below.

COMPOSER 1

He regards *kreasi baru* as the development of ceremonial (traditional) gamelan music which still retains the pattern of the original music, comprising the concepts of head, body, and feet related to the Balinese Hindu religion. This new creation comes from the composer's imagination and experimentation, as well as the influence of others (i.e. through discussions). He regards contemporary gamelan as the music for today, unrelated to the traditional ceremonial form of composition: it does not show Balinese characteristics and it is not considered to be Balinese by the Balinese. Although contemporary music is related to the types of instruments used and the culture of the composer, it does not conform to Balinese gamelan music. The composer tells a group of players his ideas for a piece of music, and they all work together at the piece, sometimes for as long as 2 months, until the result is satisfactory.

When he plays, his feelings are similar to the players, i.e. he experiences increased tension and emotional expression with improvisation when recording. He is more relaxed and free in performance. He feels engaged emotionally with contemporary music if it is on a religious topic but all such feelings disappear when he stops playing. He feels satisfied after a successful performance but quickly returns to his normal state. When playing ceremonial music, he also experiences a sensation of floating, a sense of being 'in another world' and at 'peace'. This lasts for hours or days. He prefers to play ceremonial gamelan for ceremonies because he feels that in doing so he is expressing devotion to the ancestors, to the supreme God, and to the lesser gods. He does not have these feelings while playing the other two types of gamelan music.

COMPOSER 2

He regards *kreasi baru* and contemporary gamelan as the same. To him, *kreasi baru* is related to the composer's personality and culture. He does not agree with the other composers that contemporary gamelan is unrelated to their culture. He obtains new ideas for compositions from his own imagination, and from reading, experimenting, and witnessing others perform. He believes that outside cultures have also influenced his ideas: he often mixes foreign influences with Balinese concepts for the final result. The idea is a basic framework. He communicates it to his group of players and together they work on the idea through training until they have a satisfying form. The final result comes when his players understand what he means and then improvise on it. To transmit his ideas to the players, he combines Western and traditional methods. He said that the players find it easy to deal with Balinese musical methods but difficult to use Western musical techniques.

This composer does not feel any tension when recording; in fact, he feels more relaxed than in a performance because he can repeat if he makes a mistake. To him, recording and performing are the same in terms of emotional expression and improvisation and he does not think there is a difference between playing ceremonial and contemporary gamelan. Both types of music create in him the same mood and feelings of happiness, peace, enjoyment, and freedom to express emotion and improvise, which may continue for some time at home. He does not appear to experience any changes in sensation suggesting an ASC.

COMPOSER 3

He regards *kreasi baru* as the development of gamelan with a certain amount of creativity but with the basic gamelan pattern of Bali intact. For contemporary gamelan music, he combines old gamelan instruments which are seldom used today with current gamelan instruments of Indonesia and other cultures, creating a new composition which differs from the Balinese gamelan pattern. Therefore, his contemporary music is different in composition and sound from basic gamelan, resulting in music that is not characteristic of Bali. International musicians can play the music and feel that it is familiar. It is not specific to any one culture, as it involves a mixture of instruments from different cultures with different sounds. The composer's innovative ideas come from combining information about gamelan with music or stories he has read. When he has sufficient ideas for a piece of music, he conveys them to the players and, by trial and error, both composer and players develop a new piece of music. The result derives from the composer's ideas worked on by a team of players.[5]

Conclusion: Trance with Spirituality

Composers of Balinese gamelan can use the music to express emotion, imagination, thinking (beliefs), and devotion, as manifested in the culture. All are bound together in the life of the Balinese as they are in gamelan but because the content is influenced by outside culture, changes have been effected in some respects.

The process of creation is revealed by the method of transmitting the composer's idea and framework to the players. This approach, novel to most Western musical compositions, is consistent with

Balinese character, i.e. decisions are based on consensus and co-operation by all (in this case, the players and composers).

Although the composers had received their musical education abroad and developed relationships with musicians from Western culture, they still use their own cultural patterns. Suryani, a native Balinese, knows relatively little about Balinese gamelan, but at performances she could identify elements of Balinese gamelan in *kreasi baru* and contemporary music; the characteristics are distinctive. To draw a parallel in medicine, Balinese medical science comes from the West and is influenced by Western practice but the *balian* still use traditional Balinese methods. If the two methods are combined, the basic thinking of each discipline remains. In the same way, although *kreasi baru* is influenced by the West, it nevertheless contains some basic elements of Balinese gamelan.

Both contemporary gamelan and *kreasi baru* appear to be innovations from the traditional, using part or all of the basic gamelan patterns and manifesting the cultural characteristics of the composer. There is no distinct separation in form between the two types of gamelan. It is hypothesized that each will endure for as long as it remains interesting and acceptable to the public and for as long as the gamelan still touches the people's feelings, both in terms of enjoyment and religious meaning. For example, the *kreasi baru* called *kebyar* has lasted several decades (McPhee, 1946).

This study of gamelan musicians, composers, and instrumentalists is presented to show the occurrence (and characteristics) of trance in a heretofore unrecognized setting. Balinese music alone does not appear to be sufficient to induce trance; a religious context and the devotion of the musicians are essential. This study also reveals a number of effects of Balinese music that can be conceptualized in Western psychological terms. There are two kinds of gamelan music according to usage: one—the traditional—is for religious occasions; and the other—both *kreasi baru* and contemporary—is for performances. These two kinds have different behavioural and emotional ramifications. A psychological analysis of the players' emotional responses indicated that playing the two kinds of gamelan brings out different feelings and behaviours. In non-ceremonial gamelan the players are allowed to express emotions such as happiness and anger and to feel a sense of freedom, depending on the musical content. Ceremonial music, which is repetitious with a single melodic pattern and also longer with changing rhythms and crescendos, has a special meaning: it is close to God and the gods, and the players feel a sense of devotion when playing it. Additional elements that may contribute to an ASC in the players of ceremonial music are the crowding of the people (*rame*), incense smoke in the air, blessings by the priests, and a generally heightened sense of expectancy and excitement in the air often associated with temple and other ceremonial occasions. These factors facilitate the induction of a trance state in the players. The feelings and altered sensations they reported fit the criteria for an ASC, specifically a trance/hypnotic state. Associated feelings of peace, quiet, and happiness which continue later at home and last up to several days are also characteristic of trance-possession in the Balinese. In ceremonial gamelan, the players do not express emotion as they do in the other two newer types; instead they become self-hypnotized. These data support the conclusion that playing traditional gamelan music effects a kind of self-hypnotherapy, which results in the disappearance of unpleasant feelings for a period of time. This finding also supports the hypothesis that playing gamelan contributes to positive mental health by providing an outlet for emotional expression.

It is surprising that in his otherwise thorough review of trance and music, Rouget (1985) did not describe trance in musicians. By contrast, all of the players and two of the three composers observed in this study experienced a trance/hypnosis state during traditional gamelan. The high percentage of trance/hypnosis among the Balinese musicians is about equal to the estimate of 95 per cent of Westerners being hypnotizable to some degree (Brown and Fromm, 1986).

This study raises several queries regarding self-hypnosis. Is self-hypnosis induced by the specific environment (i.e. the temple setting); the particular type of gamelan music; the players' understanding of the meaning of ceremonial music (i.e. it is for the gods); or a combination of these factors? It is known that cultural beliefs play a fundamental role in the induction of trance/hypnosis and the particular forms it takes (e.g. trance, possession, or both). Partial answers to these questions may be obtained by comparing these data with future studies of gamelan music performed by professional musicians, village musicians, Balinese in foreign countries, and non-Hindu musicians.

* * *

The discovery that gamelan musicians enter trance during the performance of religious music recalls to mind the spiritual factor operative in ceremonial trance-possession and dances; without the spiritual context, there is no trance-procession. However, it is a known fact that a spiritual context is not a necessary condition for inducing all trance or hypnotic states. The question is raised: 'Why is the spiritual/religious factor essential for trance-possession in the Balinese, and is the same true for possession in Westerners, i.e. can Westerners be possessed irrespective of a spiritual context?' This question suggests an important dimension for clinicians to explore when evaluating patients or clients for whom possession is a consideration. Clinical implications are that when the patient believes in the spiritual essence of his condition, the clinician must have a broad enough perspective to accept the spiritual factor and communicate with the patient in his or her own terms as well as in psychological terms.

1. In *kreasi baru* the shape of the piece remains, i.e. a three-part structure with the 'gong, cyclical, and repetitive' form based on the ceremonial (traditional) type. *Kebyar*, an example of *kreasi baru*, was described by McPhee (1946) as follows: 'With the popular modern *kebyar*, a brilliant exhibition dance performed by a youth or small boy, we come to the breakdown of traditional forms in both dance and music. Composition is free in structure—a loosely connected series of melodies in different moods that are given a new and glittering orchestration. The word *kebyar* itself means a sudden release of forces—an explosion, "a flower bursting suddenly open", the crash of many cymbals. It indicates to perfection the explosive energy and liberation of both dance and music. Musicians and dancer alike find exhilarating freedom in the rhapsodic music and choreographies that are composed in a spirit of creative enthusiasm, for approaching festive occasions.'

Contemporary gamelan is derived from Western music. The gong cycles are not perceptible and the metric patterns are not double or repetitive.

In ceremonial music, the basic element is a single melodic pattern of short duration repeated over and over.

These descriptions of the three types of gamelan music were provided by ethnomusicologists Linda Burman-Hall, Sue Devale, and Elaine Barkin, all professors at the University of California, who are engaged jointly with the authors in ethnomusic research in Bali.

2. Professional musicians differ from the usual gamelan players in the villages who are primarily part-timers.

3. Co-operation-devotion, which is evident in ceremonial *gamelan* music, is generally acknowledged to be one of the character traits of the Balinese people.

4. Playing gamelan is traditionally a male activity.

5. This method of composing gamelan music is traditional in Bali and contrasts sharply with a Western composer's practice of writing a complete score and presenting it to the musicians to play.

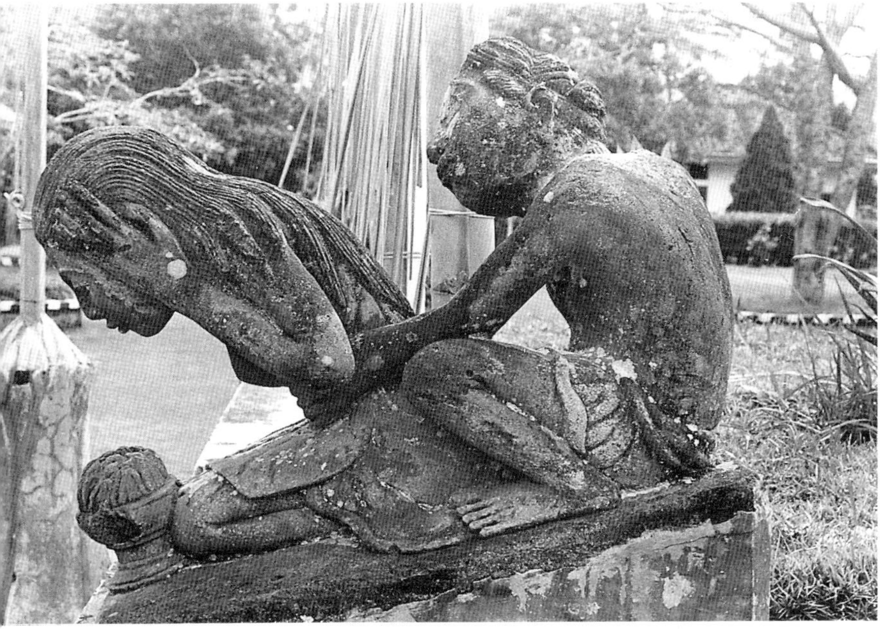

8 A carved stone statue of a *balian* using the smoke technique to treat a client in front of the Mental Hospital in Bangli. The client is shown leaning over a brazier. *Balian* do not treat patients at this hospital.

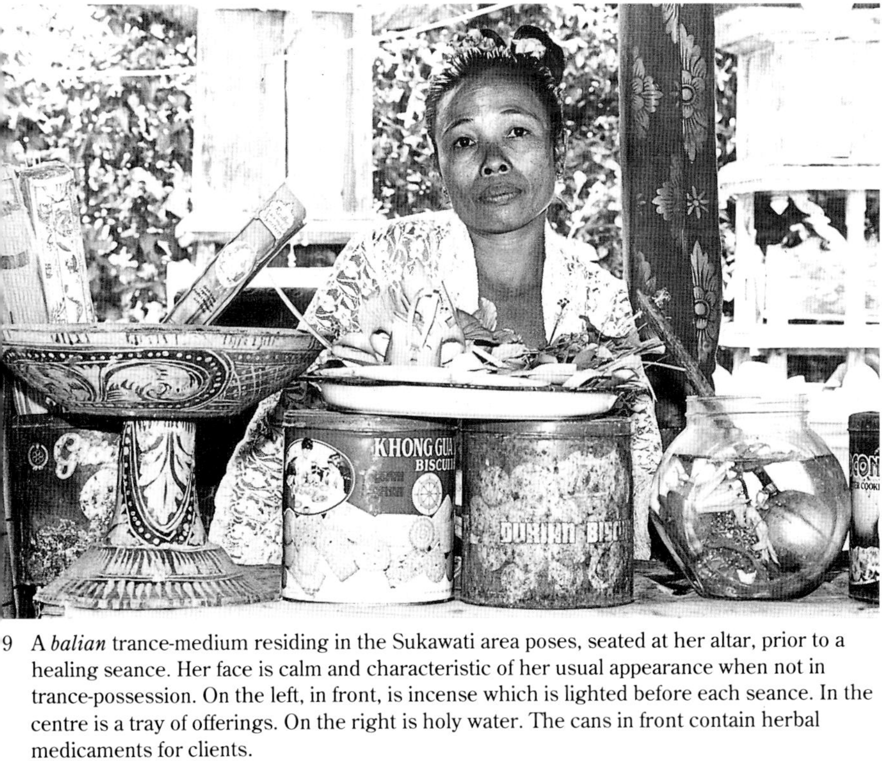

9 A *balian* trance-medium residing in the Sukawati area poses, seated at her altar, prior to a healing seance. Her face is calm and characteristic of her usual appearance when not in trance-possession. On the left, in front, is incense which is lighted before each seance. In the centre is a tray of offerings. On the right is holy water. The cans in front contain herbal medicaments for clients.

30 The *balian* in Plate 29 in a trance-possession state, in which she assumes the behaviour of the client's ancestor's spirit who possesses her. In trance-possession her eyes are always closed and she speaks animatedly and articulately at a rapid rate.

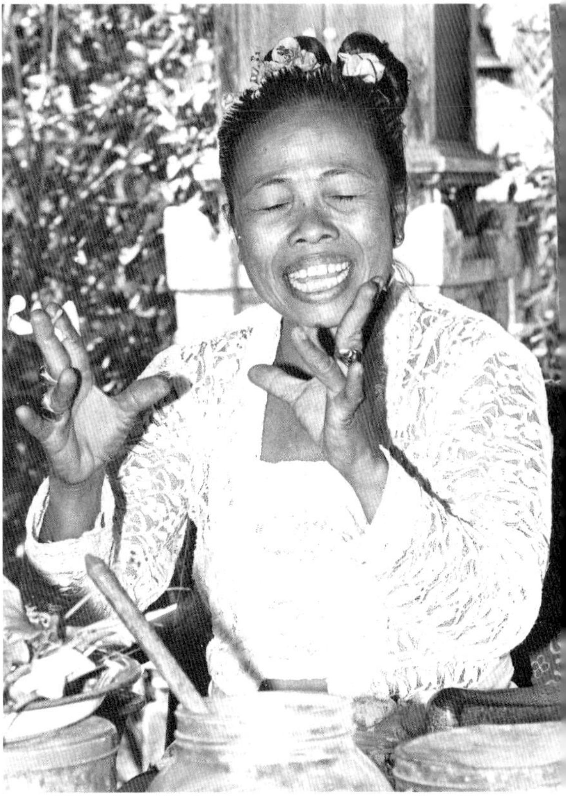

31 A *balian* trance-medium in Denpasar seated at her altar prior to entering trance-possession to treat her client.

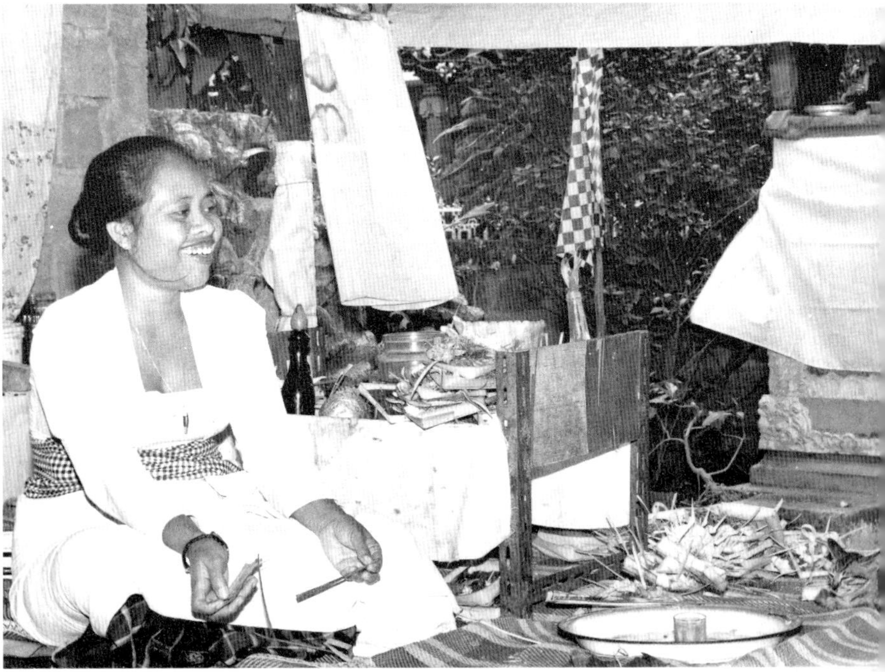

2 The shrine of the trance-medium in Plate 31 contains a Barong mask and several small statues. The statues on top represent her gods. On the lower levels are the gods' helpers, offerings, and a jug of holy water.

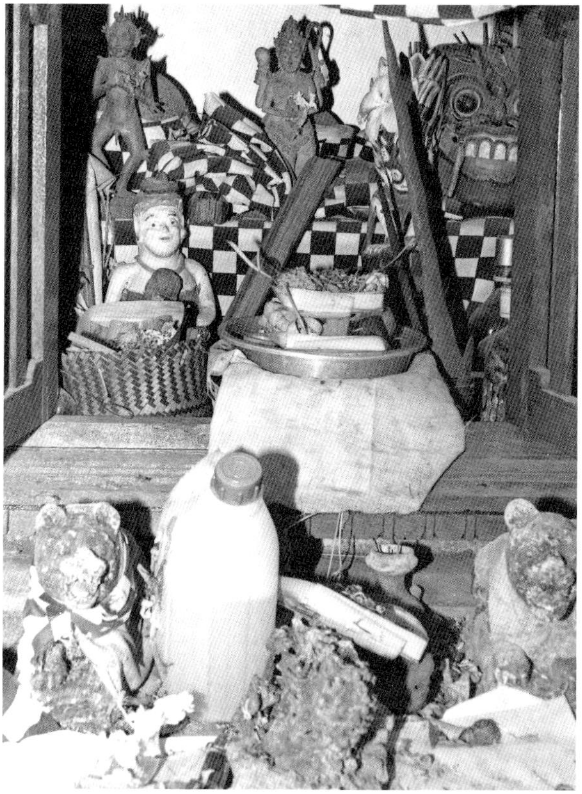

3 A client's tray of offerings for the gods of the trance-medium in Plate 31 containing a coconut, rice, an egg, money, and *banten*. Offerings of other clients are strewn on the right. The offering has to suit the type of help needed.

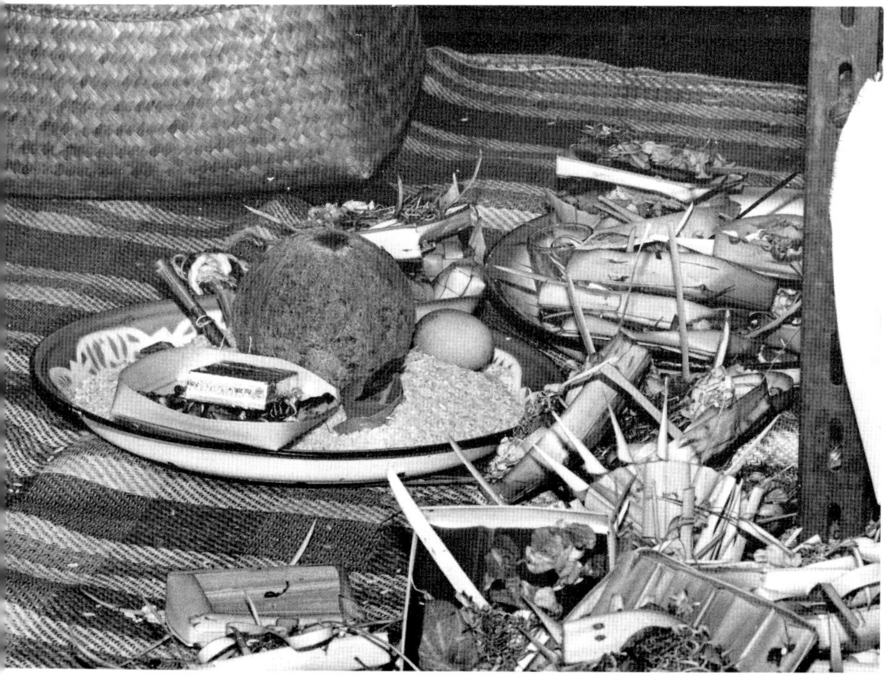

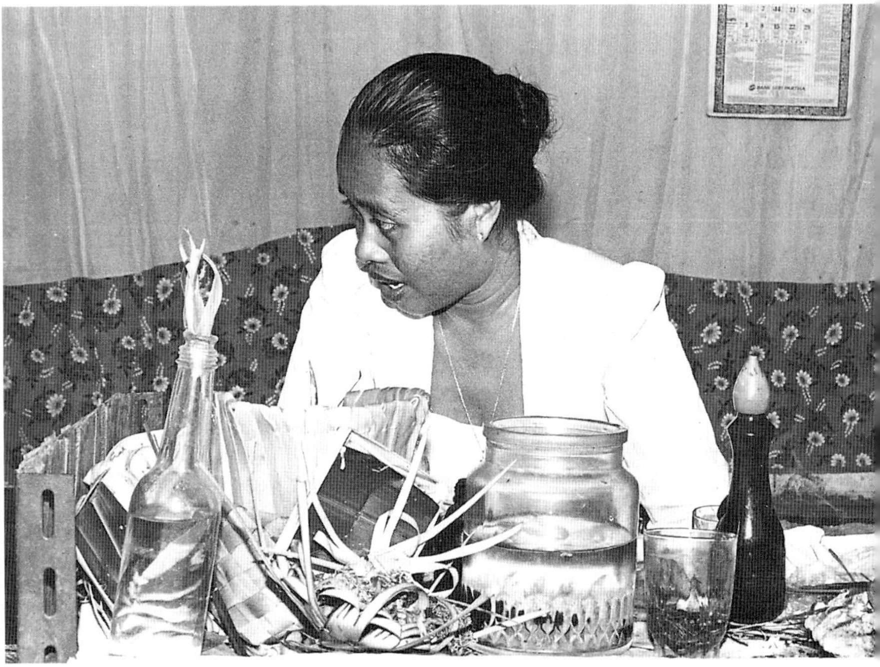

34 In trance-possession, the *balian* in Plate 31 speaks to her client with her eyes open. *Balian* experienced in possession states do not show any of the facial changes seen in ceremonial participants who are less experienced in the trance-possession state.

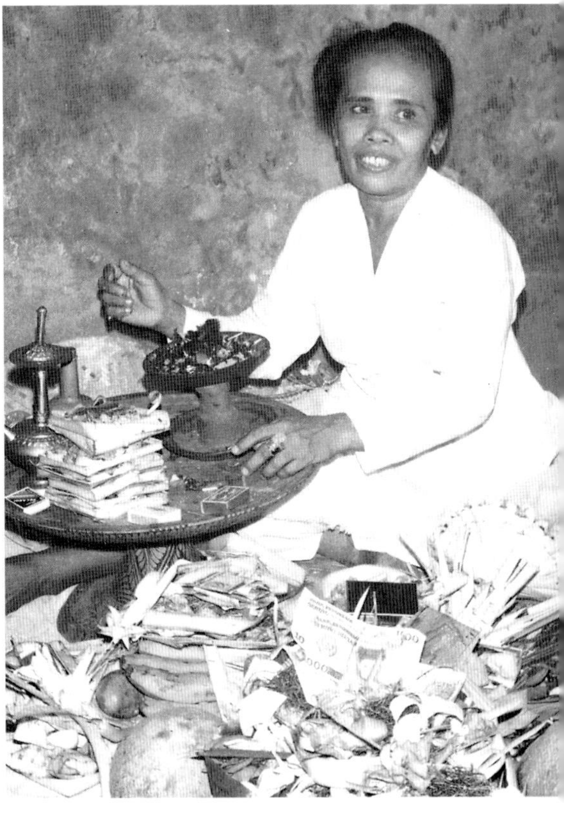

35 A *balian* trance-medium in Denpasar prior to entering the trance-possession state.

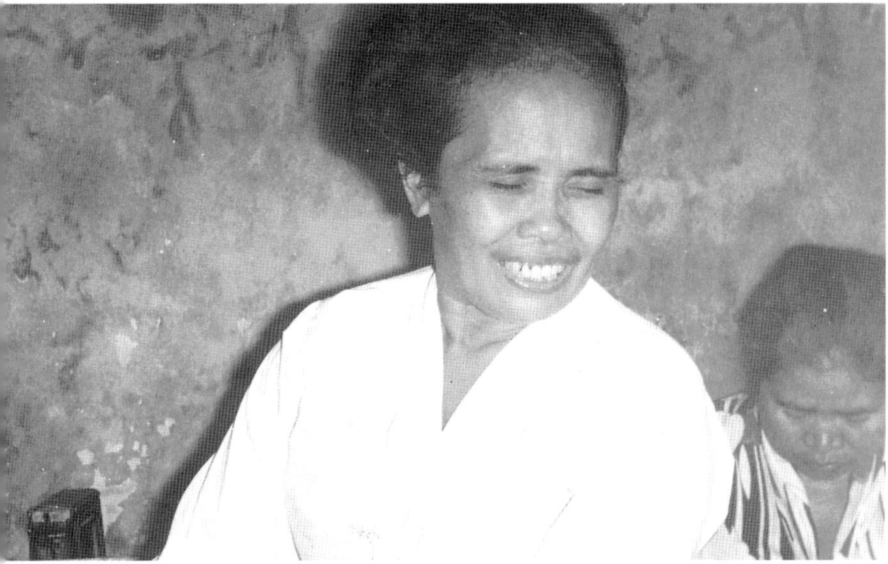

6 The *balian* in Plate 35 in trance-possession, with eyes closed and eyelids fluttering, is shown advising her client.

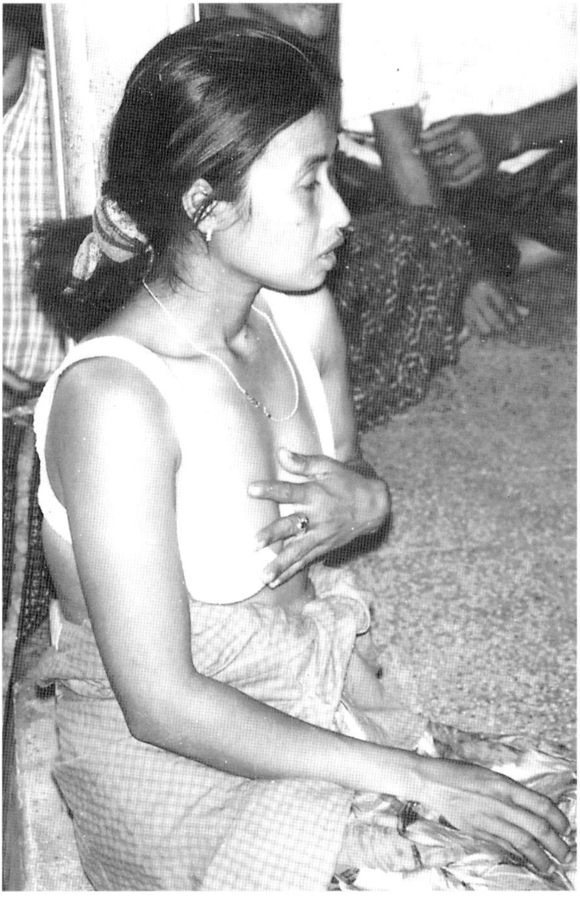

7 A client in trance-possession while under treatment by a *balian* shows some flattening of the facial muscles and expresses pain, which is believed to be caused by black magic being extruded during treatment.

38 The client in Plate 37 showing her normal facial appearance immediately following treatment.

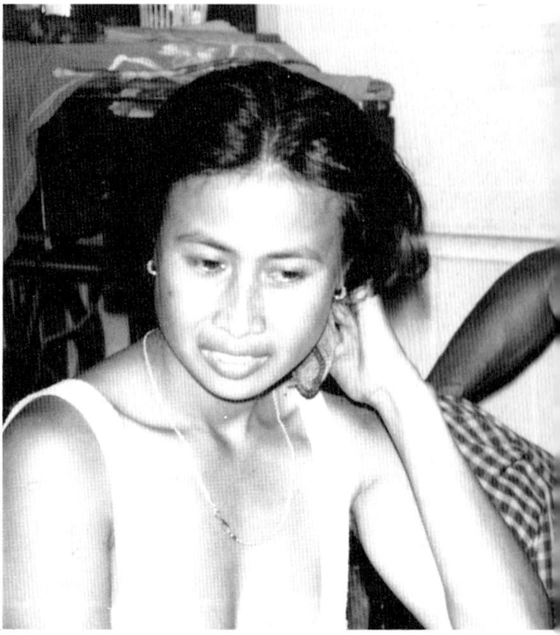

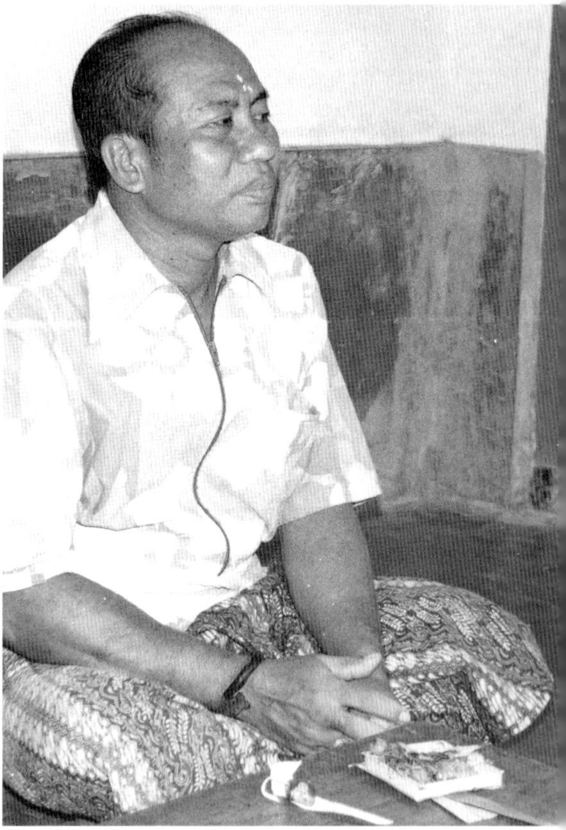

39 A *balian usada* living near Klungkung who specializes in the management of black magic spirit possession. Clients often enter into trance during his treatment. In front of him is a client's offering of money.

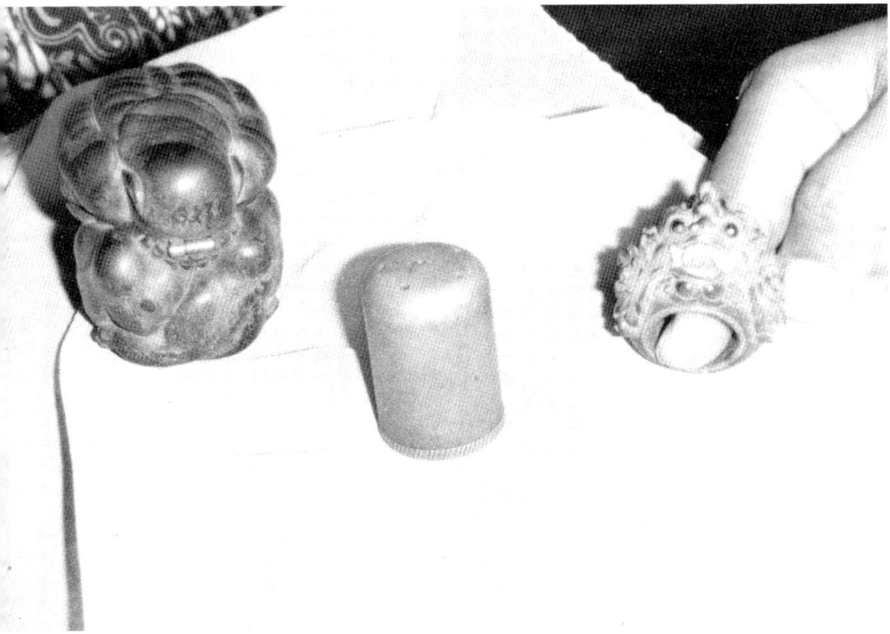

40 Paraphernalia used by the *balian* in Plate 39 to test for evil spirit possession. The pewter cylinder (centre) is held against the client's forehead for several minutes and if the client falls into trance, black magic is indicated. Black magic is also deemed to be the cause of problems if patients fall into trance at the sight of the ring.

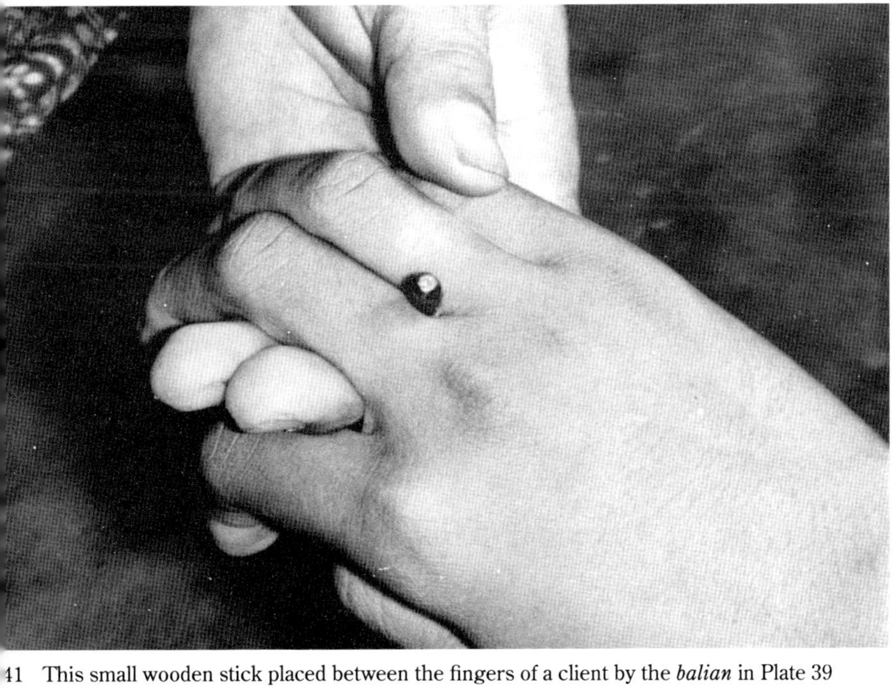

41 This small wooden stick placed between the fingers of a client by the *balian* in Plate 39 causes severe pain if the client suffers from black magic. Otherwise it has no effect.

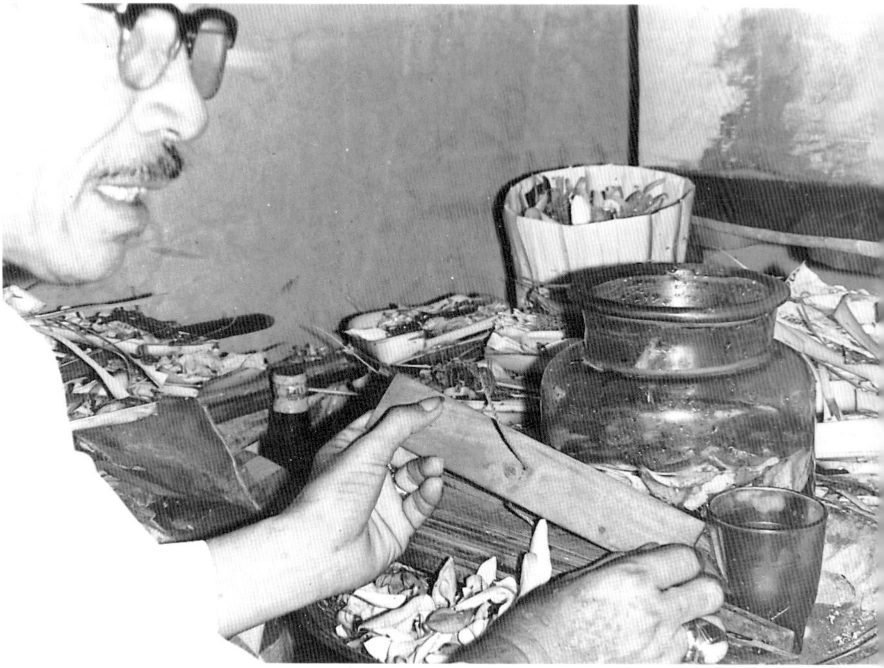

42 A *balian* in Denpasar who uses Chinese coins to discern his client's problem is shown 'reading' advice from a blank *lontar*.

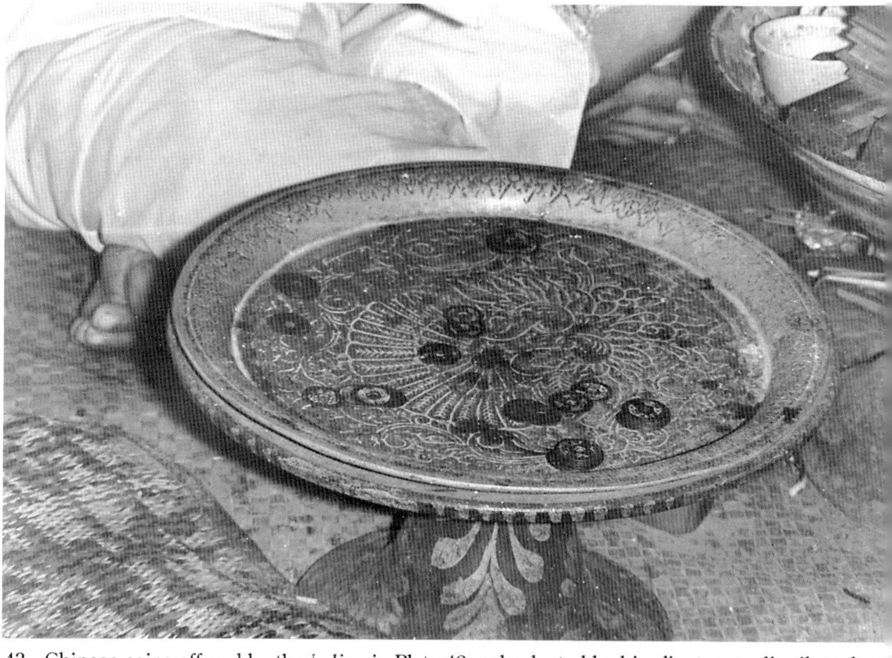

43 Chinese coins offered by the *balian* in Plate 42 and selected by his client were distributed on a plate by the *balian* in order to determine the reason for the client's visit and the nature of his problem.

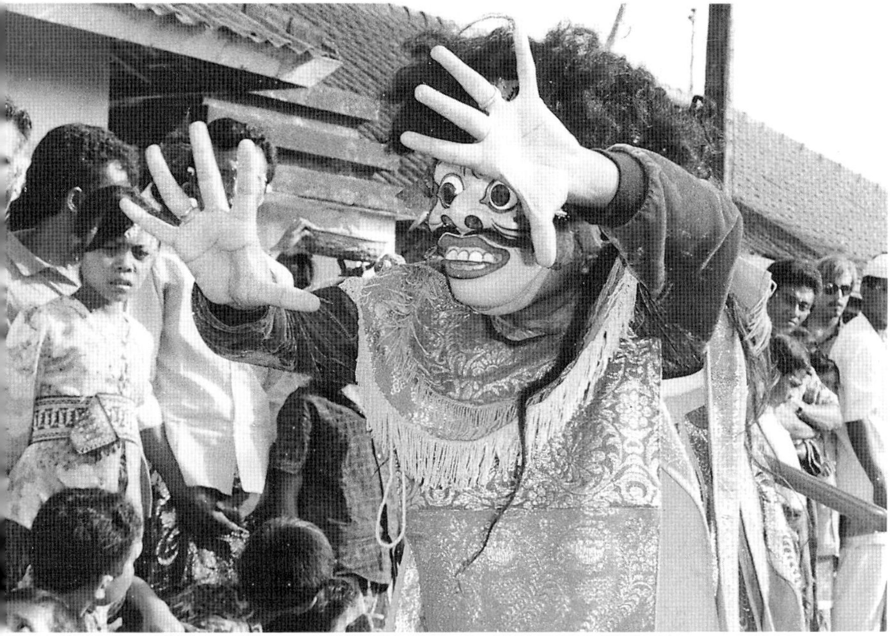

4 This masked dancer at the mass trance-possession ceremony at Jimbaran is a companion of Rangda, who acts against the benevolent Barong and his followers. The Jimbaran ceremony, a high point in the life of the village, is held to protect the villagers against disaster and illness and to promote success for everyone.

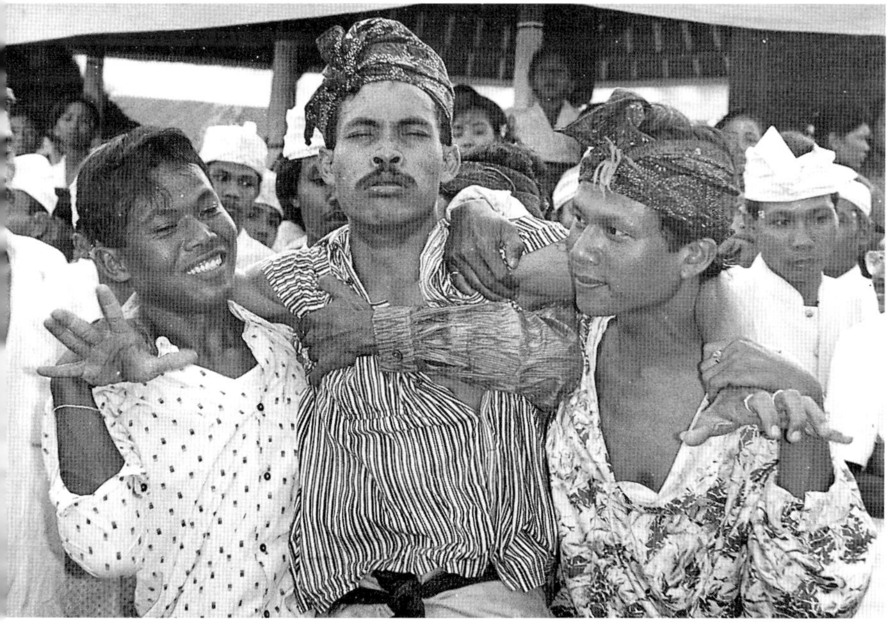

5 A trancer at the mass trance-possession ceremony at Jimbaran being guided confidently and carefully by two men who are not in trance. On awakening, this man could not recall his behaviour in the trance-possession state.

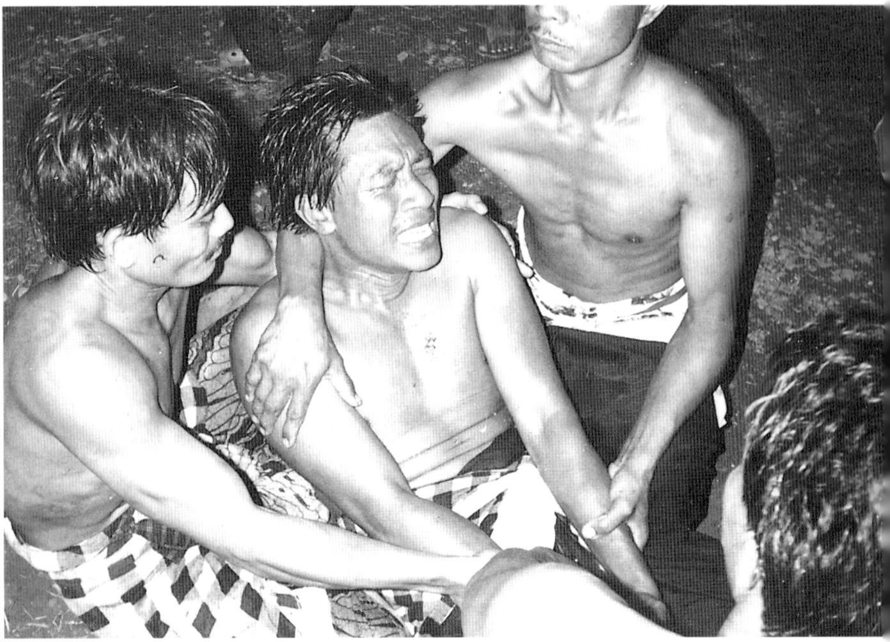

46 An unconscious trancer at the mass trance-possession ceremony at Timbrah being assisted calmly by two villagers. Following the ceremony, he was amnesic with regard to his trance- possession state.

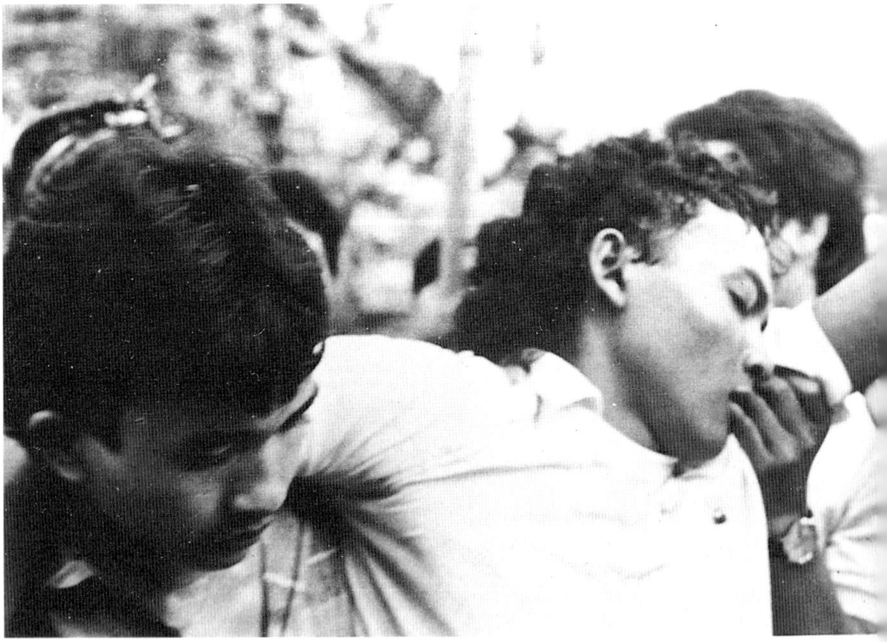

47 Another unconscious trancer, this time at the mass trance-possession ceremony at Kesiman being assisted by a villager on each side of him. After being guided into the sacred part of th temple, he was brought out of trance by the sprinkling of holy water.

8 A villager possessed by a god at the Timbrah mass trance-possession ceremony dancing with a small live chicken in his mouth. He will later swallow the chicken's blood, in imitation of what is believed to be an act of the god possessing him.

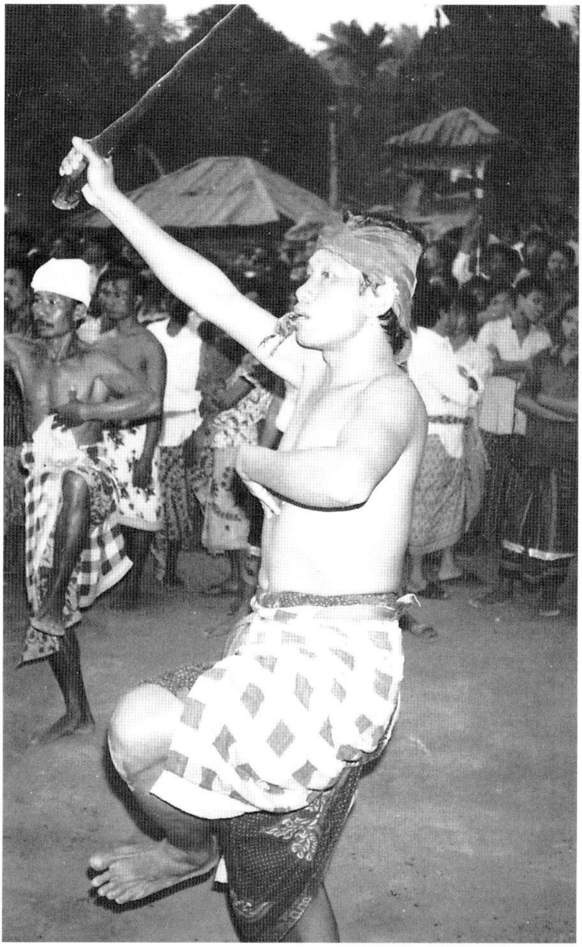

9 An unconscious trancer at the Timbrah mass trance-possession ceremony being carried into the sacred part of the temple where he will be revived by holy water.

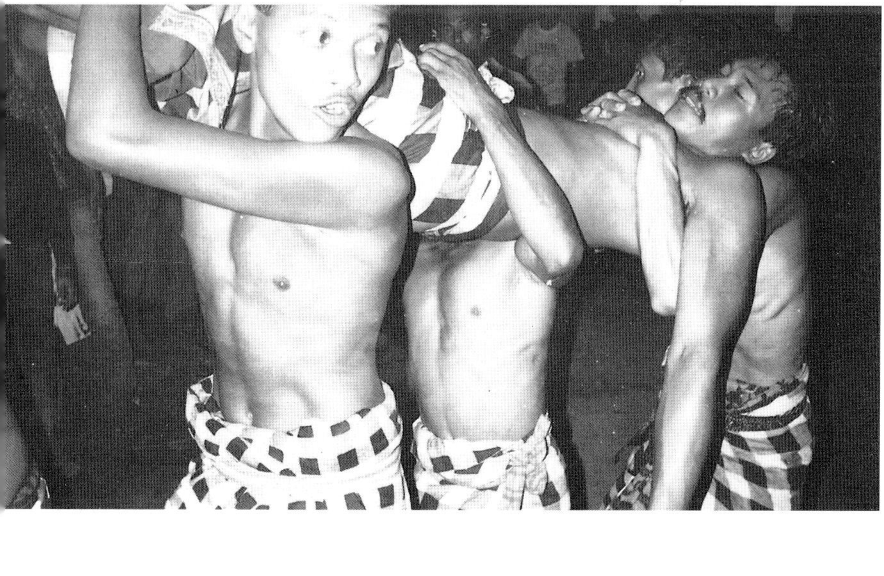

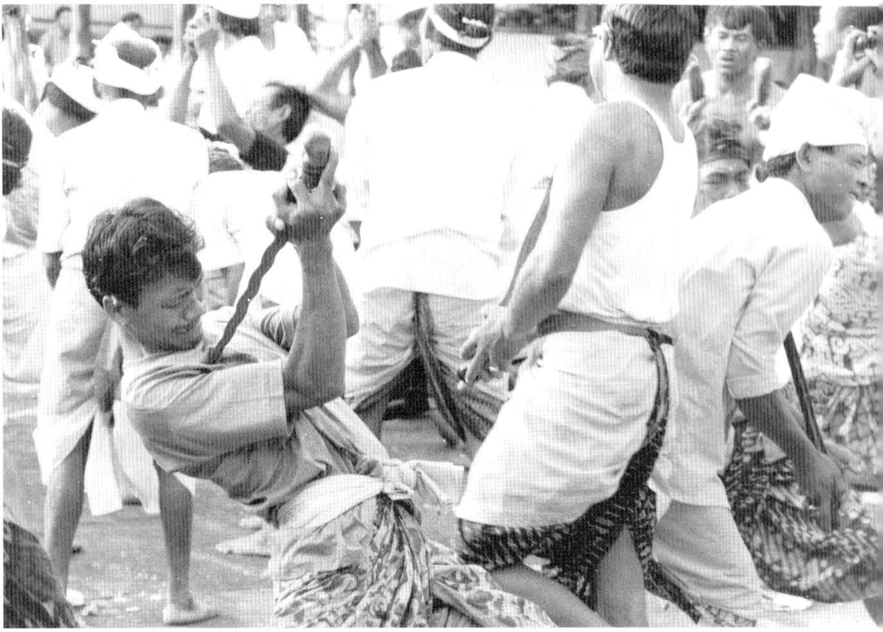

50 Men in trance-possession performing kris stabbing at the Jimbaran mass trance-possession ceremony. Considerable force is applied to the dagger, but no harm is sustained when the men are in a trance state.

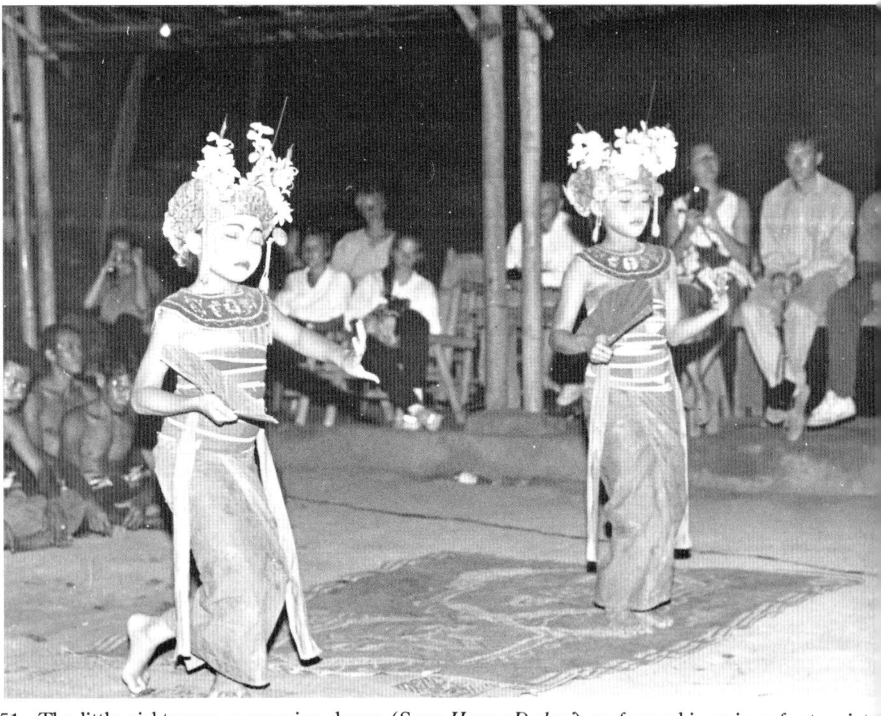

51 The little girl trance-possession dance (*Sang Hyang Dedari*) performed in unison for tourists

2 The fire/hobby-horse dance (*Sang Hyang Jaran*) performed for tourists at Bona. The fire dancer is able to touch and stand on the hot coals for several seconds without sustaining burns because of a change in sensibility caused by his trance-possession state.

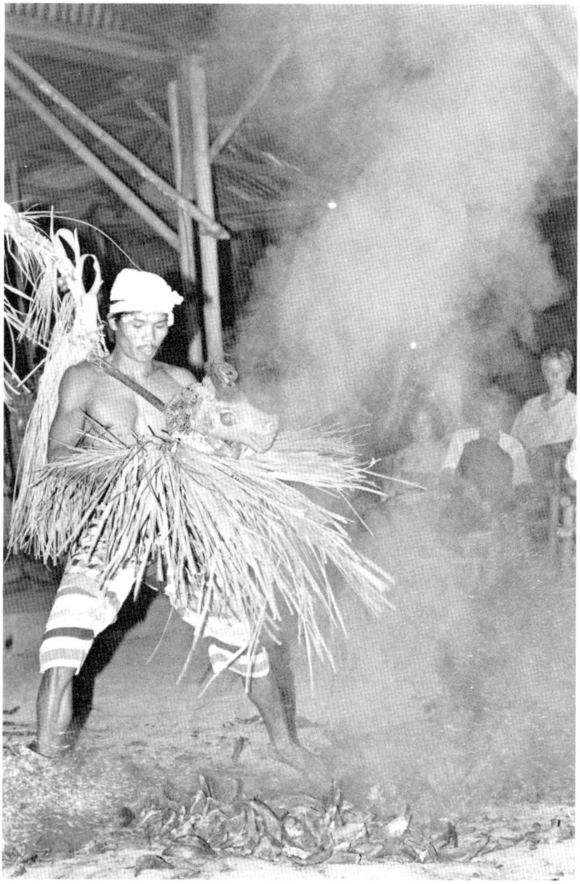

3 In the *kecak* dance, some men in the circular chorus enter trance-possession, as is evident in the two on the right. The female dancer is not in trance-possession.

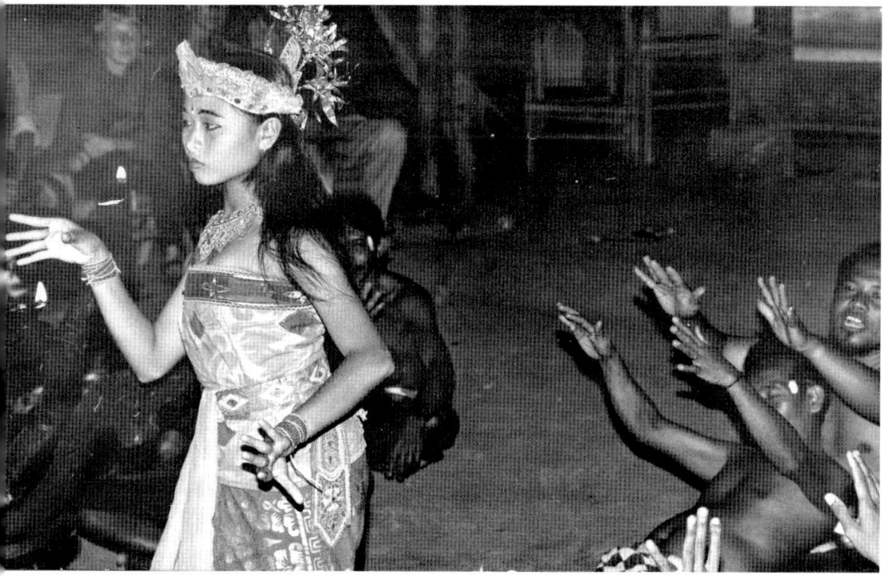

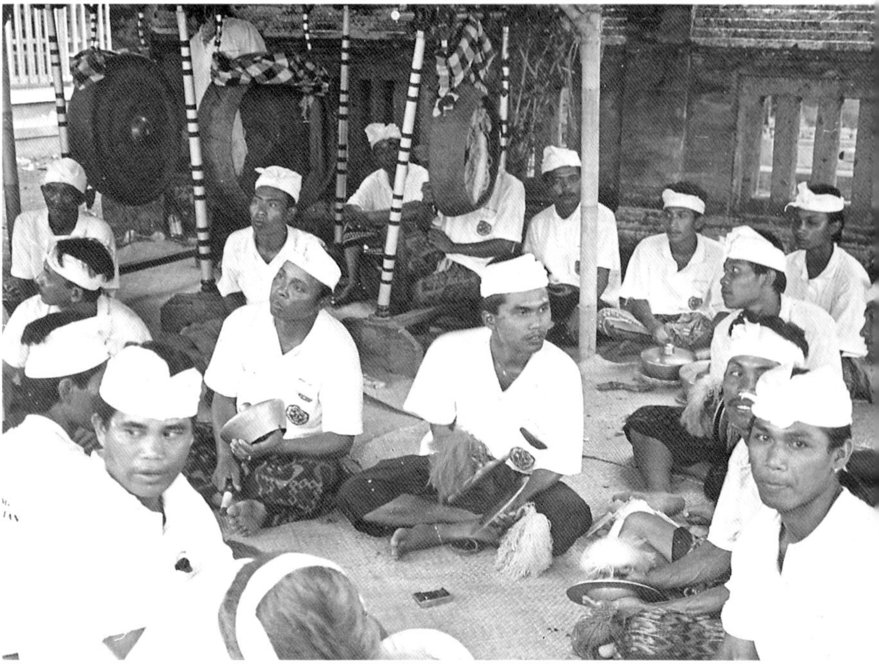

54 Gamelan musicians before a performance exhibiting facial expressions characteristic of the usual state of consciousness.

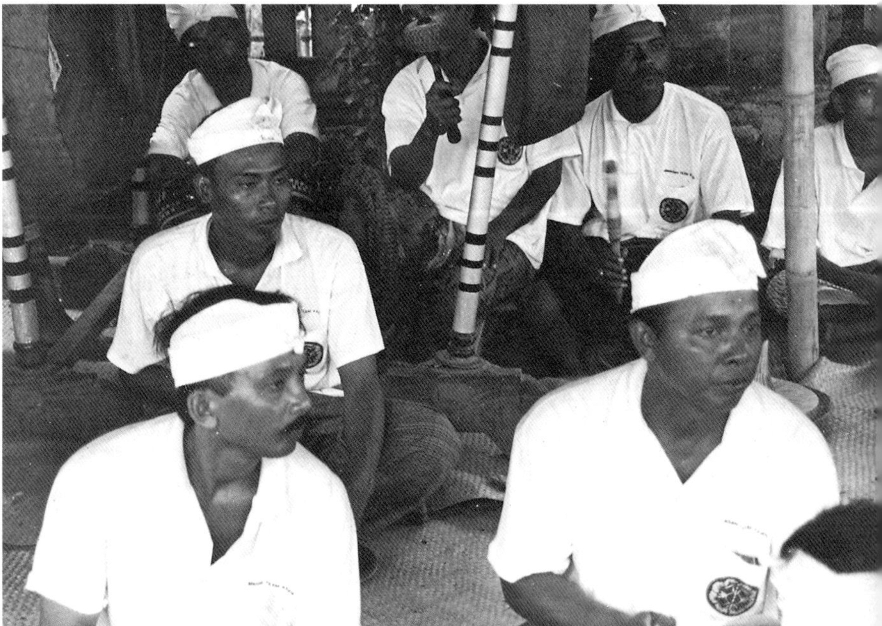

55 The gamelan musicians in Plate 54 playing traditional (ceremonial) music and showing the flattened facial expressions characteristic of a trance state.

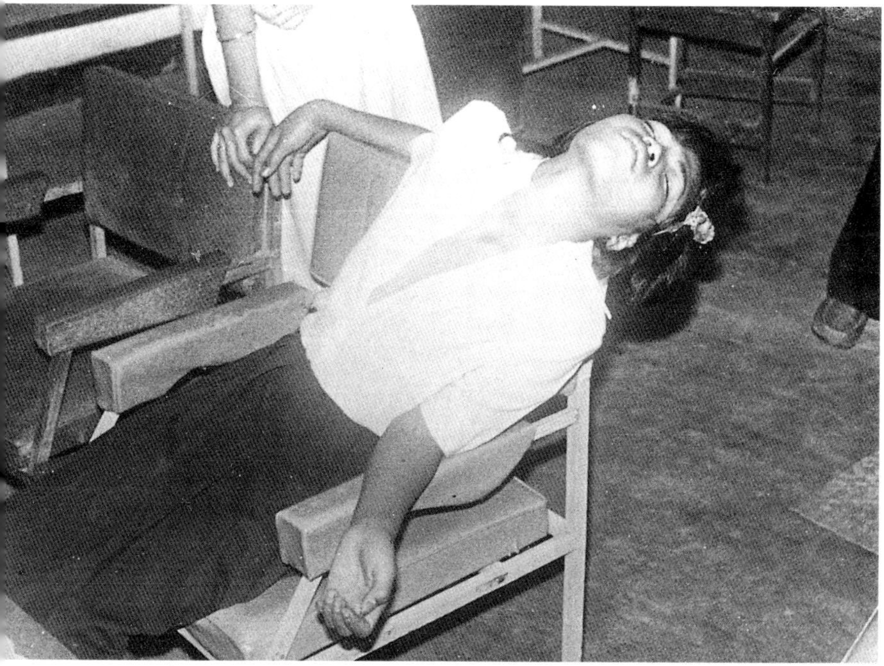

6 One of the schoolgirls who experienced trance-possession is shown in an unconscious state which lasted about 15 minutes.

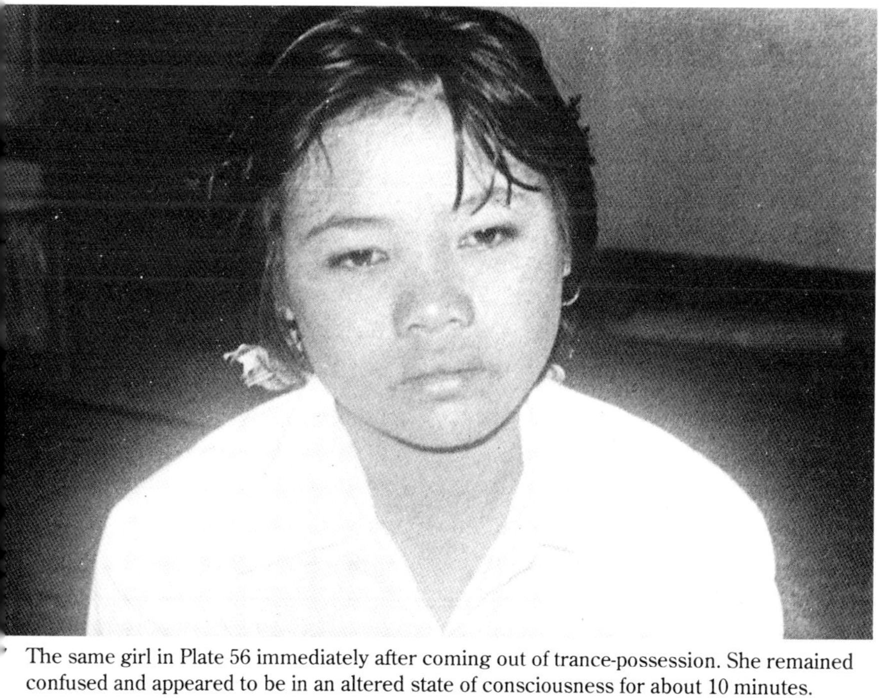

The same girl in Plate 56 immediately after coming out of trance-possession. She remained confused and appeared to be in an altered state of consciousness for about 10 minutes.

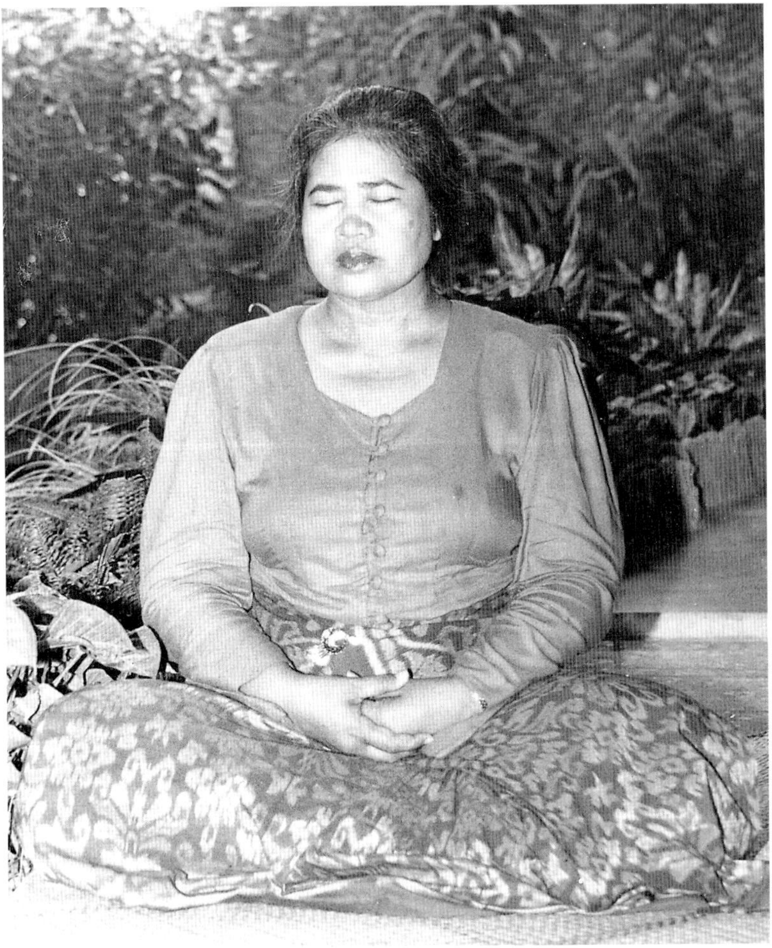

58 Suryani sitting in a meditation state which lasted about 10 minutes. Her facial musculature appears flattened compared with that of her usual state of consciousness.

Chapter 7
Dissociative Disorders, Trance-suicide, and Trance-possession Disorders

DISSOCIATION, the psychological process involved in normal trance, can also be abnormal, causing symptoms and resulting in a number of conditions or mental disorders, including psychogenic amnesia, fugue states, muscular paralysis, loss of sight or hearing, pain, anaesthesia, muscle twitching, and seizures. The terminologies for these disorders have changed over the years and can be confusing. Most of these disorders are referred to as hysterical neuroses or conversion disorders (Nemiah, 1980). Multiple personality disorder (MPD) in the West, a type of dissociative disorder, is considered by some theorists to be a form of self-hypnosis or trance (Bliss, 1984a; see Chapter 9). Most of these conditions appear under the general heading of dissociative disorders in *DSM-III-R* (APA, 1987), which also covers trance disorders. *ICD-10* (WHO, 1992) has also included, for the first time, trance and possession disorders in its listing.

All dissociative disorders (as well as hypnosis in normal individuals) involve the same underlying fundamental process conceptualized in psychiatric terms as the unconscious psychological 'defence' mechanism of dissociation. It is theorized that most dissociative disorders develop as an unconscious reaction to overwhelming situations, impulses, or feelings which cannot be tolerated by the fully conscious mind, although these are not always discoverable in therapy. It is well known that the symptoms of conversion disorders are closely related to cultural beliefs.

The following case vignettes of mental disorders (mainly hysterical neuroses of the conversion type) in the Balinese indicate that some of these disorders are similar to those in the West. The patients in these cases recovered relatively quickly after undergoing brief psychotherapy. This type of disorder is often successfully treated with hypnotherapy or Amytal interviews.[1]

1. An 18-year-old Balinese woman suddenly developed paralysis in one leg. Conventional neurological examination was negative. Supportive psychotherapy, together with the suggestion that she would regain the ability to walk, plus brief non-specific treatment with Valium relieved her symptom and feelings of tension. The nature of psychological conflict underlying her symptom was not revealed.

2. A 28-year-old Balinese woman collapsed and experienced paralysis and weakness for three days prior to her visit to the doctor. She recovered abruptly after supportive psychotherapy.

3. A young Balinese woman developed blindness seven days prior to her visit to Suryani. Medical examination was negative. Psychotherapy involved suggesting that she was not blind, that there was something she did not want to 'see', that she had some problem which she could talk about, and encouraging her to talk about it. The problem turned out to be conflictual feelings towards her father, who had three wives and who she felt did not pay enough attention to her mother. Her symptoms cleared after several psychotherapy sessions.

Trance-suicide in Bali

Suicide is a serious problem in the West and in many Eastern countries. The rate ranges from 5 to 20 per 100,000 in most countries (Murphy, 1982) but it is extremely high in certain parts of Malaysia, 157 per 100,000 (Maniam, 1988). The rates in Bali are unavailable but are believed to be relatively very low, estimated at only about 9 per cent of the rate in Singapore (a country with a population equal to that of Bali) (Tsoi and Kua, 1987).

The rates of suicide attempts in Bali for 1989 are presented in Table 7.1. The rates for the year 1990 were not significantly different for sex, age-group, and total. Each group under 20 years was overrepresented and the age-group over 60 was relatively low, about 4 per cent.

In the West, suicides and suicide attempts occur in association with a variety of mental disorders, including adjustment disorders, borderline personality disorder, depressions, and psychoses of various types. Western suicide attempters give a variety of reasons for their attempts, some rational (e.g. relationship problems, attention seeking, anger or despair at being rejected, and feeling that

TABLE 7.1
Cases of Suicide Attempts Admitted to Hospitals in Bali in 1989 by Sex, Age, and Marital Status[1]

Sex/Age[2]	*<20*	*20–60*	*>60*	*Total*
Male	45	55	3	103
Female	68	53	1	122
Total	113	108	4	225

Sex/Marital Status[3]	*Single*	*Married*	*Separated*	*Divorced*	*Widowed*	*Total*
Male	56	30	0	0	6	92
Female	62	51	0	0	1	114
Total	118	81	0	0	7	206

[1] $n = 228$.
[2] Sex and age unknown = 3.
[3] Marriage or sex unknown = 17.

life was not worth living), some irrational, and some psychotic (e.g. 'command hallucinations' telling them to do it). In the great majority of Western suicide attempts, patients report no amnesia regarding the event; they recall it fully, including their behaviour and the feelings leading up to it, as well as their feeling afterwards. They generally give rational explanations of how and why they did it. Studies of suicide attempts in Asian countries (Maniam, 1988; Tsoi and Kok, 1982; Tsoi and Kua, 1987) have pinpointed interpersonal difficulties such as marital quarrels and other family conflicts as the major cause of such attempts but generally provide no data on the thoughts, sensations, or feelings of the individuals at the time of the attempts.

A study of suicide in Toraja, South Sulawesi, Indonesia (Hollan, 1990) concluded that the primary reasons for suicide there were intense shame or remorse over any kind of wrongdoing, especially deep feelings of injustice and mistreatment. However, the data for these determinations appear to have been gained from talking with the general population and not from the persons who made the suicide attempt. It cannot be assumed that the beliefs expressed by families or other members of the culture were necessarily representative of the attitudes and feelings of the suicide victims. Ingestion of pesticides is the predominant means used for suicide and attempted suicides in a number of South-East Asian countries.

Suryani was motivated to study suicide in Bali because she was puzzled about Balinese committing suicide since it is so deeply wrong (*salah pati*) according to Balinese Hindu belief. In Bali, religious beliefs are extremely powerful in shaping and controlling behaviour. Two studies were carried out—the first from 1969 to 1974, and the second in 1988 and 1989.

Study 1

Seventy-seven case records of attempted suicide—all cases that were admitted to Wangaya Hospital Department of Psychiatry[2] from 1969 to 1974—were reviewed. Thirty-nine available subjects were interviewed regarding associated problems, reasons, attitudes, and experiences during and after the attempt. Records of the remaining 38 were also studied. Forty-six were male and 31 were female. The cases came from all over the island of Bali but mostly from two districts, Badung and Tabanan, because they have hospitals there. The age distribution is as follows: 12–20 years, 51 per cent; 21–30 years, 28 per cent; 31–40 years, 30 per cent; over 40, 8 per cent. The means of suicide attempt are as follows: ingesting pesticide poison, $n = 26$; using a knife, $n = 14$; hanging, $n = 8$; taking medication or drug, $n = 9$; jumping into a well, $n = 2$; and drinking either battery water or brake fluid, $n = 9$. These patients denied they had previous suicide attempts, and no repeated attempts were noted in the records. Twenty-one were married, 56 were never married. Psychiatric diagnoses according to *ICD-8* classification are as follows: psychoses, $n = 16$; reactive depression, $n = 60$; reactive anxiety, $n = 1$.

A number of the 23 non-psychotic suicide attempters described existing problems which were associated with relatively mild stress (e.g. father disagreed about a boyfriend) but none reported more serious stress. When queried about why they made the suicide attempt, all gave similar responses: they had a perception that the world was getting 'dark;' they were confused and unable to think; their mind felt 'empty' and a 'power' controlled and caused them to do it, i.e. a power that compelled them to drink the poison, a power that made them behave like robots. After the suicide attempt, a few recalled hearing some family commotion and crying but they did not have the energy to stand up. Then they forgot everything; most suicide attempters did not recall being brought to the hospital. When asked if they felt like attempting suicide again, they generally replied, 'I pray to God not to give me an experience like that again.' They also denied any responsibility for having done it themselves. All respondents, including the psychotic patients, said that they felt afraid to recall the experience.

When interviewed, the 16 psychotic patients said that they were confused and didn't know or could not explain why they had attempted suicide. About 30 per cent of them claimed they had responded to command hallucinations that told them to do it. None described sensations characteristic of an ASC or a trance state.

Study 2

The second study was a replication of the first because general information suggested that in recent years there may have been an increase in the incidence of suicide and Suryani wanted to know whether there were any changes since the previous study and whether the patterns of attempts were similar.

All records of attempted suicide from the Department of Psychiatry, Wangaya Hospital, between 1982 and 1989 were reviewed—a total of 315 cases, 131 males and 184 females. The age distribution is as follows: 10–14 years, n = 9; 15–9 years, n = 109; 20–29 years, n = 137; 30–44 years, n = 56; over 65 years, n = 4. The methods of attempting suicide are: ingesting pesticide, n = 281; using a knife, n = 14; hanging, n = 4; using a gun, n = 1; taking medication or drugs, n = 15. Diagnoses according to *ICD-9* are: acute reaction to stress, n = 158; depressive reactions, n= 90; confusion reaction, n = 20; conversion reaction, n = 4; anxiety reaction, n= 20; acute psychosis, n = 22; and personality disorder, n = 1.

Thirty-five patients were interviewed and asked the same questions as in Study 1. The interviews, which were conducted in a private room, were long and probing, without being suggestive, in order to obviate the Balinese characteristic difficulty in explaining their verbal and non-verbal responses. The patient's eyes were observed for responses indicative of trance. In response to initial questions about their feelings or experiences, subjects typically said, 'I've forgotten.' Further questioning of the non-psychotic patients elicited essentially the same responses: they did not know why they did it, they were unable to think at the time, they were confused, and they felt as if some thing, power, or energy had controlled them and influenced them to act as they did. The psychotic patients' experiences differed from those of the non-psychotics in Study 1; however, the psychotic patients said they were scared (*takut*) by the suicide attempt and did not want a repeat experience. None of the patients mentioned the usual reasons that Westerners give for suicide attempts.

The results of the first study were unexpected and at that time

Suryani did not know how to explain the process that could account for the data because she was not yet familiar with hypnotic states as defined and described in Western literature. After becoming a hypnotherapist, she recalled the earlier study and in retrospect recognized that the suicide attempts involved ASC.

With greater knowledge gained from interviews with *balian* and individuals in trance, it was clear to the authors that the experiences reported by the suicide attempters were those of trance-possession (*kasurupan*). This finding has not heretofore been reported in the literature for any culture. The uniformity of response of the patients was striking. All had perceptions and experiences consistent with trance-possession, i.e. the initial perception of the world getting dark, confused thinking or an inability to think, the perception of a power taking over and controlling them, automatic behaviour, and a period of amnesia regarding the events. They denied that they acted consciously of their own volition. Their conviction after recovery that they would never want to have such an experience again contrasts with the behaviour of Western patients, some of whom continue to express suicidal ideation, although most of them say they would not do it again. None of the Balinese patients described life as not worth living; nor did they want to die. None had made repeated suicide attempts.

The authors considered the possibility that these suicide attempters claimed that their actions were beyond their control in order to obviate shame or guilt about their behaviour. However, this is unlikely in view of the fact that the subjects had no contact with each other and they were interviewed in private; yet all gave similar reports, each of which contained evidence of ASC.

A few cases of attempted suicide in Bali do not involve trance and are similar to those reported in Western literature. In 1990, a 17-year-old girl took an overdose of anti-pruritic pills, but she did not know that they were non-lethal. She said she wanted to die because her father often beat her at home and objected to her lifestyle and her preference for spending time with boys. He called her a prostitute because she stayed out at night and had many boyfriends. He objected to all her relationships with boys and seemed to be jealous or somewhat paranoid about them. She reported that her parents always quarrelled with each other at home. Her mother had attempted suicide once because of displeasure with her husband.

The reasons given by the Balinese as to why their people commit suicide are similar to those reported in many cultures. They include frustration, anger, disappointment with parents or friends, feeling of hopelessncss, or insufficient money. When relatives are asked why a particular person has committed suicide, they will generally not say that evil spirits are involved even if they believe it to be so. They do not want people to think that evil spirits are affecting their family.

L. Connor (personal communication) interpreted cases in which the Balinese explained suicide by saying that 'the evil spirit did it' as a manifestation of a projective personality trait. However, Suryani's interviews with suicide attempters indicated something quite different: they were confused and a 'power'—something like an evil spirit—made them do it. These individuals indicated that they were not functioning normally at the time of the attempt, that they were unable to distinguish between good and evil, and that they carried out the act without thinking.

The question of religion as a major deterrent to suicide must be considered. The main reason for a relatively low rate of suicide among Malays is their Islamic religion; suicide is a sin for Muslims (Tsoi and Kua, 1987). One study of suicide in Americans suggested that their religions may not be a significant deterrent to suicide. American World War II veterans who committed suicide were actually overrepresented in the Catholic faith, which regards suicide as a mortal sin (Schneidman and Farberow, 1960). However, it would be a mistake to assume that the Balinese Hindu religion affects the beliefs, morals, and behaviour of the Balinese in a manner comparable to the effect the major religions in America have on Americans or the effect Islam has on Muslims. Religion in Bali has broad and pervasive effects on the mind and person. Specifically with regard to suicide, Balinese Hindus regard it as 'mis-death' (*salah pati*) with the consequence that the individual will go to hell, not heaven. The people know that suicide (1) incurs punishment from God; (2) causes God to send one to hell instead of heaven; (3) incurs bad karma resulting in a more difficult future life; and (4) causes the reincarnation process to take a considerably longer time.[3] These are considered highly effective deterrents to suicide. Suicide rates in Bali are not yet available but preliminary estimates appear to be very low compared with those of most countries.

The findings indicate that most suicide attempts and probably most completed suicides by non-psychotic Balinese are carried out during ASC, specifically a state of trance-possession. This study broadens the knowledge of the medical/psychiatric consequences of trance and identifies a heretofore unrecognized trance disorder.

The Balinese findings can be compared with data from other cultures, especially Western, in several respects, including methods of suicide, suicide pacts, trance, and other psychological factors. Suicide and suicide attempts have been reported in many countries and cultures—in the Western, Eastern, and Third Worlds—but this is not the place to review the extensive literature on this subject. Mention, however, should be made of several pertinent issues. First, the patterns and rates of suicide differ and the methods used vary according to culture. For example, in Sri Lanka (Diekstra, 1989), Malaysia (Maniam, 1988), Singapore (Tsoi and Kua, 1987), Sulawesi, Indonesia (Hollan, 1990), and in Bali, agricultural pesticides are the most common means of suicide. In the United States the use of medications or drugs is the leading method. The causes of suicide have focused on interpersonal and socio-economic causes, as in India (Bhatia et al., 1987) or on psychiatric disorders, particularly depression, as in the United States. Suicide pacts (double suicides of lovers, spouses, or friends), which occur in many countries, are the most common in Japan (Fishbain and Aldrich, 1985), but are very rare in Bali. Suicide pacts indicate premeditation and probably a conscious suicidal act. In 1991, the news media of Bali reported the case of a young couple whose parents disapproved of their marriage and who committed suicide after expressing a desire to be buried together. Because custom (*adat*) prevented this, they were buried separately with photos of each other. The generally accepted definition of suicide in Western literature includes the concept of a conscious act to end life (Schneidman, 1987). The finding of trance-suicide in Bali indicates that instead of being a conscious act, suicide may in fact be an unconscious one. A culture-sensitive definition of suicide must take this into account.

A cross-cultural comparative study found suicide to be most common in countries which are 'stable agricultural types' and which customarily expect very restrained or very open expression of emotions versus moderate expression (Smith and Hackathorn, 1982). Balinese Hindus have both characteristics. Comparisons among Balinese are not possible because of inadequate data to gauge the prevalence of suicide in the community.

The Trance-suicide Concept

There are no citations in the suicide literature that deal with ASC or the concept of trance as a significant mechanism. However, some Western and Eastern suicides suggest a trance state. One example involves individuals who have doused themselves with gasoline and immolated themselves while sitting quietly in a tower of flames, usually as an expression of political protest. Almost all of these individuals died and there are no data from interviews with survivors to ascertain their psychological state at the time.

Several mass suicide events, well known in history, have occurred in both Eastern and Western cultures. In Bali, two episodes of what may be considered mass suicide occurred in 1902 and 1908, when royal families marched ceremoniously into the gunfire of advancing Dutch troops and turned their krises on their families and themselves. At Klungkung in 1908, the entire royal family of about 200 members were killed, and only one member, a male, survived because he was out of town at the time. It was believed that the self-inflicted death was chosen by the leaders because they perceived that they would be conquered by the armed Dutch troops and as a consequence lose all they had—material goods as well as religion. The authors hypothesized that these self-sacrifices occurred in an ASC, probably in trance. Investigation of this hypothesis could possibly be pursued by studying the films taken of the massacre which now reside in Holland.

In Bali as in India prior to the twentieth century, it was the custom for a wife of a deceased royal member to throw herself on to the flaming cremation pyre of her husband and die of immolation. In Bali, this practice was outlawed by the Dutch colonial government, the last instance occurring in 1915. The authors hypothesize that this act was accomplished in a trance state.

During World War II at Saipan, Micronesia, thousands of Japanese soldiers forced their families to climb to a high cliff where they pushed them and then jumped to their own deaths on the rocks below when it was clear to them that they would be conquered and possibly captured by US Marines invading the island. In 1978 at Guyana in the Caribbean, Jim Jones, an American religious cult leader, together with about 900 followers, took cyanide in 'Kool Aid' (at his directive) when he believed that his group was threatened by the arrival of a US Congressman's delegation (Harrary, 1992). Harrary (1992) reported that many of the deaths were murders, especially in cases where children were forced to drink cyanide. For months leading to the event, Jones had prepared his followers for suicide in this manner at their religious meetings. Nearly the entire settlement of over 909 people, men, women, and children perished. It can be hypothesized that many of these people from two divergent cultures—Western, many with Black heritage, and Japanese—were in an ASC, particularly a contagious self-hypnotic state, during suicide.

After a suicide attempt, American patients generally recall their experiences. Very few cases involving amnesia have been reported. However, amnesia following suicide attempts was identified in three cases reported in Japan (Takahashi, 1988). Six additional cases of amnesia involving suicide attempts in Japan (Takahashi, 1989) recalled hallucinations of people during the attempts, while two recounted personal histories completely different from their own. The reports made no reference to dissociation, ASC, or trance. These appear to be cases of dissociative disorder and possibly multiple personality disorder.

The one case reported in the world literature of a suicide attempt while in trance was a 37-year-old American Vietnam War veteran who had post-traumatic stress disorder (PTSD). He was also diagnosed as chronically psychotic although symptoms of the latter were distinct from the acute dissociative disorder (i.e. trance) of his suicide attempt (Haberman, 1986). Two cases of Vietnam War veterans with PTSD involved self-cutting which suggested dissociation (Kim and Ainslie, 1990; Putnam, Zahn, and Post, 1990). Non-schizophrenic PTSD patients related auditory hallucinations suggesting that they commit suicide (Mueser and Butler, 1987). Vietnam War veterans with PTSD are at high risk of suicide and those who have suicide ideation or have attempted it suffer significantly from guilt over having lost control of their behaviour because of being in a state of terror and rage (Hendin and Haas, 1991). Such 'loss of control' is suggestive of dissociation and it raises the question of whether their suicide behaviour occurred in that state, possibly during a flashback experience. Like MPD patients, PTSD patients have been found to be highly hypnotizable (Spiegel, Hunt, and Dondershine, 1988). The psychological mechanism of PTSD involves an underlying dissociative process.

The following case of what was considered a suicide attempt by an overdose of Tranxene (a minor tranquilizer) and lithium (used for the treatment of manic depressive disorders) appears to have involved dissociation. The patient was a 35-year-old divorced single American White woman, who went to a general physician 2 weeks prior to the overdose episode because she showed symptoms of depression. He prescribed lithium, 300 milligrams, three times a day, and Tranxene. On the day after the overdose, the patient could recall her bottle of medication falling to the floor at her bedside and two pills falling out, but after this, she remembered nothing until she awakened in the hospital. Her boyfriend had brought her to the hospital emergency room because she could not be aroused. There she was irrational, yelling and exhibiting uncontrolled motor behaviour which required restraint. Her lithium level was 2.36, which is considered a toxic level. The toxicology screen of her blood was negative for street drugs and she denied taking any kind of street drugs for the previous year. Her blood alcohol level was zero. When interviewed at the psychiatric hospital 13 hours after the overdose, she was alert and had a clear sensorium; furthermore, she exhibited rational behaviour and her thinking was coherent. She denied that she intended to take an overdose of medicine or that she ever had any suicide ideation. She seemed puzzled as to why she had taken extra pills, which was what she was told she had done, and she had no recollection of it. She also did not recall her irrational behaviour in the emergency room. On another examination 12 hours later, there was no evidence of a personality disorder. She denied any previous episodes of loss of memory for events or of losing time. She had no history of mania, was happy to accept the recommendation that she would no longer need medication, and was discharged from the hospital to return to her home that same afternoon.

Although this patient had an elevated blood level of lithium at the time that she arrived at the hospital and was irrational, it is not possible for lithium to have produced amnesia at the point before she took the pills, and furthermore, excitable, uncontrolled, or irrational behaviour is not a side-effect of lithium toxicity. Rather, lithium toxicity is likely to produce sedation and coma. This patient's history did not reveal any reasons why she would have taken an overdose as an attempt at suicide. On the other hand, it was clear that she had amnesia regarding the overdose and for a subsequent period of approximately 6 hours. The episode would appear to represent trance disorder.

Suicide attempts and depression are reported to be characteristic of patients with fugue states, a type of dissociative disorder (Stengel, 1941). However, seemingly contradictory to this are several patients with fugue states (with amnesia) which the authors interpreted as deterrents or alternatives to suicide (Gudjonsson and Haward, 1982; Stengel, 1941).

Schneidman's (1987) authoritative book on the psychology of suicide identified twelve psychological characteristics that are present in most persons who commit suicide. Two of them suggest ASC, dissociation, or trance: (1) a perceptual state of constriction;

and (2) egression, which refers to a person's intended departure from a situation of distress. Schneidman pointed out that suicide is the ultimate egression, a desperate attempt to escape. He felt that suicide is best understood as a 'transient psychological constriction of affect and intellect'. In this state, the suicidal person totally loses the usual life-sustaining images of loved ones. The mind 'turns his or her back on the past and declares that all memories are unreal'. This type of change in thinking can occur in ASC and represent dissociation. The concept of constriction would appear to be similar to that of absorption, which is a defining characteristic of the hypnotic state (Tellegen and Atkinson, 1974). This absorption has been described as 'a disposition for having episodes of single total attention that fully engages one's representational (i.e. perceptual, enactive, imaginative, and ideational) resources' (Tellegen and Atkinson, 1974). Schneidman suggested that the concept of constriction has implications for the management of suicidal patients: there is a need to counter this constriction of thought by attempting to widen the individual's thought process and to remove him from this fixed thought or idea, a state in which there are no other considerations. He cited the case of a young, unmarried woman who was pregnant and had only one thought in mind, namely suicide, as her only option. As he talked to her about a number of other options, she came to consider these and at this point gave up her singular fixed thought of suicide.

Egression and a perceptual state of constriction and absorption appeared to have been present in the Balinese patients who attempted suicide while in trance. Their trance states, like hypnosis, were characterized by a reduction of perceptions, an ignorance of environmental stimuli, and changes in cognition. Although the Balinese suicide attempters did not describe a conscious desire to escape a stressful situation or affect, their behaviour can be interpreted as an unconscious intent and attempt to escape.

The following case of multiple suicide attempts by an American patient is an example of dissociation and in a number of respects it is similar to the Balinese cases of trance-suicide attempts and other trance-possession states.

Jane is a 39-year-old single White female, unemployed, with a history of severe and prolonged sexual abuse in childhood. She has engaged in over 50 suicide attempts or episodes of self-destructive behaviour. These have included cutting herself with knives or a razor many times, usually on the arm, wrists, back, and vagina, and taking overdoses of medications prescribed for pain, sleep, and anxiety. Some of the latter have been near-fatal episodes and many have required hospitalization. She describes the usual episode as follows: initially she gets a sensation that things look farther away, like in a fog or darkness, and then a power takes over her and carries out the behaviour, which her body performs automatically like a robot. This power has been likened to a 'very angry little girl'. She also feels that this power is 'my own demon'. It sometimes speaks, saying that she is bad and that she is going to take an overdose. She also refers to this power, or little girl, as a 'cold-blooded killer' who wants to hurt her and feels very happy about doing so. At these times her mood is euthymic; she shows no signs of depression hypomania, or agitation. When she is abusing herself by cutting her own skin, she does not feel any pain and she sees herself smiling because she wants to do it. When taken to the emergency room in a hospital, she is able to recall only small portions of events that happened during and after the suicide attempt. Generally, she only learns about what happens through someone else telling her what she did. The state may last for several hours or up to 2 days before she becomes aware of what has happened. Following this, she worries, feels frightened, and is scared because she does not want to die. She said, 'I do not know what would happen if I'm not aware of my behaviour.'

She describes the very angry little girl who enters her as being thin with brown hair and brown eyes and she claims that this little girl does not like authority. She can talk to this little girl but she cannot control her. She feels that the little girl is inside her. This experience first occurred several years ago and has subsequently happened frequently, perhaps 60 per cent of the time. The experience lasts about 1–2 hours, and she recognizes this little girl as the one who wants to hurt her and who feels glad that she is hurt. The 'little girl' admits to being scared and will not show herself very often.

The patient experienced one such episode during an interview with Jensen and, at that time, she displayed a great deal of anxiety, saying that she felt panicky and had a strong desire to hurt herself. These feelings were calmed to some extent by 2 milligrams of Ativan, a benzodiazepine. She said that she would like to be able to 'come to terms' with this little girl and even contract with her to avoid panic and danger. She felt she needed to accept the little girl as a person with rights and she believed the little girl to be 'the part of her that was abused'. That abuse led her to ignore the little girl for many years, something which she was no longer able to do.

In another type of suicide attempt, this patient felt panic-stricken and out of control, and she would do anything to stop this feeling, including cutting herself. She said, 'This is the other side of the coin. I don't want to continue and I do it to myself under self-conscious control.' At that time, she felt 'scared', and she described her thoughts as 'racing', and her mind as 'zooming'.

This patient has written suicide notes to her son on four or five occasions, stating that she is sorry, that he will not understand, and that she feels despair. At these times, she knows that she is going to make a suicide attempt and does so immediately afterwards. She describes the nature of these attempts as 'the power entering her'.

On the Dissociative Experiences Scale (Bernstein and Putnam, 1986), she scored nearly maximal—95 per cent—on the number of items endorsed. The average score of items endorsed is about 40. This number of items endorsed is comparable to typical scores for patients with multiple personality disorder (MPD). The average score of items endorsed is also comparable to the scores of PTSD patients. She probably has both conditions. She certainly meets the diagnostic criteria for MPD. Her description of the little girl taking over is similar to the Balinese experience of possession.

This case report is similar to other cases of MPD suicide attempt. Ross et al. (1989) noted that self-destructive behaviour and suicide attempts are very common in MPD patients: 72 per cent attempted suicide and 2.1 per cent killed themselves. The methods were drug overdose (68 per cent), self-inflicted burns or other injuries (56.6 per cent), and wrist cutting (49.3 per cent). In Ross's experience, cases of complex MPD involving over 15 multiple personalities with amnesic barriers were associated with histories of physical, sexual, and emotional abuse. He reported that these patients may be amnesic with regard to the suicide attempt. They may report depersonalization while harming themselves and accuse an alter of being responsible for the behaviour. Their self-destructive behaviour was not the usual 'cry for help' or 'attention-seeking'. The MPD suicide attempt group had a history of greater prevalence and more severe physical and sexual abuse, rape, and more acute psychopathology (Ross et al., 1989).

Given that the majority of these MPD patients have a history of childhood abuse, it may be expected that they would be prone to dissociation (van der Kolk, Perry, and Herman, 1991). This was supported in a study of 74 subjects with personality disorders or bipolar II disorder. Thirty-two per cent of these subjects had borderline personality disorder and 79 per cent of them reported a history of significant childhood trauma. In the overall study, childhood trauma scores (as measured by the Traumatic Antecedents Questionnaire) predicted suicide attempts, self-cutting and other self-injurious behaviour, and anorexia. There was a link between witnessing parental violence in childhood and suicide attempts. Scores on the DES were highly correlated with histories of trauma, self-cutting, and anorexia, and there was a trend towards a correlation with suicide attempts. During follow-up study of these cases, the DES scores continued to predict self-cutting and suicide attempts. The authors concluded that ongoing dissociation is directly associated with self-cutting. These results confirmed the previous studies that dissociation is associated with self-injury, and that many such patients report feeling numb and 'dead' prior to inflicting self-harm (Bach-y-Rita, 1974; Favazza, 1989; Favazza and Conterio, 1989; Gardner and Cowdry, 1985; Graff and Mallin, 1967; Grunebaum and Klerman, 1967; Leibenluft, Gardner, and Cowdry, 1987; Pattison and Kahan, 1983; Rosenthal et al., 1972; Roy, 1985; Simpson and Porter, 1981; Stone, 1987).

This study of the Balinese has implications for the management of the suicide problem in Bali. It suggests that it would be helpful for educators to include, in the regular religious teaching in public schools, concepts regarding the consequences of suicide and the attitude of the culture. Psychotherapists' realization that a dissociative mechanism operates in suicide attempts of the Balinese can provide an understanding of the need to direct efforts at increasing self-esteem and confidence in suicide attempters and to avoid implications that the patient has deliberately done wrong, while still providing education in religious belief and custom. Understanding the psychological process of suicide in both non-psychotic and psychotic patients helps therapists to provide appropriate support to the patients and their families. Since most suicides in Bali are by ingestion of pesticides and appear to be impulsive (in trance), public health authorities should consider practical techniques to make pesticides less readily accessible.

Amok

Amok is a classic example of what has been called a culture-bound syndrome;[4] that is, it is specific to a given culture and is not found generally across many cultures, as is, for example, schizophrenia. Actually *amok* occurs in a number of South-East Asian cultures, particularly Malaysia. Typically, *amok* is characterized by a person, suddenly and without provocation or warning, losing control of his actions and behaving violently. It may last minutes to hours and can result in injury and death to persons who fall victim to the attacker.

In Bali, *amok* occurs occasionally and is generally believed to be more frequent in the areas of Karangasem. Suryani (1984) noted an 11 per cent incidence of *amok* among persons affected with the possession disorder termed *bebainan*. Suryani and her husband, a general medical practitioner in Denpasar, have examined a number of *amok* cases, three of which are described below.

Case 1

In 1987, a 36-year-old policeman, off duty at home, went out into his neighbourhood one morning and shot five women on the street, seemingly at random. He was restrained by other policemen living in the neighbourhood and brought to jail. Suryani and Dr Denny Thong, then Director of the Bangli Mental Hospital, examined him, and found no psychiatric symptoms except complete amnesia regarding the event. They diagnosed *amok* (a dissociative disorder). He had no evidence of an organic disorder: EEG, psychological testing, and x-ray of the skull were negative. History revealed that for several months prior to the episode, the man had been under severe stress from his job and his wife, who had been admitted to a hospital. The patient was sentenced to 6 years in jail. In 1992, Suryani met him at her private practice when he came with a patient, a friend from his policeman days. He hoped that his friend would not experience what he did when he had severe stress. Suryani asked how he got free and he said that he did not go to jail because the highest court gave him freedom. But he felt very sad and guilty because he did not know he had killed five women. He lived for a year outside Bali. After he decided that this was his *karma*, he tried to accept what the community thought about him, and went back to Bali to become a farmer. He continued living with his wife, as he had done prior to his attack.

Case 2

In 1970, a 30-year-old male, who had no prior psychiatric history, suddenly locked his extended family in the family temple and killed the entire lot. Psychiatric examination revealed that he had visual illusions that his family members were pigs entering a temple. The police asked, 'Why did you kill your family?' He said, 'I didn't. I just saw pigs at the temple and wanted to make it clean.' He spent 15 years in jail without exhibiting any mental symptoms.

Case 3

In 1990, an adolescent took a knife and suddenly attacked and killed his father after he had quarrelled with him regarding his desire to sell their land. The young man felt that the family would not be able to survive without ownership of the farmland. On examination, he stated that he did not know why he did it. He said that the world was dark, and his thinking 'empty', and he felt as if someone controlled his thinking and behaviour. He was remorseful about the event and in jail experienced visual hallucinations of his father's face but did not manifest a psychotic disorder.

In Bali, persons who have committed serious crimes while experiencing an attack of *amok* may be correctly diagnosed as *amok* but nevertheless are given jail sentences. If *amok* or a comparable behaviour were to occur in Western society, it would fit the criteria for a court of law acquittal on the basis of insanity: the individual did not know the significance nor was he aware of his act at the time and sometimes subsequently as well. The M'naghten rule, which still governs insanity pleas in many states of America, holds that

> to establish a defence on the ground of insanity, it must be clearly proved that at the time of the committing of the act, the party accused was laboring under such a defect of reason, from disease of the mind, as not to know the nature and quality of the act he was doing; or if he did know it that he did not know that he was doing what was wrong.

During *amok* Balinese lack the capacity to appreciate the wrongfulness of their conduct.

There are no known cases of recurrence of *amok* in the Balinese except for that which occurs in *bebainan* (see below). Similarly, no evidence of recidivism was found in Malaysians who committed *amok* (Carr and Tan, 1976). This is unlike the general pattern of violence among most Western criminals in which violent behaviour is recurrent. In the West, it is well established that the best predictor of violent behaviour is a history of previous violence by the person.[5] While Suryani has not examined patients during an *amok* attack, she regards the disorder as identifiable by the symptoms of amnesia following the attack, the lack of awareness of why they had behaved aggressively during the attack, and the absence of a psychotic disorder. *Amok* fits the criteria of a dissociative state or a trance-like state. However, it belies the general rule of hypnosis that persons in trance will not do something they would not do in their usual or non-hypnotic state.

Bebainan: A Trance-possession Disorder[6]

This was an investigation of 27 cases of *bebainan*, a disorder which the Balinese believe to be caused by sorcery (Suryani, 1984). The most common symptoms were sudden feelings of confusion, crying, screaming, and shouting, followed by an inability to control one's actions. The victims, mostly female, reported suddenly 'losing control of themselves'. Some cried out continually for no reason (82 per cent), some spoke, giving voice to the *bebai* (see below) that they felt possessed them (44 per cent), whilst others were silent (11 per cent), and a few ran *amok* (11 per cent). Only a small number of respondents could not say how they felt or acted during an attack (7 per cent). In the majority of cases, attacks were brief, lasting ¼ to 1 hour.

In an attempt to control troubled and uncertain feelings during the prodromal stage, sufferers usually went to a bedroom. After lying down, they suddenly found that they could not control themselves anymore. They cried out or sobbed or talked to themselves against all attempts to calm them down. Most (81 per cent) were lying down at the time of an attack, 15 per cent were standing or walking, and 4 per cent were running around aimlessly. If restrained, 89 per cent said that the more they were restrained, the greater was their capacity to resist. None could say how they gained the extraordinary strength. For example, a female sufferer who was restrained by six men was still able to struggle free.

Bebainan is an illness which the Balinese believe to be caused by the possession of the soul of the ill individual by a malignant spirit called the *bebai*. The term *bebai* (meaning evil spirit in old Balinese) refers to both the malignant spirit and its material representation. The latter is an embodiment of Balinese belief in the supernatural characteristics of the newborn. In Balinese religion, it is believed that at conception the 'soul' of the mother and that of the father intermingle to become the foetus (*rare ring jeroning garba*) which assumes the quality of a supernatural human being (*manusia sakti*). This quality remains with the foetus until the newborn reaches the age of six Balinese months, i.e., about 210 days. Belief in the powers of the newborn has inspired some Balinese, who seek to practise sorcery or black magic (*ilmu pengiwa*), to capture those powers and transform them into those of a *bebai* (Weck, 1937).

Bebai may be made of different raw materials such as an aborted foetus, a baby which has died before or during delivery, a placenta, a bud of the banana tree, which is still very young and is commonly used in ceremonies (*pusuh*), an egg of a black hen, the water which has been used for bathing a corpse, or the brain of a murdered person. The type of material used determines the power of *bebai*. For instance, a *bebai* made from an aborted foetus of a female high priest (*pedanda istri*) would be much more powerful than another made from the foetus of an ordinary woman. A very powerful bebai is called 'king of *bebai*' (*raja bebai*).

Having found the material needed, the sorcerer then proceeds to treat the object as a baby. Like a real new baby, the *bebai* undergoes the normal series of ceremonies, performed for it immediately after 'birth', after one (Balinese) month and seven days, at the age of three months, and finally at the end of six months. Unlike a human baby, after the last ceremony the *bebai* is taken to the cemetery where a special ceremony is performed. At this ceremony, the sorcerer makes offerings to the gods, entreating them to bestow on the *bebai* the greatest powers possible. If the request is granted, the sorcerer then gives the *bebai* a name, usually simply 'human baby' or *bayi wong*. Afterward, back at home, the sorcerer prepares rice and other dishes specially for the *bebai*, which is now truly treated as a precious and precocious child. The next period lasts until it reaches the age when a normal child begins to talk. During this period, the *bebai* is not only fed regularly but is also given special offerings on *kajeng kliwon* (an important Balinese religious day which comes every 15 days). Finally, now that the *bebai* can 'talk' and 'understand', it is regularly consulted by the sorcerer to ascertain its 'maturity'. Only when it is fully mature is it ready to be used. At this stage, it is said to have acquired 30 powers or to have become 30 *bebai* in one. These powers can be used either by the sorcerer-owner, rented out, or sold.

Each of the 30 powers or manifestations of the *bebai* has a particular name and produces a particular symptom through the person it possesses. For example, *I Bebai Bongol* makes its victim unable or unwilling to talk. On the other hand, *I Bebai Sebarung* makes the person in its possession very talkative and rude. Another example is *I Rejek Gumi*, presumed to have 108 *buta* (evil spirits) under its command and therefore known as the king of *bebai*. This *bebai* attacks its victim violently in the pit of the stomach, making the victim enraged before rendering him or her unconscious. The victim is likely to die unless help is quickly obtained. Although each power or manifestation of the *bebai* has a distinct name and a distinct mode of attack, the various manifestations are supposed to be very co-operative, and to be ever ready to help one another to subdue victims.

Not every hated person can be attacked or possessed by *bebai*. The impervious individuals are those who are free of sins, who are wise, or who have powerful amulets. The vulnerable persons are those who are believed to be weak either in mind or body and those who are sinful.

Most commonly, a person falling into the possession of the *bebai* is reported to experience a sudden sense of blankness, loss of desire and will, and confusion. These feelings are accompanied by a stomachache or headache and ringing in the ears, followed by a loss of vision and a feeling of cold starting from the feet upward to the pit of the stomach. Finally, the victim loses all control and either cries uncontrollably, shouting and screaming, or incessantly talks angrily to himself or herself. Sometimes, the afflicted person becomes violent, exhibiting unusual strength.

Once in control, the *bebai* is believed to be capable of harming or even killing the individual. Usually, however, its power can be mitigated and overcome by a traditional healer (*balian*). Sometimes a spiritualist (*ahli kebatinan*) or a Balinese Hindu high priest (*pedanda*) is consulted. But since the illness is considered to be impure (that is, affliction by a lower form of spirit), help can be obtained relatively easily only from the *balian*. The high priest is usually reluctant to come into contact with this illness.

Puri Klungkung encompasses the residential quarters or compounds of the family of the former King of Klungkung. It consists of Puri Agung or the grand compound where the King and his principal wives (including the queen) live, Puri Agung Semara Negara where the younger wives reside, Puri Agung Saraswati where the still younger wives of the King have their quarters, and three other *puri* (i.e. Puri Anyar, Puri Kaleran, and Puri Semarabhawa) where the brothers and sisters of the King and their families have their residences. At the time of the fieldwork, conducted in June and July 1980, the *puri* accommodated a total of 59 families or households with a total of 296 members.

In the past, a *puri* girl would at adolescence (following her first menstruation) be taken out of school and confined to the *puri*. From then on, she would be taught to weave, prepare offerings, and behave properly in accordance with the intricate etiquette of the *puri*. For her, the outside world only appeared through the cracks and openings in the walls of the *puri*. In the past decade, however, this tradition has undergone a slow decay. A number of *puri* girls have continued their education as far as the university, and some have outside employment in government bureaucracy and in private enterprise. Nevertheless, almost all of the female members in the *puri* have been trained in the weaving of the Balinese traditional sarong (*kain songket*), the Balinese hat (*udeng*), and the shawl (*selendang*). And in general they are still unrebellious. They seem to be complacent and willing to accept the decisions of their parents and families.

In the *puri* as a whole, the older generation of men generally have more than one wife while most of the younger generation have monogamous marriages. All the wives in each polygamous marriage live together in the same compound, apparently quite harmoniously, each one putting the interest of the husband above her own. They appear to comply with the expectation that they should be completely obedient to their husband and, at the same time, be able, generally through weaving, dressmaking, or retailing, to support themselves and their children with minimum help from him. At any rate, none of the wives expressly expects to be completely supported by her husband. They accept support from him, of course, but without exception they recognize the need to be self-supporting. In effect, each wife with children is the head of her own household.

Suryani administered formal questionnaires and interviewed all of the members (296 persons) in the compound of the descendants of the former royal family of Klungkung. Twenty-seven individuals, mostly female from 16 families, had experienced *bebainan* at least once. All these individuals, who were between 10 and 76 years of age, were included in the sample. The control group consisted of 215 individuals, *puri* residents who were between 10 and 75 years of age.

When the first signs of an attack occurred, all family members who happened to be in the immediate vicinity of the victim rushed to his or her side to render assistance. As mentioned above, relatives always tried to physically restrain the sufferer who might be shrieking, writhing, crying, or running around aimlessly. At this stage, families had a lot of discussion about where to find a suitable healer to treat the victim. Close family members usually had no hesitation in making the diagnosis of *bebainan* as the symptoms were easily recognized and *bebainan* was regarded as a common illness. It was also considered a condition which must be treated by traditional healers (because of the sorcery involved) and which lay outside the power of modern doctors and paramedics to cure. In 93 per cent of cases recorded in the survey, the family immediately sought the help of a traditional healer. In 30 per cent of cases, the help of a Balinese Hindu high priest was sought in addition to, or as an alternative to, the healer's ministrations. In only 11 per cent of cases was the patient taken to a doctor or paramedic. In some of these cases, the close relative took the sufferer to a doctor (not accepting the diagnosis of *bebainan*) while other relatives sought the help of a healer as well. A mere 3.7 per cent of cases did not receive any treatment at all.

In most cases, the healer would be summoned to the house-yard of the victim. Several healers living close to the *puri* were the ones usually summoned to treat *bebainan* cases. On some occasions, close relatives would go to the house of a more distant healer for advice and medicines, but rarely was the victim taken outside the *puri* walls.

The healer usually arrived while an attack was in progress and typically the sufferer would cry out in fright at seeing the healer, and ask for mercy. In fact, it was the voice of the creature possessing the sufferer (*the bebai*) which was believed to be talking through its victim. The *bebai*'s utterances varied little in content and tone from one victim to another. Sometimes the healer interrogated the *bebai* who had possessed the victim, asking, for example: 'Where do you come from?', 'Why are you here?', and so on. After such a session, the healer prepared to exorcize the *bebai*. Some healers used holy water, or certain ritual objects. Another common technique was to squeeze the thumb of the victim, so that the *bebai* was forced to cry out in pain (through the victim), asking for mercy and promising not to bother the person again. Often the *bebai* would only leave the body of the victim after its demands for certain foods or offerings were satisfied. When food was asked for, it was not necessarily food which the victim would normally have found appetizing. After the victim had returned to normal, the healer gave the family a supply of holy water or oil, which they were advised to administer regularly so that there should be no recurring attacks. During and after the attack, several close relatives of the victim were occupied with carrying out the healer's instruction, e.g. preparing food or making the small inexpensive offerings usually required.

In cases where the healer was delayed in coming, the distressed relatives of the victim might seek help from other *puri* households in treating the attack. Close relatives sought out other residents who had experience in handling cases of *bebainan* and who might have reserves of holy water and other medicines on hand. Thus *bebainan* attacks provide opportunities for informal co-operation between *puri* households, a temporary breakdown of otherwise rigid behavioural codes. Some time after the attack, on a predetermined day, the afflicted person underwent a purification ceremony which was thought to have a calming effect on the sufferer. It was performed by a very high-ranking priest who had a special relationship with *puri* residents. The ceremony itself was small, brief, and inexpensive, and was performed at the priest's house. This ceremony provides an occasion for the former victim to leave the *puri* briefly.

Basically, the same procedures were followed for first and recurring attacks. Apart from the purification ceremony mentioned above, no special attention was bestowed on the *bebainan* sufferer when not experiencing an attack.

Analysis of the psychological and social pressures acting on these women suggested that *bebainan* attacks provided sufferers with an opportunity to release feelings of frustration and anger about conflicts engendered by their social environment which they had no means to resolve. The victim benefited psychologically from the disorder because it was one of the few ways in which women in particular might give vent to negative feelings without risk of widespread disapprobation or stigmatization. However, *bebainan* was not instrumental in altering access to resources within the restricted environment of the royal compound, nor did it empower the victim within this environment in any but the most transitory ways.

From the psychiatric standpoint, the most compelling characteristics of *bebainan* are its sudden occurrence and the temporary character of its impact. During its attack, the victim suffers a severe impairment of consciousness and sense of identity and loss of control over motor functions. But these symptoms disappear completely at the cessation of the attack. There is no amnesia for events during the attack. *Bebainan* cannot be regarded as a form of psychosis, even of the reactive or atypical type; it is neither an organic mental disorder, nor a form of neurosis. Instead *bebainan* can be considered a form of dissociation, specifically trance with possession, which is understandable only in the context of local Balinese culture. The disorder fits the definitions of trance and possession disorders in the newly published *ICD-10* (WHO, 1992).

It is highly significant that within a year after Suryani's study of this long-standing disorder, it ceased to occur in the palace population. Because of this, some families regarded Suryani as having magic powers. The authors regard the disappearance of the disorder under the circumstances as consistent with it being a community-wide culture-related dissociative disorder with possession. It is hypothesized that the families' relaxation of restrictions on adolescents took the pressure off them and decreased their resentments. Possibly this and related changes in the community, which reduced the stress-producing customs and the education which Suryani provided about the nature of the disorder, removed some of the mystery of the illness and were the primary factors responsible for its curious disappearance. It still occurs sporadically in the wider Balinese population.

Kasurupan: A Dissociative Disorder in Schoolchildren[7]

A clinical study of an outbreak of dissociative disorders (*kasurupan*) in 45 elementary schoolchildren (Suryani and Jensen, 1991) illustrates a mass or epidemic trance disorder and the need for Western-trained psychiatrists to develop an intimate and thorough knowledge of the Balinese culture as it affects behaviour, personality and mental disorders, and clinical strategies.

In January 1984, a number of schoolchildren in a mountainous area of central Bali began to experience spells characterized by sudden onset, fainting, unconsciousness, crying, visual hallucinations, anxiety, and occasionally automatic dancing (lasting minutes to hours) with complete awareness of events of the spell after recovery. The number of children afflicted (45 of the 215 schoolchildren), the frequency of the attacks (65 per cent had 6–15 episodes; one had 30; some had several per day), and the apparently contagious nature of the disorder, interfered severely with the functions of the schools and caused fear in the children and community. It was apparent that this problem touched the entire community, as well as the children experiencing the mental disorder. Treatment efforts by traditional healers and psychopharmacotherapy advised by psychiatrists were ineffective. Education and government officials from the region became concerned and involved.

The village heads and associated government officials invited Suryani to investigate the problem. She visited the village on several occasions and interviewed teachers, school officials, community members, and afflicted children, examined one child during an attack, and surveyed 19 victims by structured interview.

The spells consisted of three phases: prodromal symptoms, trance, and recovery. The prodromal phase was characterized by weakness (90 per cent), a feeling of emptiness in the head, piloerection on the neck, closing of the eyes and difficulty opening them, and intense fear of impending events. This phase lasted from 2 to 10 minutes.

The trance phase was characterized by hallucinations and dissociative phenomena. The experiences varied in details but had common elements. Many victims lost their hearing and the ability to hear voices around them. Most (70 per cent) saw a woman or a man, usually a big, 'horrible' woman with yellow or red-coloured matted hair, a red or black face, hairy arms, and long hair hanging down or fixed behind the head (45 per cent), sometimes appearing like a giant or Rangda, the witch in classical Balinese drama well known to all Balinese. Some saw a woman with light-shaded beautiful skin. Some reported that this woman took them for a walk in the forest (in front of the school) and spoke to them, but they could not speak back. In the forest, they cried from fear, saw little men and snakes with big bright eyes, and then were led back to school by the woman or man. A few experienced being taken to the forest along with another child from school to whom they were unable to speak. On one occasion when 17 girls had attacks simultaneously, two sixth-grade children suddenly sat up and told of being 'possessed' by the two women spirits who were sisters; the older one lived in a large stone, partially buried in the schoolyard, and the younger one lived in a stone hidden under a classroom of the school. The spirits asked for floral offerings to the supreme God and for a traditional Balinese gamelan orchestra so they could teach the children to dance. The teacher complied by turning on taped gamelan music. At the first note of the gamelan, all the children who were experiencing the attack suddenly arose and the two girls danced *legong*, a classical Balinese dance that most had probably seen performed in the village but had not before learned to do themselves. The other 15 children then performed *legong* spontaneously. When the music ended, all returned to sleep-like behaviour. The trance phase lasted about 40 minutes.

The recovery phase was characterized by sitting up, expressionless, confused and anxious with weakness of neck and body muscles (70 per cent). After a few minutes, most of the victims continued with their schoolwork as usual but a small number were fearful and went home.

A number of responses of the teachers and community were significant. Soon after the episode began, they recalled an episode two years before when two children suddenly lost consciousness (*pingsan*) at school, were taken home, and recovered after about six hours with several recurrences. They were treated by a traditional healer (*balian*), who said the cause was a buried small temple on the school grounds that offended the gods. At that time the community promised the *balian* they would build a new temple but had not done so because of a lack of funds. With the onset of this new outbreak of a similar disorder, the community quickly built the temple on the school grounds. This effort along with ceremonies and offerings to the gods was fruitless. The 'spirit' rock on school grounds was fenced off. Teachers became fearful and unable to teach effectively because of these interruptions. The school authorities transferred some victims to another school; however, this caused additional attacks in other children in that school and they were returned. The *balian* believed the attacks were caused by the gods who were angered by the villagers' mistakes. Non-afflicted children feared being attacked, and the news media expressed alarm.

Examination of a 13-year-old child during an attack revealed a pale face, flickering eyelids, and resistance to efforts to open her eyes. Pupillary reflexes and deep tendon reflexes were normal. Her extremities were cold, but her heart rate was normal. Fifteen minutes later, she was crying and breathing slowly (five respirations per minute). Eye movements resembling nystagmus were noted. After another fifteen minutes, she sat up, was unresponsive to questions, and had cold extremities. Fifteen minutes after this, she spoke slowly with an expressionless face. Forty minutes later, she returned to her normal behaviour and could recall her experience well.

Interviews with victims included questions about their relationships with parents, peers, and siblings, and about their life out of school. There were no reported changes at home except fear that the 'big woman' would follow them home. They typically reported a home life lacking communication with parents and with inadequate opportunities for play, because of the lack of immediate neighbours. Working or doing school homework were their chief activities. They did not report sleep problems but some felt fearful at night. At school, the pattern of play with peers went on as usual but fear of another attack persisted.

It was clear from these studies that the attacks represented a dissociation phenomenon or trance. The stressor for most victims in this study was anxiety among the children and teachers. A specific stressor for the children initially afflicted could not be identified. There was evidently a high degree of suggestibility involved as evidenced by the 'spread' of attacks to new contacts, including two adults.

Suryani observed that the temple built on the school ground was not properly oriented in its location according to the traditional Balinese Hindu religion. She became aware of the many visiting strangers (i.e. officials, news media, and curious outsiders) and their apparently disturbing influence on the village and its people who previously were relatively isolated from outsiders.

Various possible approaches to the problem were discussed. First, diagnosis was necessary. Arriving at a diagnostic term to be used in the management process with the community involved taking into account its suitability not only for individual 'patients' but for the community and even the country as a whole. It had to be acceptable to the culture if it was to be workable. For example, labelling the behaviour 'hysteria' would insult or anger the people and destroy rapport; using the term 'epidemic illness' would cause fear in the Balinese people; the diagnostic term 'dissociative disorder' would be incomprehensible and if used with the people would destroy confidence in the psychiatrists. This situation presented a dilemma to and generated conflict among the psychiatrists. The diagnostic term finally chosen was possession (*kasurupan*), a concept known to the Balinese, and understandable as well as acceptable to them. This term does not carry with it an implication of illness or stigma; rather, it is part of normal life in Bali.

Next, a treatment and intervention strategy had to be developed. There was no precedent for treatment of this kind of disorder in Bali. Pharmacotherapy was ruled out because prior experiences had shown it to be ineffective. Individual and group psychotherapy was considered but regarded as impractical in view of the urgency and extensiveness of the disorder. The epidemic nature of the problem suggested public health strategies. It was agreed that multiple aspects of the culture had to be taken into account and brought into harmony or balance with psychiatry. The final plan developed combined clinical and socio-cultural elements.

The main components of the plan were outlined to the community leaders, and to health, education, and religious officials at a meeting held in August 1984, one month after initiation of the study. The characteristics of the disorder were explained, the diagnostic label of possession (*kasurupan*) was used, and specific measures were advised:

1. The high priest (*pedanda*) was recommended as the primary healer. This decision was based on his traditional role in treatment of mental disturbances, his high status in religious matters, and the prior ineffectiveness of local *balian*. The villagers would regard the high priest's intervention as appropriate since the community believed the attacks were caused by supernatural forces (anger of the gods) and did not represent disease.

2. A new temple should be built to correct the error in orientation of the existing newly built temple on the school grounds. This rationale adhered to the concept of 'balance' of forces traditionally believed to cause mental disorder. A proper temple is regarded as the source of all community power.
3. Teachers would allay fears of the children by reading and teaching traditional stories from the Hindu epics, *Mahabharata* and *Ramayana*, which feature positive and benevolent spirits. These stories are consonant with Balinese Hindu belief.
4. The village should be closed to all outsiders including the investigators. This was intended to reduce confusion, stress, and fear engendered by outsiders.
5. Individual psychotherapy was offered if needed.

These suggestions were accepted and all were carried out immediately. The high priest directed the temple change and the ceremonies of purification. Teachers had more confidence and a fresh direction of teaching; village life returned to its usual pattern. Within one month after the initiation of the plan, all attacks ceased. At yearly follow-up visits during 1985–90, no further attacks were reported.

Spirit Possession in Other Cultures

In north-west Madagascar, two types of spirit possession have been described which manifest behaviours similar to those of both the *bebainan* and *kasurupan* types of possession in Bali (Sharp, 1990).

One type of spirit possession called *njarinintsy* is a 'sickness' occurring primarily in adolescent girls which sometimes causes violence. It may typically begin by a teacher asking a student to perform a task, perhaps an assignment at the board; instead of responding, the student suddenly starts to wail loudly, sob, scream, or yell obscenities and may stand up and run about the room. She may throw objects or swing her arms violently, and it may take four or five boys to catch her and hold her down. There have been mass outbreaks of this type of possession, which is thought to be contagious. Fifteen or twenty students, including sometimes a few boys, may become possessed at one time. It is regarded as a form of possession or as a sickness caused by a bad or evil spirit. Symptoms include shaking and chills, uncontrollable screaming and crying, loss of memory, and mental confusion. During possession, the individual does not recognize anyone and has amnesia with regard to the events afterwards. It is believed that if a healer is not obtained who can drive the spirits from the person's body, he or she may go mad or die. A study of outbreaks of the disorder among schoolchildren indicated that it was the outcome of culturally and socially alienated youth in a rapidly changing society.

Another type of spirit called *tromba* primarily possesses women, is troublesome, and makes demands on the traditional healers and others close to the individual. This altered state begins with an onslaught of chronic symptoms, including headaches, dizziness; soreness of the neck, back, or limbs; or persistent stomach pains. Whereas the possession by *njarinintsy* is regarded as a problem, possession by *tromba* is an important aspect of the cultural identity of the women, a marker of status, and a means to enhance her status locally. A woman who becomes a traditional healer for *tromba*, called a *tromba*-medium, is a powerful and respected healer in the community. Services and the techniques used by these healers (Sharp, 1990) resemble those of the traditional healers of Bali in many respects.

Demonic possession has been described as a 'frightening, negative experience of some uninvited, evil entities assuming complete control over one's body' (Goodman, 1988). Goodman described two types of possession: African and Eurasian. In the Eurasian type, the evil entities who have settled in torment their victims and attempt to kill them. The feelings are relieved by dislodging, expelling, i.e. exorcizing, the malevolent being (Goodman, 1988: 98).[8]

There are relatively few case reports of possession disorders in the West. Since possession occurs in some Western religious settings, it may be expected that possession would occur in non-religious settings as it does in Balinese and in other non-Western cultures. Only a few cases have been reported in Westerners and observed at first hand by a psychiatrist who is an expert in dissociative disorders and MPD (Allison, 1992). Five cases of possession were reported by a Jesuit priest (Martin, 1976), two cases by an anthropologist (Goodman, 1981, 1988). In the latter two cases, data and examinations could not rule out a number of other neurologic and psychiatric conditions. These included seizure disorder, bipolar affective disorder, mania, multiple personality disorder, and several other dissociative disorders. Jensen examined a patient in California in 1990 who seemed to be possessed by the Devil for a period of years and attributed his murder of an individual to the work of the possessed Devil. On psychiatric examination, it appeared that this man suffered from a psychotic delusion rather than a possession disorder. On the other hand, it can be expected that persons who have grown up in a foreign country where possession and possession disorders are characteristic are more likely to manifest possession disorder while living in a Western culture.

* * *

Dissociative disorder is a general term applicable to a number of mental disorders, including amnesia, fugue state, hysterical paralysis, deafness, blindness, and multiple personality disorder (MPD). *ICD-10* (WHO, 1992) differentiates trance and possession disorders from the others. Most types of dissociative disorders, except MPD, have been observed in the Balinese. A study of suicide attempters revealed that most non-psychotic patients were in a state of trance-possession during the attempt. These cases are classified as a type of trance-possession disorder and represent a heretofore unrecognized psychological process in suicide. Dissociation is a significant mechanism in suicide attempts of patients with MPD. Case-studies of *amok* indicate that trance is operative in an acute attack. An epidemic trance disorder (*kasurupan*) affecting schoolchildren and a trance-possession disorder (*bebainan*) which occurred in a palace population were studied and described. They revealed several cardinal aspects of the trance-possession state, including the factor of contagion, hallucinations, and wild, uncontrolled behaviour. The treatment of these two conditions involved traditional healing and a combination of traditional (religion-based) and Western psychiatric methods.

Delineation of trance-suicide has important implications for the management of suicide attempts in Westerners (see Chapter 9). The healing process used successfully with the children suffering from trance disorder is a model for treating similar disorders that occur in Balinese and other Eastern cultures, and in the West. The current operating split of body/mind in Western medicine compromises the treatment of many maladies of Westerners. To ignore the spiritual realm of life would further compromise healing. The Balinese cases of possession disorder bring into sharp focus the WHO definition of health: this would be more complete when it adds the factor of spiritual health to its current definition covering physical, psychological, and social health.

1. An Amytal interview is one conducted while the patient is in a sedated state brought on by the controlled, slow, intravenous injection of the fast-acting barbiturate, Amytal.

2. Wangaya is the only public psychiatric hospital in Bali, apart from the mental hospital at Bangli, Bali.

3. An exception to these beliefs was the ancient practice of the wives of royalty voluntarily throwing themselves and burning to death on the cremation pyres of their husbands (*masatia*).

4. An alternative term is 'culturally recognized syndrome', indicating that it may occur in cultures in which it has not yet been given the same degree of attention.

5. Single episodes of mass killing by individuals also occur in the West but are relatively rare compared with the usual types of violent acts.

6. This section on *bebainan* is reproduced from *The Balinese People: A Reinvestigation of Character* (Jensen and Suryani, 1992: 113–45).

7. This section on *kasurupan* is reproduced from *The Balinese People: A Reinvestigation of Character* (Jensen and Suryani, 1992: 163–7).

8. For a description of exorcism rituals used by Catholicism, see Martin (1976) and Goodman (1988: 120).

Chapter 8
Meditation, Meditation Healing, and Hypnotherapy

MEDITATION is an ASC (altered state of consciousness) that needs to be differentiated from trance and possession. The technique of meditation healing used in Bali may prove useful to Western practitioners. The phenomenon of possession during hypnotherapy of Balinese patients may contribute another dimension to Western hypnotherapy.

Meditation

Meditation has a long history of practice in both Eastern and Western cultures. It is an act or process of focusing one's thought to become aware or to engage in contemplation. Broadly, meditation is understood as a specific practice which achieves a number of different goals, including (1) self-development; (2) self-realization; (3) the act of experiencing oneself; and (4) the discovery of ultimate truth (Chaudhuri, 1974). In Bali, meditation is usually performed by persons who want to learn how to relate to God and by older persons who are more inclined towards the spiritual life. Balinese meditation has two objectives: (1) to become aware of and improve oneself in the natural world (e.g. increase one's ability to solve problems and diminish needs stemming from real life); and (2) to understand one's supernatural world (e.g. connect with the gods to get messages or a lecture from them). There is no mind–body dichotomy in Balinese philosophy such as there is in the West.

The various meditation techniques used for healing and promoting well-being have been described in the literature. Most of these consist of imaging or focusing on the distressed or diseased part of the body (DeBerry, 1992). It is believed that these techniques are effective in relieving pain, restoring health, possibly prolonging life in individuals with AIDS, promoting localized healing (Schwartz, 1983: 114), and ameliorating cancer (Meares, 1978). Meditation has been found to be helpful for patients with cancer in terms of improving sleep, relationships, attitudes towards death, and understanding the meaning and purpose of life (Magarey, 1988). There is experimental evidence that meditation is effective in reducing anxiety and depression (DeBerry, Davis, and Reinhard, 1989). Despite these applications of meditation to distress and illness, in a critical comparison between meditation and psychotherapy in terms of method and aims, Kokoszka (1990) stated that the aim of meditation is primarily self-development through a specific way of life and practices, whereas the aim of psychotherapy is to restore health.

All forms of meditation are characterized by an alteration of awareness of attention. There are two basic techniques of attention in meditation which produce ASC although both aim to bring the persons concerned to a better understanding of their mental function as they experience a change in the level of consciousness from their usual state. Both techniques are used in Bali. One is concentration with a single focus, using a visual object or an auditory stimulus, such as a mantra. This is analogous to using a camera zoom lens. The other technique is mindfulness, where the individual allows himself to be aware of a situation in general, such as mentally following the breath through the body. This is analogous to a wide-angle lens.

In concentration meditation, one's thinking and emotions tend to be subordinate; the focus of attention is limited to a repeated stimulus such as a word, a voice, a prayer, breath, or a visual object, and a passive attitude is maintained. Intrusive mental activities disturb concentration. If the meditator is disturbed, he must refocus his concentration on the stimulus. When meditation phenomena develop, his mood will change from relaxation to an emotional and cognitive state of ASC.

In mindfulness meditation (Delmonte, 1989; Kelly, 1955), the individual tries to observe his or her mind without ignoring thoughts, desires, and moods. Thoughts are allowed to flow in and out of the mind and the subject acts as if he is observing these non-judgmentally from outside himself. This is analogous to the hidden observer phenomenon of the hypnotic state.

In meditation, a number of psychological phenomena, which

occur in the normal non-ASC state, as well as in abnormal mental conditions, are encountered. These include hallucinations, delusions, depersonalization, and derealization (Castillo, 1990; Deikman, 1963; Kennedy, 1976).

Meditation is characterized by a number of neurophysiological changes, including lowered consumption of oxygen, decreased heart rate, slow rate of breathing, low blood pressure, and decreased serum levels of lactic acid, increased skin resistance, and changes in blood circulation. These changes are related to a decrease in sympathetic nervous system activity (see Kutz, Borysenko, and Benson, 1985). A large reduction in resting metabolism was recorded in Tibetan Buddhist monks in India during meditation (Benson et al., 1990). Experimental evidence has been found for reduced beta-adrenergic receptor sensitivity in subjects practising transcendental meditation which supports studies postulating that meditation is associated with reduced sympathetic adrenergic receptor sensitivity (Mills et al., 1990). Other evidence of the effects of meditation on the nervous system come from studies of Qi Gong meditation, which has been known for thousands of years in China and which is widely practised (Liu et al., 1990).This form of meditation causes an enhancement of brain stem auditory evoked response with a concomitant depression of cortical responses. These changes are hypothesized to be related to the healing and other health benefits of this type of meditation.

Findings of brain wave changes during meditation are not entirely consistent. Kutz, Borysenko, and Benson (1985) found a change in α and β rhythms of the EEG (electroencephalogram) during meditation. Triman et al. (1978) studied 69 meditation subjects who practised meditation for over 15 years and 69 non-meditation subjects in Surabaya, Java. The frequency of breathing and heart rate decreased in the meditators but was unchanged in the control subjects. The EEG of the meditation subjects showed a change in α rhythm, decreasing from 69.6 to 15.9 per cent, becoming more regular, and moving from the occipital–parietal towards the central area of the brain. β waves decreased (68.1 to 52.5 per cent) in the frontal–central areas. θ waves increased from 1.4 to 14.5 per cent. After a quiet period θ waves decreased from 1.4 to 1 per cent. The control subjects, who sat quietly concentrating without meditation, had increased α and β waves but in the same areas before and after the quiet period. θ waves were not increased. Respiratory rate and heart rate were significantly different between the meditators and the control subjects. Meditating Tibetan monks living in India showed a marked asymmetry in α and β activity between the hemispheres and increased β activity (Benson et al., 1990). In another study, EEGs of non-meditating subjects came into coherence or synchrony with those of meditators in the immediate area (Travis and Orme-Johnson, 1989).

It has been hypothesized that meditation has field effects that link individuals, i.e. the meditation affects non-meditators in the vicinity. In support of this, studies of population groups reported that meditation in a group of individuals decreased crime in the 99 per cent of the community who do not practise meditation (Dillbeck et al., 1989).

Meditation Healing and Possession

Suryani learned meditation from a schoolteacher when she was 14 years old. At this time she spontaneously became possessed and she knew of about 30 in several thousand in the meditation group who were also possessed and had visual hallucinations during possession. Several years after her experience of possession by a goddess, the healing component of meditation technique was revealed to her by God. For the past 25 years, she has been perfecting and improving this technique. She has used it with many patients and taught it to mental health workers, educators, medical students, psychiatry residents, and a senior citizens' group.

The technique uses a combination of both kinds of meditation. The patient must sit in a comfortable position of his choice. He is asked to relax all muscles and then focus on one point in front of him (about 1 metre) with sustained concentration. He is then asked to wait, while focused, until his eyelids feel heavy and when they do, to allow them to close. Next, he is asked to concentrate on his nose, to be aware of the sensations of breathing, and to try and feel the energy from outside (this refers to healing energy from God) pass into his body and out through his nose. If he has difficulty concentrating, he is asked to feel the energy move from the nose out through the feet, or from the nose out through the fontanelle, and finally out of the entire body, by which time all thoughts and feelings are focused only on the breathing without any change in the normal breathing pattern. When meditation occurs, breathing will decrease in volume, resulting in hypoventilation. The body will begin to feel lighter, and the person will experience a feeling of peace. In that frame of mind, he can speak silently 'in his heart' to himself according to his own beliefs, e.g. he may pray to God, saying that he wants to be healthy or that he wishes to overcome sickness. This is continued for a total of only 10–15 minutes. The purpose of this meditation is to increase one's psychic ability to understand oneself, the environment, and God. Meditation is recommended in the morning on awakening to prepare one for the day and in the evening before sleep for 'clearing' the mind of the day's conflicts or worries and burdens. It may be done at any time during the day when one wishes to resolve a problem. There are no dietary or other prohibitions. It can be performed irrespective of date, time, or place.

Suryani differentiates 'meditation healing' from hypnosis or self-hypnosis. She recognizes it as an ASC but one in which the individual mixes an outer power with his own inner power, and uses them in combination to effect the healing. The individual feels himself taking the power from the outside as he goes through the breathing exercise. By contrast, Suryani perceives the individual in hypnosis as utilizing imagination from within himself.

A state of relaxation without meditation is used for self-treatment of tiredness, sleeping problems, and also sickness. The individual sits down or lies down, relaxes all muscles, and empties his mind. The emphasis is on feeling the energy move from the feet, through the body, and out of the top of the head (fontanelle), and then feeling the energy from outside the body enter the fontanelle, go through the body, and out through the feet. This is continued until the feeling of fitness is attained. If there is pain or a problem in one area of the body, the breath is visualized and expressed as going out through that particular place, all the while focusing on that place. If this relaxation technique is used to treat a physical problem, concentration is focused on the site of the problem in the body until a feeling of relief is attained. If one feels sleepy, it is all right to sleep for a few minutes or for whatever amount of time is needed. Persons who have difficulty concentrating may be helped by another person in meditation: the individual can experience the power of helping and/or healing from this other meditator.

Following the 3-month period in Suryani's youth when possession experiences were frequent, she worked with people who came to her with problems, essentially as a *balian* works with clients, giving advice, using her psychic powers, and sometimes divining for a lost person or things. For example, her brother, who was repairing electrical equipment at a hotel, was unable to get the circuits to work. He asked her about it. She consulted God, who told her that they should make an offering at a certain place and after this was done, the electrical system began to work. She stopped practising as a *balian* when she became a medical doctor. Currently in her daily life and in her practice of medicine, she no longer talks about her *balian* powers because she does not want colleagues or patients to be confused about her role as a physician. A few close friends still come to her house to consult her about problems with their family; in such instances, she may ask God what the problem is and provide counsel in the style of a *balian*. However, in her case, she meditates only for a few minutes and the goddess uses her body directly; no special ritual is required for her to be possessed by the goddess. Most *balian* perform a ritual in order to enter into the possession state.

Suryani had an unusual experience of possession during meditation while visiting the high priest of Ubud, to whom she had gone to accompany a friend who wished to observe his technique. When Suryani asked the priest about her level of meditation, he made extensive enquiries about her experience, asking her where she had learned meditation in the beginning and so on. At the priest's request, Suryani proceeded to meditate using her own method. At that point she was suddenly overcome by a power which she felt emanated from him, a power which became so strong and highly energetic that she felt she could barely maintain her sitting position without falling over, collapsing, and possibly dying from it. In an effort to counteract this feeling, she breathed rapidly and deeply and clasped her hands together, pulling them strongly apart against resistance. The total amount of time she spent in meditation was about 10 minutes and she woke up in the usual manner. The priest commented that her level of meditation was higher than her friend's and told her not to relax her body in deep meditation. She and her friend noticed that the priest looked at her intently with open eyes. During the ensuing five days, she spontaneously experienced the high priest's appearance on each day in a number of different situations, including at her home, at work, in the car, and at a store. Each time he appeared, he spoke to her, apologizing for his comment and asking her to give him back his power. She declined and said that she did not want to give it back. Her reason for refusing was that she felt he might use the power to harm her in some way. After those five days, she no longer experienced the hallucinations. This was her first experience of a power entering her or possessing her during meditation.

In Western terms, the 'power' Suryani described during meditation can be interpreted as a possession phenomenon, but one that does not occur in a state of trance. During this meditation,

Suryani did not have any of the sensory changes or perceptual experiences that she usually observes when she enters into trance and which are typically associated with trance. The auditory and visual hallucinations of the high priest on the days following her meditation experience occurred in her usual state of consciousness, not in a trance state. This is an example of the phenomena frequently seen in Balinese: auditory and visual hallucinations during a normal, presumably non-altered state of consciousness.

Suryani's possession abilities and traditional healer techniques have affected the way she practises psychiatry. For example, after a relatively brief contact with a patient, Suryani often tells him/her what she believes the problems are and how to solve the problem with the family, based on intuition and the information she gets from the god who possessed her. She does not tell the patient where she gets her ideas from but simply presents them as part of her psychotherapeutic work, as she explains, advises, and gives support. Balinese patients find this technique familiar and reassuring because they experience something similar with the *balian*, to whom they generally go for all sorts of problems. Functionally, this technique resembles one used by Western practitioners in the sense that Western psychotherapists often resort to intuition in their work with patients.

Suryani feels that by using her psychic abilities it is possible to determine if her patients have black magic; it is not necessary for her to use any specific ritual or diagnostic techniques, as most traditional healers do. If she determines that her patients have been affected by black magic, she will sometimes advise them to meditate and may advise them to attend religious ceremonies and make offerings as well. She does not tell these patients that this is her working diagnosis because she feels it may make them upset and confused about her role as a physician. A number of traditional healers who refer patients to her tell the clients that Suryani has the skills of both a traditional healer and a psychiatrist.

A Balinese explanation of Suryani's possession states and its consequences for her and her patients is straightforward. There is no mystery about possession and it involves supernatural power. Some experience it and some do not. Western accounts of it and explanations in the literature, however, are different from Suryani's experience. For example, Connor (1984) described the case of a man who had bizarre and psychotic behaviour for some months and subsequently became a *balian*, an episode which she called divine madness (see Chapter 9). Belo (1960) described a 2½-month-long illness of a man who was subsequently inducted by a priest to become a *balian*. Suryani has known only one *balian* who began his career without such a severe and relatively prolonged illness.

It is a truism about Balinese culture that there are many variations in the cultural patterns. Villages may differ dramatically in their ceremonies. Examples presented in this book are those at Timbrah and Kesiman (Chapter 4). The gods for which ceremonies are held may differ as may the days on which special ceremonies are held. It is apparent that the patterns of trance-possession are also different to some extent. Probably no two *balian* have the same style of practice, although their beliefs may be basically the same. Each *balian* develops his/her own style; the same can be said about Western physicians and psychotherapists.

Hypnotherapy with Possession

Suryani is the only practitioner of hypnotherapy in Bali. She has found the Balinese to be easily hypnotizable using a technique with relatively little verbalization in contrast to many Western induction techniques. She has used it primarily for the treatment of patients with chronic disorders, including anxiety, panic disorder, depression, and somatoform disorders. For patients with acute disorders, she generally utilizes ordinary psychotherapy.

About 25 per cent of Suryani's patients become possessed during hypnosis. Possession in hypnotherapy has not been described in the literature. The following case is an example.

A 25-year-old Javanese woman, married with two small children and living in Bali, had suffered tics or contractions of the facial muscles, fluttering of the eyelids, and severe spasms of the jaw muscles. She was worried that she might have a brain tumour, although Western-trained Balinese physicians, including a neurologist who had carefully examined her, reassured her that this was not the case. She also had episodes of collapsing on the floor (about three times a day at home), chronic headaches, and a sleeping problem. All these symptoms, present over a 4-year period, had been treated by many different traditional healers and a number of Western-trained physicians. One of the latter referred the patient to Suryani.

A programme of psychotherapy at weekly visits was instituted and carried out over a 3-month period. It was revealed that several of her problems were related to her lack of understanding of Balinese culture:

1. She felt she was in a disadvantageous and unfair position at

home because her mother-in-law, who visited her every other week, complained to her whenever her husband refused to give her the money she requested for ceremonies. The mother-in-law claimed that she and her husband cared more about themselves than about his parents. (In Balinese culture, a son is responsible for his parents.) She did not like her mother-in-law and her behaviour but was unable to express her feelings, and she could not tell her mother-in-law that she did not want to see her.

2. Her husband seldom talked to her about any of her problems and he was unwilling to discuss them.
3. She felt disappointed that her husband was more attentive to his parents than to her. She also felt bored. She merely stayed at home, did not work, and had few personal relationships outside her home. Over time, she took progressively less responsibility for the care of her children and husband.

Psychotherapy included couple therapy and prescription of a minor tranquilizer for the facial tic, anxiety, and sleep problem. As a result of these treatments, she started to show improvements. She began to sleep better; she no longer had her episodes of collapsing; she stopped worrying about the possibility of a brain tumour; she developed better relationships with her mother-in-law and her husband; her headaches disappeared; she felt she could take better care of her children; and her mood improved. However, the disfiguring rigid facial muscle spasms continued.

At this point in therapy, Suryani instituted hypnotherapy. The patient readily went into hypnosis and on the first session became possessed by her dead mother's soul. It was then revealed for the first time that the patient was conflictual and guilty about her change of religion from Islam, which she had grown up with in Java, to Hinduism, her husband's religion. Her dead mother's soul told her that she and her husband should go to Java to undergo a ceremony which would absolve her from guilt and assured her and her husband, who was present, that this would not be an elaborate or expensive ceremony. Under hypnosis and immediately following the hypnosis, Suryani discussed this with her patient and her husband, and it was agreed that she would travel to Java for this ceremony.

During the second hypnotherapy session, the patient was possessed by her husband's dead grandfather's soul, who spoke to her about her illness and told her that she should make offerings to God and take holy water in the husband's family temple so that she would gain power from it to help herself. Suryani discussed this recommendation with her and her husband during hypnosis, and they agreed to carry it out.

During the third hypnotherapy session, the patient was possessed by the soul of a neighbour, a woman who she believed was trying to take her husband away from her. The soul said that she did not want to continue to love her husband and asked for help to leave the patient's body. Suryani asked the soul why she had come and why she loved the patient's husband, and advised the soul not to disturb the patient further. The patient made spontaneous hand gestures as if to remove the soul from her body. She awakened from the hypnotherapy session in a relaxed and pleasant mood. By the end of this session, her facial muscle spasms had completely disappeared and they did not subsequently recur.

In this case a number of Western techniques were combined: psychotherapy, pharmacotherapy, and hypnotherapy. However, the psychotherapy and hypnotherapy incorporated cultural concepts of illness: religious healing ceremonies were incorporated as adjuncts.

Yoga in Bali

There are several types of yoga practised in the East and West. A form currently taught in Denpasar utilizes some techniques, similar to those of meditation, which may lead to an ASC. This form of yoga purports that learning how to concentrate by breathing correctly is one of the most important parts of yoga practice. It teaches diaphragmatic breathing, with each breath 'absorbing the universal energy', called prana in India, which is regarded as the origin of all forces. By breathing correctly, exponents of this type of yoga believe that they are maximizing the amount of vital energy absorbed and feel filled with inner power. They practise slow, gradual movements which are conceived as accumulating energy in the person rather than expending it, as in vigorous exercise. They believe that these exercises (*asana*) affect the internal organs, especially the endocrine glands. They relate the endocrine glands to the *chakra* or subtle energy centres located along the spine. The physical poses taken during yoga, such as sitting with the head down, are believed to affect the pineal gland and develop memory power and higher consciousness. A deep relaxation pose relaxes muscles and reduces blood pressure.

* * *

Meditation is an ASC employed widely in the East and West to promote healing, relieve pain, restore health, and combat disease. However, the basic aim of meditation is to enhance self-development, self-realization, and self-experience. In Bali, the general aims of meditation are to become aware of oneself in the natural world and to understand the supernatural world. Objectives of meditation differ from those of psychotherapy. The Balinese use two basic techniques: (1) concentration of awareness on a specific stimulus; and (2) mindfulness of one's entire situation. Meditation is associated with numerous changes in psychobiology and neurophysiology.

Meditation healing is a specific technique developed and taught by Suryani. This technique includes awareness of breathing, appropriation of spiritual energy, and conscious focus on aspects of life in which changes are desired. A similar breathing and concentration technique is used for relaxation only and also for treatment of troubles or illness. Meditation healing is not the same as hypnosis. Suryani has utilized meditation, psychic abilities, and possession abilities in psychiatric practice.

Hypnotherapy is particularly effective for the Balinese because they find it difficult to verbalize feelings, emotional states, and problems. Balinese patients are easily hypnotized and about 25 per cent experience possession under hypnosis. This possession state can be utilized in psychotherapy.

Some of the techniques of yoga and exercises practised in Bali are similar to those of meditation (i.e. relaxation and breathing) and may result in an ASC. They are useful for attaining feelings of peace and well-being.

Meditation and yoga are integral treatment modalities in some mind/body healing clinics in American medical centres, especially in cardiac disease reversal programmes. Meditation has great potential as an adjunct to modern medicine. The phenomenon of possession with hypnotherapy is little recognized in the West but an awareness of it may expand the healing techniques of Western hypnotherapy.

Chapter 9
Conclusions and Implications of Trance and Possession for Western Concepts of Multiple Personality, Possession Disorder, Suicide, and Mental Health

THE foregoing chapters presented descriptive data on several ASC in the Balinese, including meditation, trance, and trance-possession, (*kalinggihan, kasurupan*), both normal and abnormal. They also delineated the psychosocial characteristics of these states and drew relationships to Western psychological concepts. These analyses will facilitate the recognition of similar normal and abnormal states involving trance and possession in the West. This final chapter draws generalizations about the trance-possession state,[1] conceptualizes two continua of dissociation phenomena, advances a theory of possession, and presents diagnostic criteria for possession. Based on this information, guidelines are presented for differentiating possession from psychiatric symptoms and the newly recognized condition called possession disorder is discussed. A primary objective of this book is fulfilled by comparing Balinese possession with the predominantly Western disorder, MPD. This leads to insights into the psychobiological mechanisms of MPD and carries implications for therapy. Finally, diagnosis and therapy for suicidal ideation and attempts are viewed with ASC in mind.

Trance and trance-possession are different states (Langness, 1976). Trance can occur alone or in association with possession (Bourguignon, 1976). However, Bourguignon has added a classification of possession without trance. In this regard, the authors have seen patients in Bali and America who claimed to be persistently possessed, who were not in trance, who showed no evidence of

ASC upon careful psychiatric evaluation, and also proved to be delusional and psychotic. The only documented instance of possession without trance in Bali is that of Suryani's personal experience. Although MPD patients appear to be possessed without trance, MPD can be regarded as a self-hypnotic state (Bliss, 1986) or as trance-possession as noted in analyses below.

Characteristics of Trance-possession

The most salient characteristic of trance-possession in the Balinese is the meaning it has for the culture. It is always linked to the Balinese Hindu religion and the supernatural is paramount in the forms it takes. Possession has also been noted to be connected with religion in the many cultures studied. Almost exclusively, all trance-possession states known to the Balinese are associated with positive possession by gods, spirits, or souls. The exceptions in Bali are the trance-possession states of mental disorders, such as *amok* and trance-suicide. The Balinese do not have a specific word for trance. The words they use to designate trance-possession phenomena literally mean 'coming down' (of the gods or spirits). This fact emphasizes the cardinal role played by cultural beliefs in trance-possession in Bali.

Balinese society has its own, and in many respects unique, repertoire of beliefs, values, and customs. Many of these are related to the Hindu religion but some are specifically Balinese. It is the particular religious customs and beliefs of the society which give trance-possession its characteristic patterns or forms in Bali.

However, in spite of the cultural patterning of the trance-possession state in the Balinese, most trancers experience the core 'symptoms' of dissociative disorders in the West: amnesia, depersonalization,[2] derealization,[3] and identity alteration (Cardeña, 1989; Saxena and Prasad, 1989; Steinberg, 1991b). Amnesia is variable, with some trance-mediums professing complete amnesia and others none at all. Most persons unconscious in trance (in ceremonies) have only partial recall. It is clear that amnesia is not a necessary requirement for possession (Noll, 1989).

Among the various types of behaviours observed in possession states, there are probably some aspects which are common to most cultures. One is the pattern of falling down unconscious, and another is shaking and crying out as if in a convulsive seizure. The latter behaviour is easily distinguished from a generalized epileptic (*grand mal*) seizure. It does resemble it in terms of the unconscious state, the arched posture with head falling back, and the occasional trembling of hands and legs, but the writhing body movements, facial expressions, and vocalizations are unlike a true epileptic seizure of any type. In addition, *grand mal* epileptic seizures are less variable in form than unconscious trance-possession (behaviour) and epileptic seizures may include bladder or bowel incontinence and salivation with foaming at the mouth. On the other hand, hysterical seizures, currently called conversion disorders or hysterical neuroses (APA, 1987), a dissociative phenomenon, may closely resemble epileptic seizures.

The quality of involuntariness is also present in the Balinese during trance-possession states. Spiegel, Hunt, and Dondershine (1988) have identified involuntariness as a quality of experience common to dissociation, hypnosis, and trance. Writing about PTSD, they stated, 'The kinds of events that mobilize dissociation as a defense also seem to be those in which the patient's volition is physically overridden.' Whether it is consciously desired, as in the case of dancers, ceremonial participants, and traditional healers, or unexpectedly experienced, as has occurred occasionally, it is regarded as being caused by forces other than one's own will, i.e. God, the gods, spirits, or some such power.

The content and form of thought of the Balinese in trance-possession sometimes resembles that of Westerners in hypnosis. For example, they may speak clearly and coherently and/or may reveal cognitive material that is best understood as coming out of their unconscious mind.[4] A related pattern of thinking in the trance state has been called trance logic (Orne, 1959) or tolerance of incongruity. Orne (1959) believed that trance-logic is the 'essence' of hypnosis. He referred to it as 'the ability of the S [subject] to mix freely his perceptions derived from reality with those that stem from his imagination and are perceived as hallucinations. These perceptions are fused in a manner that ignores everyday logic.' Trance-logic is just one aspect of deep hypnosis. E. L. Bliss (personal communication) regards realistic fantasy as the predominant essence of hypnosis.

Many Westerners are reluctant to be hypnotized because they fear that they will give up conscious control of themselves, particularly to the hypnotist. The sense of being in control of one's self is prominent and highly valued in Western personality and thought. This trait is not characteristic of the Balinese, whose lives have in the main been controlled by their families, their ancestors, and the supernatural. The normal Balinese expecting or experiencing possession gladly and completely gives up control of himself.

The basic psychobiological processes of trance may well be universal for mankind, regardless of culture. This is in keeping with the theoretical understanding of trance as a form of hypnosis involving dissociation, the ubiquitous normal psychological activity of the mind by which it separates or splits off one kind or aspect of thinking, behaviour, or affect from a situation and from one's usual pattern of conscious behaviour and thinking.

Possibly other pan-cultural or universal characteristics of trance-possession are psychic or parapsychological, such as the possession of clairvoyance, ESP, the ability to divine, predict, or know aspects of a person's life and problems without having heard of them. All these phenomena are commonly observed in the various forms in which trance and trance-possession occur in the Balinese, especially in traditional healers.

It is clear from interviews and observations that most possessed trancers experience the 'power' of the gods, and this power takes over the mind and the body, resulting in changes in sensory perceptions and motor functions which are generally out of keeping with the individual's normal and usual behaviour. This switch into the possession state generally occurs instantaneously or in a matter of seconds, and is often dramatic. (An instantaneous shift into hypnosis may also occur in excellent hypnotic subjects.) It is a step beyond hypnosis or trance without possession. Possibly it occurs only in states of deep trance.[5]

It is perhaps striking that the involved spirits in possession of the Balinese are always positive and welcome spirits, except in the case of dissociative disorders such as *bebainan* (see Chapter 7). Although the dancers donning the Rangda mask are possessed by Rangda who represents evil in the Calonarang drama, Rangda is nevertheless highly valued by society. The authors looked for evidence of evil spirit possession, particularly by *buta-kala*, the evil spirits known to all Balinese, but could not find any. Annual ceremonies in the village of Jimbaran in South Bali involve these two bad spirits but they do not possess the trancers: rather it is the gods of the *buta-kala* spirits that possess them.

In contrast to the ritual possession in Bali which involves positive entities, most of the possession states described in non-healer individuals in many cultures throughout the world involve malignant spirits except in religious groups such as the Shakers (Henney, 1973). Malignant spirit possession also occurs in many cults in Africa; for example, Lewis (1971: 75, 82) has noted the possession of Somalian women by malignant spirits which cause a range of illnesses and bodily symptoms, such as 'hysteria or light depression to actual organic disorders'. Similarly, women in China and Ceylon are frequently beset by demons which cause sickness (Lewis, 1971: 84–5). These differences between Bali and other cultures point up the factor of cultural determination in the forms possession takes.

Trance-possession in Bali is not only common, but desired, and it serves a number of diverse functions useful to society. In cultures where it has been studied, possession is usually associated with religion or with healing by the shaman or 'medicine man,' which may be considered a religious function. The social role, meaning, and value of possession are significant factors in its occurrence world-wide. In Bali, the traditional healers, especially the trance-mediums, use trance with possession very effectively in their religion-based therapeutic techniques. Trance-possession in Balinese dance generally has a religious function, as in the ceremonies which involve Rangda (see Chapter 4). Sometimes trance-possession takes on a public health function, as in the little girl trance-possession dance which is traditionally believed to protect the village from epidemics, pestilence, and illnesses caused by evil spirits. Dances involving trance-possession include the 'Barong' (kris dance) and the 'Calonarang', which, in addition to being presented for entertainment, are sometimes performed to honour the gods in religious ceremonies such as those in Kesiman (see Chapter 4). The trance-possession of musicians (see Chapter 6) and ceremonial participants serves a mental health function (see Chapter 4).

In sharp contrast, possession states in Western societies are relatively rare. They occur as isolated events, and have never been associated with any particularly useful social function, except in the case of some channellers (Hastings, 1991) and relatively small religious cults or groups such as the Holy Rollers, Jumpers (Linton, 1956), and Shakers who perceive that the Holy Ghost or Spirit enters them and shakes them from within (Henney, 1973).[6] Speaking in tongues, or glossolalia, occurs in religious contexts world-wide and conforms to the pattern of possession in that the practitioners report that the Holy Spirit, or the spirit of an ancestor or a deity, enters their bodies, 'possesses' them, and uses their tongues to utter messages. Interestingly, their utterances are not related to their mother tongues: Americans, Japanese, and Maya Indians all exhibit the same patterns of speech (Goodman, 1972). When possession occurs in individual Westerners, especially outside of a religious context, it is almost always unwanted, relatively long-lasting, and usually regarded as pathological. Some authorities of the Catholic Church and other denominations recognize possession (disorder) and still utilize lengthy ritual exorcistic techniques to terminate states which may be prolonged and which they regard as possession by undesirable demons or the Devil.

Most possession states in Bali do not present any problems to the individuals or society because they are always rather easily and reliably if not spontaneously controlled or terminated by public ritual behaviour. The authors know of no instances in which trance-possession in the Balinese persisted for prolonged periods; it usually lasts no more than several hours with a maximum of 20 hours. This is also true of possession in other cultures where it is common.

There are no clear data on the sex distribution of trance or trance with possession in societies world-wide. Bourguignon (1976) gained the impression from the literature that possession-trance is more widespread among women while trance without possession is more likely to occur among men. In Bali, contrary to Bourguignon's observation, the persons in trance-possession in the communal ceremonies are predominantly men. A large percentage of trance-mediums who utilize trance and trance-possession are women (see Chapter 3). Therefore, it appears that the sex distribution of trance and trance-possession in Bali is governed more by social considerations (i.e. healing or religious ceremonies) than by the form the trance takes (i.e. with or without possession).

Pathology is often mentioned by authors discussing trance and possession. A number of scholars consider these phenomena abnormal while others consider one or the other normal within a given culture. In Bali, the matter of the normality of these altered states is based upon society's beliefs and upon Western-derived psychiatric definitions of normal and abnormal. Trance-possession can represent an abnormal condition as illustrated by an epidemic in schoolchildren (see Chapter 7), or it can be, and usually is, entirely normal, culturally appropriate, and institutionalized as exemplified by the trance-mediums and the communal trance ceremonies. Whether trance-possession is deemed normal or abnormal in Bali is related to the social context and to whether or not it is a problem for the individual or the community. It does not depend specifically on the state of trance-possession *per se*. Trance and trance-possession are normal capacities of the brain/mind, probably in part genetically based.

The thoughts and behaviours by persons in the trance-possession state may reflect those from normal consciousness or the unconscious mind.[7] Examples of the former are the coherent and logical verbalizations of some trance-medium *balian* while examples of the latter include automatic dancing of the schoolchildren in trance-possession (see Chapter 7) and the particular hallucinations of the little girl trance-possession dancers (see Chapter 5). Just as the data presented on trance-medium *balian* demonstrate conscious and unconscious mental processes, the material expressed by MPD alternative personalities indicates both processes at work. Thus, the two different types of expression are possible in dissociative states.

The Dissociation Continua

Because the psychological process of dissociation[8] is manifest in many different conditions, both normal (i.e. everyday behaviour and thinking, meditation, hypnosis, and possession) and abnormal (i.e. dissociative disorders or hysterical neuroses, PTSD [Spiegel, Hunt, and Dondershine, 1988], and MPD), it would be useful to clarify the concept by reconciling all conditions as manifestations of a single basic process.

Bernstein and Putnam (1986) and Putnam (1991) reviewed the historical development of the concept of a dissociative continuum and traced it back to the work of nineteenth-century clinicians, including Pierre Janet, Morton Prince, and William James. For example, M. Prince (1909:123) characterized dissociation as a general principle governing normal psychology but abnormal when in an extreme form. More recently, a number of others (Ludwig, 1983; Orne, Dinges, and Orne, 1984; Shor, Orne, and O'Connell, 1962; H. Spiegel, 1963; Tellegen and Atkinson, 1974) conceptualized dissociative disorders as forming a spectrum of increasing psychopathology.

Given similar basic mechanisms of normal and abnormal dissociative conditions, two parallel continua are proposed. Manifestations of normal dissociative phenomena may be conceptualized on one continuum, ranging from everyday normal dissociation at one end, such as fantasy and separation of one's ongoing perceptions from one's environment, to possession at the other end, with meditation and trance in between (Figure 9.1). Each of the conditions on this continuum has a spectrum: e.g. light to deep trance with amnesia or light to deep hypnosis (Brown and Fromm, 1986: 46–7). Those normal states of trance and hypnosis may be regarded as representing varying degrees, depths, or intensities of the dissociation, or self-hypnotic[9] phenomena, to use Bliss's term. Similarly,

FIGURE 9.1
Parallel Continua of Dissociative Phenomena[1]

Normal Dissociation		Meditation		Trance (light to deep)	Trance-possession
Depersonalization Disorder	PSTD	Other Dissociative Disorders[2]	Fugue	Possession Disorder[3]	MPD

[1] Normal states above the line and abnormal conditions below.

[2] *DSM-III-R* (APA, 1987: 277) includes the following under other dissociative disorders (Dissociative Disorders Not Otherwise Specified): fugue without assumption of a new identity; more than one personality but these never assume complete executive control; and dissociation associated with prolonged and intense coercive persuasion, e.g. brainwashing.

[3] Possession disorder is newly included in *ICD-10* and is proposed for *DSM-IV,* to be published in 1993.

dysfunctional, symptomatic, or abnormal dissociative conditions can be placed on a continuum in terms of severity (mild to maximum or severe), with depersonalization disorder at one end and MPD at the other. There is consensus that MPD is the most severe of the dissociative disorders (Putnam, 1985; D. Spiegel, 1984). These disorders also have their own spectra, e.g. transient, brief episodes of depersonalization to quantitatively and qualitatively different, recurrent, and prolonged episodes (M. Steinberg, personal communication).

Writing about the relationship between hypnotizability and dissociation, Frankel (1990) pointed out that there is a lack of clarity on dissociation and questioned equating measures of hypnotizability with dissociative capacity. He (1990: 828) also questioned the perspective that dissociation lies along a continuum: 'Dramatic amnesia and clear-cut changes in or discontinuity of consciousness, control, or identity make compelling arguments for the presence of both the hypnotic state and dissociation. It is considerably less clear that other, milder experiences with some resemblance to the core event are qualitatively similar.' Suggesting that the numerous implications of dissociation could be a detriment to the concept and might eventually render it useless, Frankel (1990: 825–6) noted that 'common' hypnosis is different qualitatively from the 'somnambulistic trance that yields a post-hypnotic amnesia'. He regarded the two dimensions as related but distinct and stated that it may be an oversimplification to 'regard all hypnotic behaviour and experience as evidence of trance'. Such comments emphasize the lack of precise operational definitions of a variety of related terms.

In the proposal presented here of continua for both normal and abnormal dissociative phenomena, dissociation is regarded as the basic psychological mechanism. It is recognized that in the Balinese, the differences between mild and maximum dissociation are not only quantitative differences but also qualitative. The characteristics of possession suggest that there is a qualitative difference between it and trance, analogous to the difference that Frankel (1990) has observed between light hypnosis and trance with amnesia. However, in view of the awareness that dissociation is multifaceted, such differences do not necessarily vitiate the application of the general concept of dissociation to all these conditions. The qualitative difference between trance and possession parallels that between low levels of anxiety and panic or fear. Although the latter two states are phenomenologically different, similar elements occur in both and they are linked by a common, basic, psychobiological, or neurophysiological process (Barlow, 1988: 206). The variety of behaviours, symptoms, or clinical manifestations of a single psychobiological process need not detract from its conceptual and heuristic value. Psychology, psychiatry, and cultural anthropology are replete with illustrations of this principle. Such unifying concepts are extremely useful clinically and are particularly desirable when they are scientifically researchable, as is the case with dissociation and the forms in which it is manifest, especially hypnosis/trance and trance-possession.

While both the normal and abnormal manifestations of dissociation take a variety of forms, the psychobiological mechanism in all is postulated as a related process and more importantly, the process serves the same psychological function: namely, a split or switch out of a conscious state into a state of thinking, behaviour, and feeling that is quite different, more comfortable or enjoyable, and/or protective. The switch into dissociation wards off conflict, anxiety, or terror and/or provides an outlet for behaviour or emotions that are not acceptable to or permitted in the usual state of consciousness.[10]

Professional Recognition of Possession

It is astonishing that Western psychiatry and psychology have not recognized, defined, or given a name to the psychobiological phenomenon of possession since it consists of objective and subjective behaviour that is describable, relatively consistent in manifestations, and known to the laity and public at large for millenniums. One hundred years ago, William James wrote (in Oesterreich, 1974): 'The refusal of modern enlightenment to treat "possession" as a hypothesis to be spoken of as even possible, in spite of the massive human tradition based on concrete experience in its favor, has always seemed to me a curious example of the power of fashion in things scientific.' Only since 1992 has psychiatry considered a category of possession disorder (WHO, 1992). That possession phenomena has not become a subject of study by modern psychiatry and psychology is all the more puzzling when one considers that for nearly a century Western psychiatry has professionally recognized the phenomenon of depersonalization,[11] a behavioural state or symptom that in some respects resembles possession in types of behavioural and emotional manifestations (Levy and Wachtel, 1978; Mayer-Gross, 1935), is no less mysterious in origin (Steinberg, 1991a, 1991b), and appears similar to ASC. Perhaps the reasons for this blind spot of Western science relate to a widespread perception that possession lies in the realm of metaphysics, magic, occultism, religion, and 'unscientific' thought, areas from which Western psychiatry and psychology have endeavoured to separate themselves.[12] The great psychoanalyst, Carl Jung, who maintained an interest in the occult throughout his lifetime, wrote as follows in 1931 with regard to religion and parapsychology: 'The European of yesterday will feel a slight shudder run down his spine when he gazes more deeply into these delvings. Not only does he consider the subject of this so-called research obscure and shuddersome, but even the methods employed seem to him a shocking misuse of man's finest intellectual attainments.' (Campbell, 1975: 468–9.) An unfortunate consequence of the professional avoidance is the failure of mental health professionals to recognize possession in most cases. It is unfortunate when possession disorder is wrongly diagnosed or, worse, treated inappropriately as a psychosis, with antipsychotic medication. There is no question that Western psychiatry and psychology need to recognize the possession state, identify its characteristics, and study its clinical forms. It is time that they accord professional recognition to possession and catch up with the growing public awareness of the condition, especially as it occurs in religious groups, trance-mediumship, shamanism, channelling, and mental disorders.

Possession is an appropriate term for use in Western psychiatry because it is the word that best denotes a natural, culturally diverse psychobiological process associated with trance, as well as with certain symptomatic conditions in the West. On the other hand, possession is considered a lay term and until recently was not found in the professional lexicon. The term 'dissociation' is correct but non-specific.

Perhaps an alternative term should be used to denote the phenomenon of possession. The authors suggest, as a possibility, the term 'intracorporal influence' which conveys the meaning of an identified entity, force, or alternative personality, perceived by the individual as coming from outside the self, or an entity aside from the self or usual personality (perceived as coming from within the self), operating and exerting influence within the body/mind of the individual. This idea of entities is not incompatible with the psychological concept of dissociation.

Possession Disorders: Balinese and Western

Possession disorders have been known for centuries and have been described in several cultures, particularly non-Western ones (Jensen and Suryani, 1992; Metraux, 1959; Suryani, 1984; Suryani and Jensen, 1991; Yap, 1960). They were the focus of interest 300 years ago in connection with the fits of New Englanders who were subject to the witch trials at Salem, Massachusetts (Hansen, 1969: 36–8). One case—that of Anne Cole in 1662 (Hansen, 1969)—was described in some detail. It was characterized by fits of violent bodily movements and voices coming from her that were clearly not her own and that seemed to be plotting to further harm her. She had amnesia with regard to these episodes but confessed 'that the Devil had frequent use of her body with much seeming but indeed horrible, hellish delight to her' (Hansen, 1969: 37). After the hanging of the woman accused of witchcraft, her fits ceased and did not return for at least 20 years. Crabtree (1985) reviewed several reports of possession in Westerners who did not desire or consent to be possessed, dating from the 1860s up to the present. Some of these were exorcised[13] by religious figures and were reportedly cured.

Since possession disorder is to be included in the latest revision of *ICD*, *ICD-10* (WHO, 1992),[14] as well as in a separate entry under dissociative disorders in *DSM-IV*,[15] it is important for mental health professions to master the clinical presentation of the disorder. As the new diagnostic category of possession disorder gains recognition among the professions and many more cases are identified and reported, it will be possible to develop more comprehensive descriptions of the disorder's clinical presentation in the West.

The possession disorders in Bali, which predominantly involve evil spirits, are of two main types. One type is well-recognized and includes *bebainan*, described in the members of the royal household, and *kasurupan*, described in the schoolchildren (see Chapter 7). These are of sudden onset and termination; they tend to be of relatively brief duration (less than 5 hours) and involve a complete takeover of the individual, along with aberrant, seizure-like, sometimes violent behaviour apparent to all during the acute attack. A second type is the possession disorder that becomes evident in seizure-like behaviour only during treatment sessions by *balian* which are declared to be responsible for a variety of persistent somatic symptoms, some of relatively long duration (up to four years), during which time the possession is not evident. The same long duration of symptoms is true of Suryani's case of possession revealed during hypnotherapy (see Chapter 8). In such cases, the patient complains of possession by an evil spirit, the soul of a relative, or some other person during treatment but is unaware of this possession prior to treatment. Possession is revealed only in hypnosis induced by the therapist. The first type of possession disorder is called overt, while the second is called covert or obscured.

As in Bali, possession disorder in the West usually involves a devil, a demon, or a malevolent spirit, although relatively few cases have been described (Allison, 1980; Crabtree, 1985). Probable cases of the overt type of possession disorder have appeared in the literature but have been labelled as psychotic disorders (Blacker and Wong, 1963). A few cases of the covert type of possession have been identified through hypnotherapy (Allison, 1980).

The following is a case of possession disorder and related dissociative symptoms in a Westerner. The patient was a 32-year-old divorced female, a devout Christian, who began hearing voices of 'evil spirits' approximately two months prior to admission to the psychiatric hospital in 1992, which she attributed to having had sex prior to wedlock, listening to rock and roll music, and other such activities that she considered wrong according to her religion. The voices were clearly perceived as coming from within her and speaking and behaving through her. They made 'faint, growling noises'. There was perhaps more than one voice telling her, 'You are going to commit suicide because I've got you. You can't do anything about it.' She felt very suicidal prior to coming to the hospital. She had no other symptoms of psychosis. Haldol medication was prescribed. At the same time she was praying to the Lord to 'deliver' her and confessing her sins. The voices became weaker and finally ceased in five days. They did not recur in the subsequent two months after the patient's discharge from the hospital despite her not taking any medication. This patient had two other similar experiences. One day while walking down the street, she felt 'uneasy', as if the Devil (Satan) were creeping up on her and trying to scare her or 'take her'. She put her Bible, which she regarded as a shield against the Devil, in front of her chest, and the sensation she had of 'a power of the enemy' immediately disappeared. She attributed this riddance to the Lord. The other episode occurred when she was sitting in church. She felt she was being spiritually attacked by the Devil as she watched the ceiling fan above her turning around. She believed that she could put a stop to this by praying silently to herself, 'Satan, you have no hold over me. I am a Christian. I can stop this by the power of the Lord.' At this point, 'the force' which threatened to 'take over' her disappeared. This type of experience did not recur. The patient felt that her sensation of these two experiences was similar to that of the evil spirit possession but not as severe.

The patient's hospitalization experience meets the criteria for possession disorder. In view of her subsequent success in controlling dissociative symptoms through prayer and religious ritual, it seems possible that her possession state was also relieved by the same means and this raises the question of whether—and if so, how—the antipsychotic medication helped. The patient was convinced that it was her prayer and strong religious belief that delivered her from the evil spirit. Such a termination of dissociative symptoms by religious ritual may be considered self-exorcism.

Crabtree (1985: 210) indicated that most cases of possession disorder present with three types of symptoms: (1) the hearing of voices; (2) a sense of something residing in the body; and (3) a feeling of regularly not being oneself. While identification of these symptoms in a patient points to the existence of possession disorder, more specific information is required for diagnosis because these symptoms are also characteristic of MPD.

Diagnostic Criteria for Possession Disorders

Based on 66 cases of possession disorders admitted to a hospital in Hong Kong, Yap (1960) gave the following operational criteria for what he referred to as the possession syndrome:

(1) short periods (a few minutes to a few hours) of change in the person's identity manifested by change in voice, mannerisms, and behaviour—the

new identity may be of a known person already dead or of a culturally accepted spirit, demon, god, or mythical figure; (2) sudden onset and termination; (3) partial or complete amnesia regarding the new identity and events that occurred during the possession episode; (4) disturbance not due to an organic mental disorder; and (5) associated features: attention seeking and dramatizing behaviour during the possession episode—may occur during religious ceremonies.

Based on the Balinese data and the literature on Western cases, the following diagnostic criteria for possession disorders are presented:

1. There is an experience of unpredictable, uncontrollable, unwanted, and sudden takeover of the subject by a generally malevolent entity.
2. The observer(s) and the subject believe that the entity is the Devil, a demon, a spirit, or a person.
3. The entity speaks and acts through the subject who may exhibit changed affects.
4. The entity speaks of itself in the first person and of the subject in the third person. It may argue and carry on a dialogue with the subject. The discussion loses normal progression, and becomes illogical and incoherent.
5. The possession may be preceded by a brief period of perceptual changes in the subject such as a sensation of darkness or constriction (i.e. the subject experiences loss of awareness of aspects of the immediate environment or focuses on restricted stimuli).
6. During the possession, one or more of the following behaviours are observed:
    (a) Level of awareness and psychological function ranging from conscious to unconscious.
    (b) Falling or losing voluntary motor control, or manifesting assaultive, violent, or convulsive-like behaviour without incontinence.
    (c) Unusual speech (i.e. different in tone or content).
    (d) Inability to hold the eyes open.
    (e) Physical movement perceived as automatic or not controlled by the subject.
    (f) Hallucinations, auditory and/or visual.
    (g) Unusual physiological phenomena such as feats of balance, touching fire without feeling any pain or burning, and loss of allergic reaction.
    (h) Unpremeditated behavioural actions totally out of character for the person or different from his or her usual state.

7. Following the possession, the changes that had occurred completely disappear and the subject may experience:
   (a) Amnesia, partial or complete, with regard to the episode, and
   (b) A sensation of calm or an absence of *usual* thought lasting a few hours to several days.
8. There is no evidence or presumption of an organic factor initiating the possession.
9. The possession is not regarded as a normal aspect of the culture or religion in the society.
10. The possession results in social, occupational disruption, and/or personal distress.
11. The possession does not stem from a psychosis and is not due to a substance-induced disorder.

Differential Diagnosis of Possession Disorder

In Western psychiatric classification (APA, 1987), symptomatic 'trance states' are included under the category of 'dissociative disorders not otherwise specified'. However, in a majority of cases, Balinese trance (which is usually associated with possession) is not symptomatic nor does it represent a mental disorder. Rather, the individual and his society consider the behaviour normal, and it does not result in his being brought to a traditional healer, a psychiatrist, or a mental health clinic. These reasons explain why it would be inappropriate to apply the *DSM-III-R* (APA, 1987) nosology to most trance states in Bali.

If one looks at Balinese trance-possession from the viewpoint of American psychiatric diagnostic classification (APA, 1987), it appears to meet the criteria for depersonalization disorder. The latter include a sensation of not being in complete control of one's actions, an alteration in perception of oneself, and a feeling of being like an automaton (APA, 1987; Castillo, 1990; Steinberg, 1991b). The Balinese in trance-possession describe such sensations. However, examination of the data in Bali in a variety of situations, both normal and pathologic, shows a number of differences between trance-possession and depersonalization disorder. The most significant difference is that the trancer does not feel estranged or separated from himself. The trancer also does not exhibit associated features of depersonalization disorder, including dizziness, anxiety, hypochondriasis, fears of going insane, or disturbances in sense of time (Nemiah, 1980). In addition, trance-possession is marked by altered outward social behaviour (e.g. stabbing oneself in ceremony, and dancing automatically), as well as inward social behaviour (e.g. falling unconscious, changing one's voice and facies) which does not occur with depersonalization (Levy and Wachtel, 1978: 292). According to M. Steinberg (personal communication), patients with depersonalization described changes in behaviour associated with feelings of 'going through the motions' and 'lack of affect' which could be similar to automatic behaviour of the possessed. Patients experiencing depersonalization do not report the post-possession feelings of calmness and peace. These differences separate trance-possession from depersonalization disorder, even though the two conditions have some features in common and share a basis in dissociation. Possibly depersonalization, which is experienced by a high percentage of normal young adults, up to 46 per cent (Dixon, 1963; Trueman, 1984), and occurs during meditation (Castillo, 1990) becomes distressing and symptomatic only when the individual experiences it repeatedly, over a prolonged period, and cannot assimilate it into a framework of his or her society's beliefs or acceptable myths (Castillo, 1990).

During Jesus Christ's time, it was believed that possession by evil spirits, sometimes representing malevolent human beings, caused madness and that Jesus could 'throw out' these evil spirits (Clark, 1977: 778). Since 500 BC, madness has often been confused with possessed trancers (Rouget, 1985). Some early anthropologists studying witch doctors, medicine men, or shamans who were believed to possess magical or paranormal powers in their cultural roles concluded that they must be delusional, schizophrenic, or suffering from some mental disorder (Devereaux, 1956; Silverman, 1967). Such views are no longer held (Lewis, 1971). However, even in Bali and in the West in the early 1990s, trance-possession is sometimes confused with psychosis. Some Balinese psychiatrists have difficulty in distinguishing trance states, including *amok*, from psychoses. This is understandable, particularly since trancers sometimes hallucinate. When a Balinese develops a psychosis for the first time, especially in connection with religious delusions, the people assume that it is a trance-possession state. Only when the symptoms persist do they realize that it is not. Some psychotic Balinese have the delusion that they are possessed by gods. Although some psychotic patients in the West profess that they are possessed by the devil (Berwick and Douglas, 1977) and other mentally ill patients have attributed their episodes of violent behaviour to a possession state, they are not truly possessed. Western psychotic patients may also suffer from the delusion that they are God. The latter complaints and symptoms need to be differentiated from possession.

There are several keys to differentiate psychosis from possession: the abrupt and sharply delineated shifts in and out of the possession (dissociated) state; the duration, which is generally not more than several hours for possession states but lasts days in the case of psychosis; the retention of reality orientation when the possessed person returns to his usual non-ASC state[16] in contrast to the psychotic's longer-term or persistent disorder of thinking and loss of contact with reality; and the possessed person's lack of other associated symptoms of psychosis such as persistent delusions, hallucinations, and sustained social decompensation. Balinese trancers may feel that gods have entered them or say that they are God in the trance-possession state but when they are out of the state they retain their sense of reality and do not believe that they are God; they only believe that God or a god used their body in the state of possession. Confusion of cases of possession with psychoses has occurred largely because literature reports and case-studies of possessed individuals have seldom included psychiatric evaluation by experienced clinicians familiar with possession as well as the full range of psychiatric disorders of the West and the non-Western cultures under study.

The diagnosis of possession disorder is sometimes difficult to sort out from a number of possibilities; it may be easily confused with both MPD[17] and psychoses, particularly schizophrenia and mania.

A case of probable possession disorder, originally diagnosed as a psychosis, involved auto-castration by a 42-year-old White, single, Catholic male (Blacker and Wong, 1963). For 13 days, he was unable to sleep and was tortured by 'evil spirits' who, he reported, used his body to 'perform unnatural acts'. On hearing both male and female voices planning to possess his genitalia for their own purposes, he experienced a 'burning sensation' in his penis and became anxious. 'Then, panic-stricken, he ligated his scrotum with string and proceeded to incise his scrotum in an effort to free himself of the "spirit's" influence. Still not satisfied, he had begun to amputate his penis with a razor when he was discovered by his sister.' At the receiving ward of the hospital, he seemed confused. However, the amputation act effected a permanent removal of the feeling of being tortured by evil spirits, and subsequently he did not have further hallucinations or psychotic symptoms (N. Wong, personal communication). As an illustration of the diagnostic confusion in this case, Blacker and Wong (1963) reported in the same paper several other cases of auto-castration that appeared to be psychotic disorders.

If other mental disorders, including MPD, coexist, even greater confusion may arise. The problem of differentiating between possession disorder and MPD was brought to the fore by a 27-year-old exotic dancer[18] who was brought to a psychiatric hospital in Sacramento, California, in 1992, after she was found sitting down in church speaking loudly and incoherently. She complained that she was possessed by devils and she desperately wanted a priest to exorcize them. She had a history of child abuse, but she was amnesic with regard to the actual molestation, although she could recall the events surrounding it. She also had amnesia regarding her own behaviour that resulted in her children being removed from her custody several years earlier. She described the devils as having been present for 17 months, and as being very distressing. She had never had such an experience or heard voices before. At times during interviews, she appeared to dissociate as she broke into outbursts of loud, rapid, unintelligible speech, doubling over at what appeared to be hallucinations which she was unable to describe. These episodes appeared to be provoked by her frustration at her inability to explain the nature of her symptoms but they also occurred throughout the day without any obvious provocation. She was able to identify one of the voices as that of her deceased father. She also described hearing mumbling voices as if there was an argument going on inside of her. At intervals during the interview, when she was able to recover from these distractions, she was calm and her thinking was logical and clear. In psychotherapy over a period of several days, she was able to comprehend the concept of an entity taking over her and the possibility of learning to control it or prevent it from possessing her. After her discharge from hospital, she persisted in her desire to find a priest to exorcize the entities.

It was not possible to determine if this woman was suffering from a possession disorder or had MPD of the possessioniform type described by Kluft (1991c) in which the alter that is most evident, or the sole one, presents itself as a demon or the Devil.

The difference in the course of symptomatology of MPD and possession disorder is helpful in distinguishing the two conditions. MPD generally has a chronic and unremitting course (although the alter states may be intermittent). Possession disorder is subacute with intermittent episodes, often terminates abruptly, and may not recur.

Connor (1984), an anthropologist, described a man who fell ill for two and a half months prior to becoming a *balian*. Her description of the man's behaviour, which she termed 'divine madness,' fits the Western psychiatric criteria for a psychosis. He had both delusions and hallucinations and in that sense, the lay term 'madness' is apt. The man's behaviour after becoming a *balian* was no longer psychotic and he continued to have possession experiences. In such an instance, other *balian* may consider the person mad during the acute manifestation of the psychotic behaviour but if he subsequently becomes a *balian*, they regard his condition as madness conferred by the gods, who are testing him to see if he is strong enough to bear the burden of becoming a *balian*.[19] If so, they view the 'madness' in retrospect to be normal possession. This revision of an assessment of mental phenomenon or illness, depending on the subject's subsequent choice of social role or occupation, illustrates how confusion can arise as regards an actual mental state.

Western-trained psychiatrists in Bali can make a clear distinction between psychosis and possession, a distinction not always clear in the minds of *balian*.

The following case of a Balinese illustrates how psychotic disorder can resemble in some respects the type of illnesses which afflict *balian* prior to becoming *balian*. A 20-year-old woman with a psychosis of three years' duration, diagnosed as schizophrenia, had delusions that other people were in love with her, that she was pregnant, that she had intercourse with others, and that she masturbated in a way that everyone knew what she was doing. She had auditory and visual hallucinations as well. At home, she was afraid to leave the house; she also slept a lot and was very lazy. Psychiatric treatment included a number of psychotropic medications including Haldol, Clopromazine, Trilafon, Tegretol, tricyclic antidepressants, and citicoline. All were given with very little response. She was last seen one year prior to a visit in 1990, at which time she returned by herself to visit Suryani and tell her that she had recovered in January 1990. She described the recovery process as the consequence of an auditory hallucination telling her to work, not to care about what others say, to go out of the house regardless of what the neighbours say, help her mother, and take a cooking class. She did all of these things and expressed a desire to go to computer school. She appeared to be establishing better interpersonal relationships over the past months and seemed much brighter. She still had auditory hallucinations which asked her to find the voice that said 'I want to marry you; try to find me.' She believed that it was a doctor's voice and asked Suryani if she knew the person. It is clear that this patient had auditory hallucinations and an ongoing schizophrenic process, but the recent hallucinations apparently helped her recover her social adaptation in a remarkable way. Aspects of this illness that do not resemble the illnesses of *balian* are the long duration of symptoms and the residual psychotic symptom (hallucinations) following improvement.

Hallucinations: Normal and Abnormal

The foregoing patient's psychotic hallucinations are similar to the auditory hallucinations of *balian* who are not psychotic and in daily life act normally in all respects. To correctly interpret hallucinations, it is imperative to look at context and meaning. The authors estimate that about 1 per cent of normal Balinese in the population have experienced auditory hallucinations. During meditation, people who are not psychotic may also have visual and auditory hallucinations. Suryani frequently encounters Balinese with visual hallucinations who are asymptomatic and functioning normally. Her cook could literally see spirits that keep the house safe. Another servant reported hearing people coming to the door of the house but found no one there.[20] A person may report an awareness of a very bad smell, such as that of a decaying corpse or animal, but cannot locate it and then the smell disappears. Normal Balinese people have reported visiting and seeing people who have died, apparently hallucinations.

Three factors may contribute to the hallucinatory abilities of normal Balinese: (1) in their belief system they form a close relationship with God and many can see Him and hear His voice; (2) the supernatural is very much 'alive' and perceivable; (3) they may have abilities on a genetic basis. In support of the last is the fact that psychotic Balinese frequently have visual hallucinations, while Javanese psychotics seldom do. (Java is geographically close to Bali and the two islands are also historically close in customs but not in religion.) This was Suryani's experience during the year when she was a resident psychiatrist treating psychotic patients in Java and was confirmed by Dr W. Maramis, a lifelong practising psychiatrist in Surabaya, Java. Psychotic Javanese do, however, have auditory hallucinations. Some cultures differ in manifestations of hallucinations. For example, in Mexico, visual hallucinations of religious figures are relatively common in the normal Mexican population. A large-scale survey in England in 1890 found 9.9 per cent of 17,000 subjects had at some time in their lives experienced at least one hallucination that was not accounted for by illness and in 1948, a smaller follow-up study confirmed these findings.

Hallucinations in trance and hallucinations of normal people seemingly not in trance may appear to be similar to psychotic hallucinations, but differ in a number of respects (Table 9.1). Differences distinguish the hallucinations of different states and suggest different psychobiological bases. Conversely, the differences may help in clinically distinguishing hallucinations as manifestations in normal persons not in trance, possessed persons, or psychotics.

Theories of Possession

There have been few psychological explanations of the mechanism of possession or theories of possession. Janet (1898) regarded possession phenomenon as comparable to hysteria and claimed dissociation as the crucial psychological process (van der Kolk and van der Hart, 1989). Sargent (1974) proposed classical (Pavlovian) conditioning as a mechanism. Several authors and scholars on trance (Brown and Fromm, 1986; Fromm, 1979; Gill and Brenman, 1961; Walker, 1972) have elected to explain it by use of the psychoanalytic concept of 'regression in the service of the ego', originally proposed by Kris (1952) to explain the ability of artists to access symbolism from their unconscious for use in their creative work. This concept itself, however, has been subject to controversy over whether the phenomenon actually involves regression or is more a type of 'relaxation of other ego functions' (MacKinnon, 1980). Bourguignon (1976) suggested a similar concept as a theoretical explanation of 'possession-trance', termed 'regression in the service of the self'. However, many of the trance states of the Balinese, for example, the musicians' and various kinds of trance-possession, which are regarded as normal in Bali, do not appear to involve regression at all in the sense of the definition of that defence, i.e. 'a partial or symbolic return to more infantile patterns of reacting or thinking' (APA, 1984). This would appear to be the case with the Balinese trance-mediums. Persons in a trance-possession state at communal ceremonies may be dependent in the sense that they rely upon persons in their immediate environment to assist them in order to function properly and safely, but it is questionable if their behaviour qualifies as regression. For those who lean towards psychoanalytic concepts, it would be appropriate to use terminology such as 'dissociation in the service of the ego' to connote a

TABLE 9.1
Characteristics of Auditory and Visual Hallucinations in the Balinese under Three Different Conditions

Normal (Not Possessed)[1]	*Normal (Possessed)*[2]	*Schizophrenia (Undifferentiated)*
Not in trance	In trance state	Not in trance
Auditory and visual	Auditory and visual	Mostly auditory; some visual
Religious meaning	Religious meaning	Often no religious meaning
Some have a religious context not related to to stress	Religious context not related to stress	Some may but often do not have religious meaning; may or may not be stress-related
Exaggerated in size or features, or diminutive, or unlike real life	Structured and appear as if in real life	Incompletely structured; may be fragmentary; lacks reality
Transitory; associated with coherent thoughts	May be lengthy and associated with socially acceptable thought content	Thoughts about hallucinations often idiosyncratic, incoherent or unintelligible
Thought associations normal	Thought associations normal	Thought associations may be loose (disconnected)
No related delusions or other psychotic symptoms	No related delusions or other psychotic symptoms	May be associated with persistent delusions and other types of psychotic symptoms

Normal affect	Normal affect	Affect likely abnormal
No social impairment	No social impairment	Generally associated with social decompensation
Associated thoughts connected to reality of cultural beliefs or religion	Associated thoughts connected to reality of cultural beliefs or religion	Unrealistic content of behaviour and thought
No change in social behaviour	Individual operates within socially accepted standards	Associated social decompensation
Considered normal by the society	Considered normal by the society	Considered abnormal by the Balinese
Person deemed normal by peers	Person deemed normal (not crazy) by peers	Person regarded as crazy by peers
Within socially approved and expected bounds	Within socially approved and expected bounds	Outside of society's approval and expected bounds
Relatively common in general population	Common in some villagers and in some *balian*	Less than 1% of population

(*continued*)

TABLE 9.1 (*continued*)

Normal (Not Possessed)[1]	*Normal (Possessed)*[2]	*Schizophrenia (Undifferentiated)*
Dealt with rationally by the individual	Dealt with rationally by the individual	Not under rational self-control
Transient	Transient	Often persist for days, weeks, or months
No amnesia	Mostly partial or complete amnesia; some, no amnesia	No amnesia
Normal facies; no paleness	Flat facial expression; pale lips and mouth	Expressionless face; no paleness
Normal eye appearance and expression	No focusing of eyes (looks into distance)	Eyes focus but may appear as if looking into own world

[1]Examples are *leak* (witch-like spirits) phenomena and seeing religious spirits.
[2]Examples are traditional healers (*balian*), dancers, and ceremonial participants.

theoretical concept of trance with possession.

Devereaux's (1956) theoretical concept of the 'ethnic unconscious' appears to have merit in describing and understanding the forms possession takes in various cultures. The concept holds that 'conflicts are part of the ongoing but unrecognized cultural tradition, they occur in the "proper reactions" and can become stereotyped, and are unconsciously learned by everyone'. As Langness (1976: 60) pointed out, 'Unconscious motives may well be involved in shamanism also; indeed it was in a discussion of shamanism that Devereaux first invoked the notion of the ethnic unconscious.' The conflicts regarding good and evil, as espoused in dramas involving Rangda and the Barong, are possible examples of an expression of the ethnic unconscious of the Balinese.

Rouget (1985), a French ethnologist, proposed a theory that possession is a 'conjunction' of several constituents: (1) an innate structure of the consciousness, making it susceptible to being invaded by an emotional event that submerges its normal state; (2) social perpetration of the event as a sign of the will of the presence of a spirit or divinity; (3) domestication of the event with the intention of establishing it as a mode of communication with the divine; (4) identification of the entranced subject with the divinity held responsible for the trance; and (5) theatricalization of the identificatory behaviour.

The data presented in this book lead to a theory of possession (not including disorders) which contains one of Rouget's constituents and several in addition: (1) a genetic or innate degree of hypnotizability of the individual; (2) a religious context; (3) entry into trance; (4) dissociative transformation into another spirit or power; (5) in trance-possession, semi-automatic actions of the person with behaviour and emotions appropriate to cultural patterns and enabling communication between the divine and the people; (6) expressed behaviour and emotions which go against the rules of the society governing everyday life; (7) overt or covert expectation, support, and encouragement by the society or group and the individual's environment; (8) institutionalized or self-imposed controls on the duration of trance; (9) often partial or complete amnesia with regard to the possession state. The authors agree with Rouget that the behaviour of the possessed one is often theatrical in the sense that it is dramatic. Rouget's idea that the trancer identifies with the divinity held responsible for the trance is conceivable as an unconscious process. It should be borne in mind the above theory utilizes Western psychology only and does not incorporate the Balinese religious belief and concept of an outside force or supernatural entity, which takes over and controls the individual.

Multiple Personality Disorder (MPD) Conceptualized as a Trance-possession Process

It is important for comparisons of behavioural phenomena in one culture with those in another culture to be clear that the things compared are of the same categories of discourse. Confusion could arise for some readers, when comparing normal possession in Balinese with MPD which is regarded primarily as a mental disorder (and, indeed, it is considered a disorder by psychiatry). However, persons with multiple personality are not affected by their condition for certain periods, especially early in their lives, in any case not in a manner or to an extent that it results in psychological and/or social disability, nor does it interfere significantly with their functioning. Nevertheless, in Western practice, all such persons are conveniently and conventionally labelled as manifesting a disorder, MPD. Hence, the term MPD might be confused with the phenomenon of multiple personality. In the following discussion, the traditionally accepted term MPD will be used to designate both multiple personality in non-impaired people and the clinically manifest disorder.

It is not difficult for psychiatrists and psychologists to reconcile many of the psychological commonalities of mentally normal and abnormal conditions because both non-symptomatic individuals and patients often manifest some of the same psychological mechanisms, differing only in the degree of distress that is incurred by the individual or the situation. Examples are dissociation and other psychological mechanisms operative in a number of psychological conditions such as some forms of depression, compulsive behaviour, phobia, addiction, and anxiety; the mechanisms involved in each condition are the same, whether the individual is symptomatic or not. The data presented in this book indicate that normally occurring possession (e.g. in ceremonies) and the possession disorders in Bali (e.g. *bebainan* and evil spirit possession) manifest what appears to be the same psychobiological processes. Trance in Bali is the same psychobiological process in both normal and abnormal conditions and it is the same throughout all cultures. A similar statement can be made about possession.

A number of dissociative disorders seen in Balinese are similar to those in the West. These include the psychogenic amnesias, conversion disorders (e.g. paralysis, blindness, and deafness), psychogenic fugue states (abrupt unannounced travel away from one's home town with assumption of a new identity and amnesia regarding one's real identity), possession disorder, and depersonalization disorder (a perceived experience of feeling detached from one's mind or body or feeling like an automaton).

One dissociative disorder seen in the West that does not occur in the Balinese, or at least that has not yet been determined, is multiple personality disorder (MPD), defined as the existence within the individual of two or more distinct personalities, each of which at some time takes full control of the individual's behaviour (APA, 1987).[21] The authors have looked specifically for MPD cases at the psychiatric hospitals, as well as in private practice, and have asked other psychiatrists in Bali about possible cases. No clear-cut cases have yet been identified. Suryani has not identified a single case in the psychiatric service of the major hospital in Denpasar in the past 10 years. It is curious that multiple personality has not occurred in Bali, since trance is so common there and MPD has been regarded as a form of self-hypnosis (Bliss, 1986).

MPD, formerly regarded as rare, has recently been recognized as relatively common in Western countries and it has a relatively stable set of case symptoms in North America (Ross, 1989). Bliss (1984a) reported on over 100 cases; Putnam et al. (1986) reported 100 cases; Kluft (1984a) reported 171 cases; and Ross, Norton, and Wozney (1989) reported on an assembled group of 236 cases. Multiple personality disorder was found to be relatively frequent, 3.3 per cent, in a survey of general psychiatry inpatients (Ross, Joshi, and Currie, 1990). This is quite high, considering the fact that MPD has been traditionally considered to be relatively rare and by some perhaps as infrequent as 1 in 100 patients admitted to a psychiatric hospital. For every case of MPD there is probably at least one individual in society who has multiple personality and has not been identified as having a disorder.[22]

The fact that there are only rare reports of MPD in persons from cultures other than Western (Martinez-Tuboas, 1989; Putnam, 1989; Steinberg, 1990) suggests that it may go unrecognized or may be a culture-related syndrome of Western cultures.

The mental health profession has a history of scepticism about MPD based on ignorance and cognitive errors (Ross, 1990). Physicians frequently fail to recognize and diagnose it and it is commonly misdiagnosed as affective disorder, personality disorder (especially borderline personality disorder, which may also coexist), anxiety disorder, and schizophrenia (Ross, 1989). Coons, Bowman, and Milstein (1988) found that MPD patients averaged 7 years in mental health systems before the diagnosis was made. Although MPD generally arises in childhood it is not usually recognized clinically until adulthood (Bliss, 1980; Braun, 1984a). Typically MPD patients are diagnosed after having received various prior psychiatric diagnoses over a number of years. To complicate diagnosis, MPD patients can be associated with any of the 11 personality disorders described in *DSM-III-R* (APA, 1987; Fink, 1991).[23] Symptoms of psychosis such as hearing and talking with other voices and various psychotic disorders must be differentiated from MPD which is not a psychotic condition.

Although, classically, MPD has been described as occurring with rather clear-cut and even polarized personalities, Kluft (1991c) has explicated how the majority of patients represent a wide variety of clinical pictures. For example, most alters exert influence without fully taking over the individual, the entities (alters) may not be overt, and personalities may keep their existence secret from their host. Kluft (1991c) described more than a dozen different forms taken by MPD patients, each of which characterizes the clinical picture. In one type called switch-dominated, the switching process occurs very frequently and/or rapidly so that no clear alter dominates the patient at any one time and the patient may appear bewildered, confused, and forgetful. This type of patient may be misdiagnosed as having an affective disorder, a psychosis, an organic mental syndrome, or a seizure disorder (Kluft, 1991c: 625).

To further complicate diagnosis, numerous symptoms are presented by MPD patients including anxiety, depressions, somatoform symptoms, sexual dysfunction, suicide attempts, self-mutilization, eating disorder, sleeping disorder, or symptoms of post-traumatic stress disorder (Kluft, 1991c).

The psychological or scientific view of multiple personality has a long history dating back nearly two centuries, beginning with the concept of 'divided consciousness' which arose from demonstrations of hypnosis, then called 'artificial somnambulism' (Puysegur, 1784). This view recognized two consciousnesses of the mind, separate from each other, each having its own memories. The concept was applied to MPD as early as 1816, with the idea that the case of Mary Reynolds (Crabtree, 1985) was a matter of her entering and leaving a state of somnambulistic trance. Pierre Janet, a French psychiatrist in the late nineteenth century, developed a model of 'consciousness and subconsciousness' and the notion that subconscious fixed ideas such as a frightening experience could be cut off, or 'dissociated'[24] from consciousness, and continue to exist with an autonomy of their own and with thinking ability. Janet (1898) explained multiple personality this way.

At the turn of the century, Jean-Martin Charcot, a famous French psychiatrist, and Janet developed a concept of split-off fragments of the personality which they attributed to constitutional factors (Crabtree, 1985: 239). In 1894, Freud identified hysteria as one of four types of symptoms representing an outcome of 'neuropsychoses of defence' against a memory of a traumatic sexual event in early life. Somewhat later, Freud formulated dissociation as caused by a conflict and representing a psychological defence.

In 1888, Robert Louis Stevenson (1937) produced his literary *tour de force*, the tale of Dr Jekyll and Mr Hyde. It is a brilliant depiction of MPD, with some literary licence, particularly the aspect of switching personalities brought about by ingestion of a drug. Dr Jekyll's explanation in his 'full statement of the case' referred to 'dissociation' phenomena (Stevenson, 1937: 80) resulting in two persons with opposite morals, good and horribly bad, stemming from a lifelong conflict. This is typical of MPD and illustrates the ethnic unconscious as well, i.e. the Christian moral polarities of good and evil. An atypical aspect of Dr Jekyll's story of his early childhood as far as MPD is concerned was his report of an entirely happy childhood with no evidence of child abuse. (Biographers of Stevenson indicate that he himself did not have an abused or neglected childhood.) Dr Jekyll explained:

> The worse of my [childhood] faults was a certain impatient gaiety of disposition, such as has made the happiness of many, but such as I found it hard to reconcile with my imperious desire to carry my head high, and wear a more than commonly grave countenance before the public. Hence it came about that I concealed my pleasures; and that when I reached years of reflection, and began to look around me and take stock of my progress and position in the world, I stood already committed to a profound duplicity of life. Many a man would have even blazoned such irregularities as I was guilty of; but from the high views that I had set before me, I regarded and hid them with an almost morbid sense of shame. It was thus rather the exacting nature of my aspirations than any particular degradation in my faults, that made me what I was, and, with even a deeper trench than in the majority of men, severed in me those provinces of good and ill which divide and compound man's dual nature. In this case, I was driven to reflect deeply and inveterately on that hard law of life, which lies at the root of religion and is one of the most plentiful springs of distress. Though so profound a double-dealer, I was in no sense a hypocrite; both sides of

me were in dead earnest; I was no more myself when I laid aside restraint and plunged in shame, than when I laboured, in the eye of day, at the furtherance of knowledge or the relief of sorrow and suffering. And it chanced that the direction of my scientific studies, which led wholly towards the mystic and the transcendental, reacted and shed a strong light on this consciousness of the perennial war among my members. With every day, and from both sides of my intelligence, the moral and the intellectual, I thus drew steadily nearer to that truth, by whose partial discovery I have been doomed to such as dreadful shipwreck: that man is not truly one, but truly two.

... even before the course of my scientific discoveries had begun to suggest the most naked possibility of such a miracle, I had learned to dwell with pleasure, as a beloved daydream, on the thought of the separation of these elements. If each, I told myself, could be housed in separate identities, life would be relieved of all that was unbearable; the unjust might go his way, delivered from the aspirations and remorse of his more upright twin; and the just could walk steadfastly and securely on his upward path, doing the good things in which he found his pleasure, and no longer exposed to disgrace and penitence by the hands of this extraneous evil. It was the curse of mankind that these incongruous faggots were thus bound together—that in the agonized womb of consciousness, these polar twins should be continuously struggling. How, then, were they dissociated?

Possibly Stevenson's creativity and inspiration for this work owed something to what appeared to be an MPD phenomenon in himself. He experienced a curious 'other personality' throughout his life, which helped him in his creative writing (Crabtree, 1985: 87–8). He described a conscious awareness of 'little people' or 'brownies', as he called them, and, writing about himself in the third person, he stated, 'For the most part, whether awake or asleep, he is simply occupied—he or his little people—in consciously making stories for the market.' 'Who are the little people?' 'What shall I say they are but just my brownies, God bless them! ... who do one-half my work for me while I am fast-asleep and in all human likelihood do the rest for me as well, when I am wide-awake and fondly suppose I do it myself.' He also referred to these 'brownies' as 'unseen collaborators whom I keep locked in a back garret, while I get all the praise and they but a share of the pudding'.

In 1880, Breuer (Breuer and Freud, 1955) began the psychiatric treatment of a young woman, Anna O., who had a hysterical illness of two years' duration. This was an excellent example of a hysterical (conversion) disorder including symptoms of paralysis and loss of speech, and probably, in addition, MPD, with the patient referring to these episodes as 'absences' and recognizing them as autohypnosis with total amnesia. Breuer (Breuer and Freud, 1955: 24) perceived these as self-hypnotic or hypnoid states.

> Two entirely distinct states of consciousness were present which alternated very frequently and without warning and which became more and more differentiated in the course of the illness. In one of these states she recognized her surroundings; she was melancholy and anxious, but relatively normal. In the other state she hallucinated and was 'naughty'—that is to say, she was abusive, used to throw the cushions at people, so far as the contractures at various times allowed, tore buttons off her bedclothes and linen with those of her fingers which she could move, and so on. At this state of her illness if something had been moved in the room or someone had entered or left it [during her other state of consciousness] she would complain of having 'lost' some time and would remark upon the gap in her train of conscious thoughts. Since those about her tried to deny this and to soothe her when she complained that she was going mad, she would, after throwing the pillows about, accuse people of doing things to her and leaving her in a muddle, etc.
>
> At moments when her mind was quite clear she would complain of the profound darkness in her head, of not being able to think, of becoming blind and deaf, of having two selves, a real one and an evil one which forced her to behave badly, and so on.

Breuer (Breuer and Freud, 1955: 45), observing that in her waking state the patient was totally unaware of what had been going on during her absences, noted:

> ... throughout the entire illness her two states of consciousness persisted side by side: the primary one in which she was quite normal psychically, and the secondary one which may well be likened to a dream in view of its wealth of imaginative products and hallucinations, its large gaps of memory, and lack of inhibition and control in its associations. In this secondary state, the patient was in a condition of alienation.

Breuer described one aspect of her condition as similar to depersonalization or possibly the phenomenon Hilgard called the hidden observer in hypnosis:

> Though her two states were thus sharply separated, not only did the secondary state intrude into the first one, but—and this was at all events frequently true, and even when she was in a very bad condition—a clear-sighted and calm observer sat, as she put it, in the corner of her brain and looked on at all the mad business. Anna O. was successfully treated with psychotherapy involving expressing her feelings. She had been severely physically impaired as a result of her muscular paralyses. Her ideas

during her 'absences' were 'disposed of by being given verbal utterance during hypnosis'. (Breuer and Freud, 1955: 46.)

McDougal (1926), eminent Professor of Psychology at Harvard, described how a person may succeed in getting rid of undesirable fantasies or drives and splitting them off from conscious awareness, which he called dissociation. He believed that these dissociated units could break through ordinary consciousness into a 'psychic automatism', which resulted in either a 'hysterical fit' or multiple personality. Early psychologists described in detail the case histories of a number of individuals with fugue, conversion disorder, and multiple personality (Crabtree, 1985).

Any scientific consideration of MPD must take into account the occultists'[25] views of multiple personalities (Crabtree, 1985). These have a long history dating from the ritual practices of ancient Greek cultures, extending through eras of witchcraft, and up to present-day channellers. Occultists' views cover a large number of religio-philosophical traditions and explain all human mysteries including disease in terms of 'hidden' mystical forces in the individual and the universe, which operate according to well-defined laws. They believe that 'life-forces' such as God and human-created objects and human thoughts or 'thought-forms' have power which can produce effects on others. Perhaps the Balinese beliefs in malicious black magic and *bebainan* (Chapter 7) are comparable to occultists' concepts of human-created objects and their views of power which can produce effects on others.

Occultists have held two views of multiple personality, both involving possession. According to Crabtree (1985), the occultists' general concept of possession is that an individual spirit or centre of consciousness leaves the body to make room for another entity to enter, who then takes full control and leaves the individual amnesic. However, the occultists also postulate a 'lucid possession' in which the individual has full memory of the possession event. They believe that the intruders are generally malevolent. Possession in Bali differs in several aspects: the Balinese do not believe in a leaving of the individual's spirit to make room for the possession, the possession is often positive, and, generally, the amnesia may be partial or complete.

Occultists see multiple personality as a special case of possession. Although it is usually considered an outside intruder, it can also be 'a fragment of the individual's own psyche unconsciously crystallized around some thought-form'. 'The victim may have given some interiorly produced thought a specific personification and charged it with such energy that it has the power to periodically break through into consciousness and take control of him.' (Crabtree, 1985: 234.) This 'thought-form' or fragment of the personality may be harmful to the individual or positive and sympathetic. The occultists' treatment methods aim to remove these creations but consider it essential that the individual participate lest he simply unconsciously recreates the situation. 'Only if the victim recognizes his part in their production and claims the hidden thoughts which were the seeds of their formation can the personalities be prevented from reforming.' (Crabtree, 1985: 237.) In contrast, if the occultists believe that the alter personalities as possessions have moved in from the outside, they take a different therapeutic approach, believing that these spirits must be removed.

Possession in states of trance has been considered operative in some MPD patients (Ellenberger, 1970). Throughout the ages people have encountered ghosts, divine spirits both seen and heard (DeBoismont, 1855), some of which may well have been due to what is now called MPD (Bliss, 1984a). Kluft (1991a: 161) noted that MPD provides a secular expression of many of the same mental structures found in possession syndromes. It is interesting to note that many patients with MPD complain of feelings of being possessed or in trance (Kluft, 1991a: 173). Kluft (1991c: 622) described a 'possessioniform' type of MPD in which the alter presents as demon or devil. MPD and possessed individuals have been noted to have similar switching behaviour, personality changes, and amnesias (Krippner, 1987; Ravenscroft, 1965). An anthropological review of several case reports of MPD and similar states led Kenny (1981) to conclude that MPD and possession are phenomenologically similar, particularly in the aspect of amnesia.

The etiology of MPD is currently disputed. A generally accepted theory is that MPD is post-traumatic in etiology secondary to child abuse, particularly sexual abuse, essentially PTSD (D. Spiegel, 1984; Wilbur, 1984). Sexual abuse has been documented in 79–83 per cent of MPD (Ross, Norton, and Wozney, 1989). A second theory is spontaneous self-hypnosis (Bliss, 1984a). A third theory emphasizes MPD as created by repeated dissociations which utilize state-dependent learning (Kluft, 1984b).

State-dependent learning is a notion that what individuals learn and experience in one state of consciousness may not be readily transferable to another state of consciousness (Weingartner, 1978). Several studies support this concept as a contribution to the amnesias and impairments of memory across alter states (Ludwig, Brandsma, and Wilbur, 1972; Nissen et al., 1988; Silberman et al., 1985). Work on state dependent memory (Bower, 1981) has shown that memories can be more accurately retrieved when the person is in a mood state similar to that in which the event or learning took place originally. Hence, memories associated with strong feelings might resurface only in a situation or psychological state in which the individual could tolerate experiencing these strong feelings.

D. Spiegel (1984) formulated the PTSD theory of MPD as follows:

> Patients with multiple personality disorder can be seen as having had multiple stresses in their early lives, and therefore this style of defense against trauma becomes institutionalized through the need for repeated use. Such patients defend against the demoralization, fear, anxiety, and depression of the unpleasant world to which they are unusually sensitive by saying metaphorically, 'I know it is happening—but not to me.' The hypnotic dissociation becomes an attempt to anesthetize the pain by seeing it inflicted on a separate part of themselves. Frequently, they internalize the role of aggressor in the second and generally hostile personality in an effort to control the inflicting of physical and emotional pain and thereby preempt the external source of discomfort.
>
> The connection between high hypnotizability and multiple personality symptoms has been repeatedly documented. The personality dissociations have been frequently reported to have begun after the occurrence of physical or emotional trauma. Initially, in fact, the dissociated personality may comfort the primary one, offering solace and consolation wished for but unavailable from the parents. These dissociated aspects of the patient can be seen as efforts to preserve some form of comfort, safety, and identity in the face of overwhelming stress.

A good example of this type of dissociation is a case of child abuse described by Terr (1991: 17):

> Jamie was repeatedly abused by his alcoholic father. He had also repeatedly observed his father beat his mother. At age 8, he witnessed his mother shoot his father to death. When he was 9, the child was psychologically evaluated. At that time he told me, 'I started some planets. I made my planets up as a game. But it's real now. It's no game anymore.' Jamie described a safe planet he had invented long ago, his own planet. He also had invented a number of very unsafe planets where people 'got killed'. He said that he had come to achieve invisibility by repeatedly visiting his own safe planet and avoiding the unsafe ones. 'Starting when I was 6,' he said, 'I began to feel invisible. When my Mom pointed a gun at my Dad . . . I was thinking like "I didn't see it", like "This didn't happen." I blinked to see if I was dreaming. . . . I remember at first pretending I wasn't there—that I was on my own planet. I had gone there a lot before.

When Mom and Dad would fight, I would try not to hear, not to see. I'd try to go to sleep. Normally I couldn't. I'd try to get out of the room where they were. I'd try to visit my planet. But now my mind, yes, it just goes blank. Mostly it happens at home. A few minutes at a time.'

Jamie repeatedly dreamed by night about his father's death. And he visualized the killing by day. But from the moment that his dad was shot, Jamie wondered if he himself could turn invisible. 'I know I can,' he said, 'I do it here on earth. I do it all the time on my planet. You're just going to have to believe me. My friends believe it.... When my father was being shot I felt invisible. But if I turned invisible in front of everybody, they'd take away my powers.'

Balinese mental disorders involving trance-possession, such as in the schoolchildren and the women living in the palace compound (Suryani, 1984; see Chapter 7) who entered into trance states at unpredictable times but in certain situations (i.e. school and palace), may have been precipitated by anxiety, stressful events, or recall of such events. Memories of or associations with anxiety-laden or traumatic events are hypothesized to be the triggering factors in transformations of the personalities of MPD patients.

Bliss (1984a, 1986: 136) proposed that personalities of MPD patients are simply one among many possible products of hypnosis and that the basic process underlying the clinical syndrome of MPD is spontaneous self-hypnosis: 'a rapid unpremeditated withdrawal into a trance, a dissociation, a primitive reflex that they experience when anxious or fearful in response to some psychological or physical threat'. Bliss's work on MPD gives compelling evidence for the key role of self-hypnosis in MPD and is supported by other authors (Braid, 1899; Moll, 1902; D. Spiegel, 1990: 139; Sutcliffe and Jones, 1962). In addition to a high degree of hypnotizability, MPD patients have an extreme range and high degree of common dissociative experiences (Bernstein and Putnam, 1986). Hypnosis is a common and very effective treatment technique. MPD patients frequently recognize that they have spent a large part of their lives in altered states of consciousness (Bliss, 1984a). These spontaneous transformations of the patients can be swift, with some patients explaining that their personality simply disappears and the alter ego assumes the body. Bliss (1984a: 138) asserted that the process begins early in childhood and that afterwards, self-hypnosis becomes a dominant mode of coping with unpleasant experiences: 'The crux of the syndrome of MPD seems to be the patient's unrecognized abuse of self-hypnosis.'

Several facts may argue against both the child abuse and the self-hypnosis theories of MPD. Self-hypnosis has been learned and practised by multitudes of Westerners and in that state very few switch into another personality. Self-hypnosis as a process could account for a number of aspects of multiple personalities but perhaps not explain its major difference from hypnosis, namely being taken over and controlled by an entity. Child sexual abuse is not specifically characteristic of MPD; it occurs with a high prevalence in borderline personality disorders without MPD, 71 per cent in one series of patients (Ogata et al., 1990). In a survey of 960 women in San Francisco, 38 per cent reported sexual abuse before age 18 (Russell, 1983) but a minuscule proportion of these would be expected to develop MPD.

Nevertheless, data presented in this book and other reports of trance with possession in Bali (Belo, 1960) indicate many similarities in the characteristics of MPD and hypnosis as reported by Bliss (1984a, 1986) and others (Bateson and Mead, 1942; Coons, Bowman, and Milstein, 1988; Gill and Brenman, 1961; Hilgard, 1965; Jensen and Suryani, 1992; Kluft, 1991b; Putnam, 1988; Ross, 1990). These include the following:

1. Patients with MPD have unusual hypnotic abilities. It is hypothesized that this is present in normal Balinese who enter into trance-possession at community festivals and ceremonies. About 15 per cent of Western adults are excellent hypnotic subjects (Hilgard, 1965). Western writers have believed that most Balinese are highly hypnotizable (Gill and Brenman, 1961).
2. MPD patients switch rapidly to their alters, many in less than five minutes and most in a matter of seconds (Coons, 1986; Coons, Bowman, and Milstein, 1988; Putnam, 1988; Putnam et al., 1986). Observations in Bali indicate that villagers who participate in ceremonial trance, trance-mediums, and hypnotherapy patients enter trance-possession with similar rapidity; the switch to the possession state appears to be instantaneous.
3. Almost two-thirds of MPD patients report auditory hallucinations (Kluft, 1991a) and also vivid visual hallucinations which may involve complex scenes (Ross, Norton, and Wozney, 1989; Putnam, 1991). Possessed Balinese report similar experiences.
4. Amnesia or loss of time is typical of MPD, in which the patients have no memory of performing complex behaviours (Putnam, 1991), as well as other dissociative disorders. This is a prominent aspect of possession in Bali.
5. Putnam (Goodman, 1988: 20) regarded increased muscle

tension as one of the most telling observable signs of MPD patients switching into or out of alternate personalities. Similarly, a marked increase in muscle tension accompanies the possession states occurring in religious ceremonies in Bali.

6. A multitude of hypnotic-like episodes of MPD patients have included almost every classical hypnotic feat (Bliss, 1980). For example, an adolescent alter of a middle-aged adult may be excellent at an athletic sport. Balinese in trance demonstrate a variety of unusual hypnotic feats, including automatic or synchronized dancing, putting hot coals in their mouths, dancing on hot coals, incredible balancing, and self-stabbing, all without bodily injury (Belo, 1960).
7. It is not uncommon for family members and/or those involved in traumatizing the MPD patient to be represented in direct, derivative, or symbolic fashion within the system of personalities (Kluft, 1984c). Similarly, Balinese traditional healers (*balian*) and a Balinese patient in hypnotherapy were possessed by the spirits of more than one family member.
8. Some MPD personalities have included animals (e.g. birds and dogs), Jesus, sister Mary, devils, ghosts, and God. Balinese in trance are possessed by evil spirits, God, and sometimes animals.
9. Statements by MPD patients show that one personality using the pronoun I talks about the other one in terms of the pronoun she or he (e.g. 'I'm a whore but she is very moral', or 'I'm a tease but she is very solemn'). The same type of address has been observed in Balinese hypnotherapy patients when they become possessed by spirits or other souls.
10. MPD personalities may appear only once for a single mission or they may continue to function. In Balinese under hypnotherapy, possession may appear only a single time in therapy or may reappear in subsequent therapy sessions. Individuals who experience spontaneous possession may have only one or two such experiences in a lifetime or they may have them frequently, even daily.
11. Individual MPD personalities have specific and limited functions, and their repertoire remains static. Similar characteristics are true of Balinese possessed in trance (e.g. the trance-mediums and kris dancers).
12. MPD personalities have an 'unswerving dedication to their missions' (Bliss, 1984a) and they are consistent (e.g. one laughs but cannot cry, one is promiscuous, and another is violent).

Balinese in trance show a similar dedication to their missions. This is particularly evident in the trancers of the kris dance in which individuals undergo self-stabbing precipitated by the wave of a witch's (Rangda's) cloth (Belo, 1960). All trance dancers perform similar bodily motions in trance and behave similarly during revival from trance.

13. In therapy, MPD patients' feelings need to be recalled, remembered, and processed consciously if they are to recede into the past as memories. Suryani encountered the same process when utilizing hypnotherapy with Balinese who were possessed under hypnosis.
14. When MPD patients switch from one personality to another, they undergo a process identical to that in hypnosis; specifically, the individual goes into hypnosis and the personality seems to disappear as if hidden, like a second personality. The second 'personality' (comparable to the possessed entity) then appears or emerges into the 'real world' as if he is no longer under hypnosis. In Bali this phenomenon is observed in persons in trance at ceremonies, in trance mediums, and in hypnotherapy patients.
15. MPD patients are often aware of detachment or a depersonalization experience as if they are observing the behaviour of the second personality. Out-of-body experiences are reported by patients with MPD (Ross et al., 1989). The same phenomenon is observed in Balinese trancers and patients possessed in hypnotherapy: they are aware of the possessed 'person' (spirit), and they may converse with him/her and report their observations of the possessed entity.
16. The alters of MPD serve a variety of functions for the person, including acting out repressed or split-off desires or impulses that would occasion guilt or shame (e.g. aggression, suicide, and sexuality). Possession in the Balinese and other cultures demonstrates similar psychodynamics and probably serves similar functions.
17. Possessed Balinese who are aware of their behaviour or who are amnesic may feel compelled to behave in ways that are contrary to their values, wishes, or ordinary judgement as seen in individual and ceremonial trances. Similar 'influence' experiences are very common in MPD (Kluft, 1987a; Putnam, 1991; Ross, Norton, and Wozney, 1989).
18. MPDs regard alters as taking over, or sharing their bodies. The Balinese view possession similarly.

19. The personalities may have considerable investment in their own separateness and express a pseudo-delusional degree of conviction about their being separate and autonomous (Kluft, 1984b). The same quality is prominent in the Balinese trance-mediums.
20. The alters of MPD may be subtle, barely noticeable, or clearly evident and dramatic as in the case of possession.
21. Patients' recognition of their personalities is variable: 'Some are known to patients, but usually they exist in a twilight zone of dim consciousness or are totally out of awareness.' (Bliss, 1986: 149.) The Balinese are generally only dimly aware of the possessions and often not at all until asked about them.
22. Events experienced under hypnosis, such as a vision or a ghost, if remembered after coming out of hypnosis, may be believed by the subject. This was true of the Balinese school-children who experienced visual and auditory hallucinations during a trance-possession epidemic.
23. MPD patients come into therapy disavowing responsibility for the actions of their alters (Ross, 1990). Similarly, the Balinese believe that their behaviour during a possession is the responsibility of the entity.
24. As many as 80 per cent of patients known to have MPD have periods (sometimes a year or more) in which their symptoms are suppressed, or disavowed, and thus unrecognized (Kluft, 1985, 1987a). Intermittency is a characteristic of possession.
25. Only a small proportion—10 per cent—of MPD patients are exhibitionistic in their condition (Kluft, 1985). Similarly, only a small percentage of Balinese in possession show exhibitionistic behaviour.
26. MPD patients have been described as influenced by the cultural patterns and beliefs of Western historical times when life was replete with mysterious spirits, deities, and powers in the world (Frazer, 1935). The world of the Balinese is similarly populated with spirits, deities, and other powers (Bateson and Mead, 1942; Jensen and Suryani, 1992).
27. 'Characterological factors, cultural influences, imagination, intelligence, and creativity, make powerful contributions to the form taken by [MPD] personalities.' (Kluft, 1991a: 166.) The same factors shape the forms of possession in the Balinese.
28. The Balinese frequently report that preceding trance-possession they perceive a darkness, as well as a narrowing of awareness of stimuli in their environment, which is characteristic of the

hypnotic state. A patient with MPD studied by Bliss (1986: 125) reported a feeling of 'being pulled into darkness' as the alter took over. She stated, 'In deep hypnosis you give up, are calm, totally numb, your body is relaxed and you can't move. The next and final step is you are gone—everything is black. When Lisa (a personality) takes over it is the same thing.' Bliss regarded this switch to an alter as a self-hypnosis phenomenon. One of Jensen's MPD patients described a sensation of 'darkness like a curtain' falling in front of her for a second or two with switches to some of her many alters: 'It feels cold, dark, and forbidding. Everything seems to be in darkness, even on a bright sunny day.'

29. Many alters reveal their names consciously, and MPD patients often give names to each of their alters, similar to the way a child names favourite dolls who possess animate or lifelike qualities and familiar 'personalities'. A god who chooses to possess a *balian* is eminently familiar to the *balian* and he/she may know it by its common name or the name it reveals to the *balian*.
30. The Balinese hypnotherapy patients resembled MPD patients in the manner of resolution: the possession states in hypnotherapy disappeared after the individuals became aware of the nature of the possession and assimilated its demands and wishes into their conscious activities.
31. The possession state of the Balinese often provides secondary gain to the person, as for example by serving as an outlet for emotions and behaviour not permitted in the ordinary lifestyle of the culture. Similarly, the alter personality of MPD brings secondary gain in the sense of avoiding pain or unbearable distress to the individual (e.g. it allows the person to act out behaviour not acceptable to his conscious self).
32. The gods or spirits of possessed Balinese speak and/or act through the individual and may give the appearance of a personality very different from the individual's usual one—characteristics sensed inwardly by the individual. This was evident in the trance-mediums and some dancers. The alters of MPD share these characteristics.
33. MPD alters (Kluft, 1991a) and possessed Balinese may experience and represent themselves as being of different ages, genders, races, religions, sexual orientations, and as holding contrasting values and belief systems.
34. Typically alter personality and possession state switches of

Balinese are accompanied by changes in facies, speech (pitch, rate, accent, and language usage), motor activity, cognitive processes, affect, behavioural repertoire, memory retrieval, and sense of self (Krippner, 1987; Pattison and Wintrob, 1981; Putnam, 1988, 1989, 1991: 152; Ravenscroft, 1965).

35. Severe headache is a common symptom of MPD patients, and it usually becomes worse during personality changes (Coons, 1988). A few Balinese reported experiencing headaches during the onset of possession states.
36. The triggering stimulus for the actual switch of the Balinese into the possession state is not generally clear to the individual, although it is evident in cases involving the voice of Rangda or prayers used by the *balian* and priests. Similarly, the trigger for MPD patients' switches into alters is also not usually clear to the individual. Often, it is as if they were taken over by surprise and unaware of the internal or external stimuli precipitating the switch.

In the Balinese possession state an entity takes over the person and they believe that it is God, a god, or a spirit. In MPD an entity takes over the person and he and his society believe that it is another 'personality'.[26] It is evident that the conventional cultural beliefs play a large role in the form of expression of the two similar conditions.

The foregoing similarities support the contention in this book that normal Balinese in trance with possession, persons with possession disorders, and patients in hypnosis with possession share many of the same experiences and consequences characteristic of MPD alter states.

However, while personalities of MPD patients in many ways resemble Balinese in trance states with possession, it is important to note a number of differences between MPD and possession:

1. MPD alter states sometimes last longer than the Balinese possession states. An alternate personality may last a month or sometimes a year or more (Bliss, 1984a).
2. In the Balinese, the duration of the state is controlled (terminated) by traditional techniques.
3. MPD alters are generally children or people and MPD rarely involves supernatural entities as does possession. This characteristic of MPD is understandable since the alters generally developed in childhood or youth as split-off parts of the individual's personality, whereas possessions generally manifest themselves in adulthood in religious contexts.

4. MPD is believed to be created out of repeated dissociation experiences that occur under extreme stress, whereas possession in the Balinese appears to be a process that can spontaneously and suddenly appear without apparent previous dissociations due to stress. A possible explanation is that spirits have already been created and they exist in the 'ethnic unconscious' (Devereaux, 1956) and in each Balinese unconscious over a lifetime.
5. The possession state is often followed by a period of peace and calm, an experience infrequently noted and/or of shorter duration than that felt by MPD patients after switching from their alters.
6. Possession occurs in a much higher proportion in the Balinese population than does MPD in Western populations. This may be explained by the society's facilitation and support, and the value and usefulness that it serves in Balinese society. By contrast, in the West, possession and MPD are considered pathological and undesirable. The only exceptions to this are the arcane Western trance channellers, Western trance-mediums, and some religious cults.
7. Possessions are generally believed by the person to come from outside her/himself, whereas most MPD patients perceive that most of their alters are harboured within themselves.[27] This difference appears to be primarily a function of personality development and cultural beliefs: most possessed spirits exist in the supernatural world 'out there'; and the alters of MPD have developed over time (as dissociations) within the individual. Western psychological theory can regard entities in both cases as dissociated components of the personality.
8. Possessed trance-mediums demonstrate psychic abilities such as clairvoyance and extrasensory perception,[28] whereas MPD patients do not.
9. Most possessed Balinese are not self-destructive or suicidal, whereas MPD alters frequently are.
10. MPD patients show a degree of impairment from minimal to profound (Kluft, 1991a), although in earlier stages there may be no impairment. With the exception of possession constituting a disorder (e.g. *bebainan* and *kasurupan*), possession does not result in impairment.

While alter personalities in MPD and Balinese in possession are in many aspects similar, phenomenologically, the psychosociocultural causes of each and the ways in which each culture regards them are different.

1. In the West, the alter of MPD is regarded theoretically as a defence (i.e. dissociation) against or a psychological response to affects associated with emotional traumas; in the Balinese, possession is a response to (and is expected by) the culture. It is conceivable that possession in some Balinese, particularly when it represents a disorder such as ***bebainan***, may be a mechanism or 'defence' to deal with fearful beliefs or anxiety-laden conflicts.
2. In the West, most types of possession represent a symptomatic state, whereas in Bali most represent normal behaviour, either in ceremonies or as used by ***balian***.
3. The Balinese have socialized the phenomenon of possession occurring in the presence of others, whereas in the West, the alter of MPD remains a socially isolated phenomenon, generally expressing itself within the individual.

Similarities and differences in the psychological processes of MPD and trance-medium possession are listed in Table 9.2.

TABLE 9.2
Psychological Process Similarities and Differences in Trance-medium Possession and MPD Alter Personality

Trance-medium Possession	*MPD Alter Personality*
Occurs in religious contexts	Occurs in non-religious contexts
Enters trance by self	Enters self-hypnosis
Power or spirit takes over	Alter personality 'comes out'
Possession perceived as coming from outside self	Alter usually perceived as existing within self
Believed to be chosen by gods; may be unpremeditated	Chosen by alter or unpremeditated
Psychic abilities	No psychic abilities
Accesses individual's conscious and unconscious	Accesses individual's conscious and unconscious
Acts through the individual's body	Acts through the individual's body
Switches at will with prayer	Occasionally may switch into an alter at will but generally not consciously controlled
Not self-destructive or suicidal	Often self-destructive and suicidal
Duration of minutes to hours	Duration of minutes to hours but may last for days
Abrupt onset and termination	Abrupt onset and termination
Terminated by the possession and/or by conscious will	Terminated by the alter; generally no conscious control of termination

If MPD is posited as a process similar to possession, the question about duration arises: why would some MPD dissociative episodes last so much longer than trance-possession, sometimes weeks or months?[29] The answer may lie in the lack of institutionalized socio-cultural control of possession in the West and of dissociative disorders in Bali and the West. In Bali, the person is generally brought out of trance-possession by ritual sprinkling of holy water over him by a socially recognized spiritual person, such as a priest. Because trance-possession is socially and publicly controlled, everyone present, including the person in trance, trusts, expects, and is aware of the termination. *Balian* have practised bringing themselves out of possession at will, just as they have learnt to fall into trance-possession, essentially at will. They enter trance-possession by ritual prayer, mantra, and incense smoke and terminate it when the possessed God or god says he is finished by carrying out a brief ritual with prayer. By contrast, persons with MPD have developed relatively little conscious control over their alter states. Rather, the unconscious mind controls coming out of an alter state, in the same way that it generally controls switching to an alter. Although some of Jensen's MPD patients could switch to an alter at will, only one was able to terminate them at will, i.e. to consciously and reliably switch back to his/her usual personality. MPD patients are at the mercy or behest of the alter(s). One adolescent MPD patient could switch out of some alters at Jensen's request or suggestion. Two adult patients could sometimes prevent an alter from taking over by exerting great conscious effort or by getting support from the therapist. It can be hypothesized that if the patients with MPD had the internal ability, or if there were institutionalized (culturally accepted) standard procedures to terminate MPD alter states, they might not necessarily last so long. With regard to duration of alter episodes, MPD can be considered a possession process out of control, both societally and individually. Hindrances to assisted termination are that often the MPD herself/himself is the only person who is aware of the manifestation of the different personality states, and conversely, some MPDs are not consciously aware of their alters.

The fact that there are a number of phenomenological differences noted between MPD and possession in the Balinese, in addition to the broad array of symptoms and wide variations in the clinical presentation of MPD patients, does not detract from the hypothesis that both represent fundamentally the same psychobiological process. It must be borne in mind that MPD represents the outcome of a basic psychobiological process overlain with complex psychosocial, developmental, personality, and cultural factors. The cultural overlay and psychological factors determining the behavioural patterns of possession in the Balinese are much fewer and simpler than those of MPD patients.

Although MPD does not appear to occur as a clinical disorder in the Balinese at the present time, such cases probably exist; however they are likely to be regarded as possession. One type of *balian* that might appear to be a multiple personality is the trance-medium described in Chapter 3. This woman takes on a totally different but consistent personality as manifested by her behaviour, speaking voice, and attitude on a regular basis when she is invited by her god. She has a special name for the god that takes over in her trance-possession state. When she comes out of trance-possession, she is amnesic with regard to the episode. In her usual state, she knows that she is a *balian* and she and her assistants make elaborate preparations for her work in healing but she does not know what she does in trance-possession. Similarly, most MPD patients have 'named' personalities and many are amnesic with regard to them. In contrast to MPD, however, this *balian*'s switches to her possession state are very predictable, structured, and socially congruent, and she is rewarded by her clients in the form of offerings of money and status. These factors distinguish her possession state from that of MPD, in which personalities generally switch unpredictably without preparation and engage in behaviours which do not have a socially sanctioned and institutionalized role in the society. This *balian* is not regarded by the Balinese as having a mental disorder. Nevertheless, she fits the *DSM-III-R* (APA, 1987) diagnostic criteria for the mental disorder called MPD: specifically, the existence within her of two distinct personalities or personality states (each with its own relatively enduring pattern of perceiving, relating to, and thinking about the environment and self) which recurrently take full control of her behaviour. It is obvious from this incongruity that the Western psychiatric definition of MPD is not completely appropriate for Balinese culture. In such cases of seeming multiple personality and possession states in Balinese, the culture as etiologic and the cultural context as determinant of form must be taken into account in order to correctly comprehend them in Western terms.

Since self-hypnosis or spontaneous trance is very common in the Balinese, and their trances generally include possession, the authors hypothesized that, if self-hypnosis is the cause of MPD as proposed by Bliss (1984a), it would be very common among them. Therefore, it came as a surprise not to find any cases of MPD in Bali.

One possible explanation for the apparent absence of MPD in the Balinese derived from a study of juvenile delinquency in Bali (D. Rosenthal, personal communication). In a survey of all juvenile delinquency cases in 1990 and from interviews with counsellors of schoolchildren, no cases or even indications of child abuse were found. It appears that this abnormal child-rearing practice, which is a common underlying etiologic factor in MPD, is extremely rare in Balinese society. This finding indirectly supports the theory that MPD is commonly an outcome of traumatic child sexual abuse. However, not all cases of MPD have a history of sexual abuse; the abuse can be sexual, physical, or psychological, considered separately or together. A few cases are just unhappy children with excellent hypnotic capabilities who feel estranged and periodically turn to their hypnotic world and/or imaginary playmates for social interaction (Kluft, 1984c).

It has been noted in India that the possession syndrome is very common (Varma, Srivastava, and Sahay, 1970) while MPD is very rare (Adityanjee and Khandelwal, 1989: 1610). The hypothesis was advanced that 'possession syndrome in India and multiple personality disorder in the West represent parallel dissociative disorders with similar etiologies despite some major differences in clinical profiles'. The cases of MPD reported in Indians differed from most Western cases in that they experienced only minor stress in adolescence and had not suffered massive trauma or child abuse.

The question of the existence of MPD in Bali remains open. The Western experience may be illuminating. Western psychiatrists who would have assumed that MPD is rare 20 years ago have now come to see it as being more common. It is no longer unusual in the United States. To date, most cases have been identified by using descriptive phenomena. An objective assessment instrument to help diagnose MPD, the Structured Clinical Interview for DSM-III-R Dissociative Disorders, is now available (Steinberg, Rounsaville, and Cicchetti, 1990). Another scale that can corroborate the diagnosis of MPD is the Dissociative Experiences Scale (Bernstein and Putnam, 1986). This provides quantitative measures of 28 common types of dissociative experiences and MPD patients score in the range of 40–50 per cent, significantly higher than normal subjects. These instruments could be translated into Indonesian and used in Bali to better identify now obscure cases. Loewenstein (1991) described an interview protocol for assessment of dissociative disorders, including MPD, which greatly increases the probability of clinicians identifying them.

Given that it is common for the Balinese to be possessed and that some trance-mediums when possessed act like alter personalities of MPD, the question of whether the psychological processes of possession and MPD are alike was asked. The answer is 'yes' in the Western sense that both are similar forms of dissociation in which the individual changes into and temporarily acts as another entity, personality, or spirit. But one wonders why the Balinese have one characteristic pattern of dissociation, i.e. trance with possession by gods or spirits, while Westerners manifest another, i.e. an alter personality. The answer to this question lies partially in the significant differences between the characteristic personality structure of Westerners and that of the Balinese.

An apparent absence of MPD in the Balinese would suggest that Westerners have certain psychosocial characteristics necessary to manifest MPD. One such possible characteristic to be considered is the psychological concept of a 'unitary' personality. A 'unitary' personality may be necessary for the emergence of multiple personalities, i.e. the emergence of an alter personality depends on the concept of a personality unit from which it can separate. In the case of the Balinese, C. Geertz (1966), a cultural anthropologist, theorized that the concept of personhood, or personal identity, which may be synonymous with personality, is concealed, anonymous, and 'depersonalized'; thereby, individual 'personality' is submerged, unidentified, muted, or concealed. Geertz believed that social interaction of the Balinese is highly ceremonialized, and feelings of *lek* (fear of embarrassing oneself or an ever-present concern about making a *faux pas*) tend to keep individual 'personality' or personal identity of the Balinese from showing. Based on his view, it could be hypothesized that a factor responsible for MPD being virtually absent in the Balinese is a 'personality' that is not readily accessible to them. However, questions can be raised about the validity of C. Geertz's view of Balinese 'personhood' on the issue of *lek*. There is no doubt that *lek* exists but it probably does not play a pervasive or dominant role in everyday social interaction (Jensen and Suryani, 1992).

Connor (1984), a cultural anthropologist, set forth a relevant view in her analysis of Balinese 'personhood' (personality). She proposed the concept of 'unbounded self': i.e. Balinese personhood is not unitary, as in the West, but a personality composed of a fusion of self and macrocosmos (*buana agung*), both natural and supernatural, e.g. sibling spirits or souls and an intermediary spirit (*taksu*). Such an 'unbounded' self would constitute a significant difference between Balinese and Western personality.

The authors' data from persons in trance-possession raise questions about whether the consciously expressed personality of the Balinese is entirely 'unbounded' with respect to some spiritual experiences. For example, persons with trance-possession experience spoke of a force, spirit, or god, outside of themselves, who 'comes down', influences their behaviour, or acts for them but who is not part of them. Consistent with this is the fact that *balian* and the society in general regard the acts of a person in trance-possession as being done not by the person but rather by the possessor for whom the individual has no responsibility. In Suryani's view, the Balinese consciously consider most aspects of the macrocosmos as parts of their world and as influencing them but not as aspects of their own personality. The authors' data indicate that *balian* can access their own intermediary spirit (*taksu*), who may help them communicate with the gods, but contrary to Connor's view, they do not regard their *taksu* as part of themselves.

Nevertheless, it is true that the Balinese live in an interconnected world and universe of all things and, in this sense, they are less separate from and are more accessible to both nature and the spiritual world than are Westerners. This psychosocial difference between cultures is significant and is difficult for most Westerners to fully comprehend because they have not grown up with (and thus internalized) such religious beliefs. The authors view the Balinese as having boundaries in some respects, but as being closer to the natural world than Westerners and more susceptible to shifts into the supernatural world, as may be seen in their possession experiences.

In support of the unbounded self concept, the Balinese personality can be described as non-unitary in that it incorporates many supernatural entities. From birth to six months of age, a person is a supernatural human; he/she has an ancestor's spirit, as well as spirits of his/her own (i.e. sibling spirits; see Chapter 1), and throughout life he is an integral part of various groups and his community. The Balinese have long perceived spirits as being part of the self in a manner comparable to the MPD's perception of alters. The sibling spirits offer a good example. The infant is born with four 'sibling spirits' which after the 6-month ceremony unify and become one with the spirit of the soul. The 'siblings' then become two kinds of spirits, Kala and Dewa. The spirit Kala is responsible for a person's bad thoughts, emotions, and deeds; if a person is angry, it is believed that Kala has influenced him. Good emotions, thoughts, and deeds are attributed to the other spirit, Dewa: when one is calm, Dewa is in the ascendant. These spirits of the individual continue to influence the soul throughout life and they have the power to help him at work and guard him against his enemies. They are given care and offerings by the individual. Failure to do so properly could result in the spirits causing illness. At death the individual's soul (*atman*) becomes unified with God or awaits reincarnation and the sibling spirits of the individual return to their source (i.e. water, fire, soil, and air). A Balinese traditional healer or an individual dissociates in trance and, in Western conceptualization, accesses entities like the lifelong personally known aspects of themselves, such as spirits or gods, and other culturally respected spirits which have always been integral and intimate parts of their personal world.

The theoretical concept of multiple 'ego states' of Westerners discussed by Klemperer (1965) and Watkins and Watkins (1979) is relevant to the concept of unitary and multiple personalities. They viewed certain ego states (i.e. certain configurations of thinking, feeling, and perception integrated around a common principle) as repressed, dissociated, or split off from consciousness but exerting influence over behaviour and feelings of the main ego state. Some of these ego states may be involved in symptom formation and in the case of MPD, such a dissociated ego state may act autonomously. These ego states may be contacted during trance/hypnosis.

What may be termed the unitary and the non-unitary personalities of the Westerner and Balinese respectively could be crucial in the processes of multiple personality and possession. Given that the personality in Westerners is unitary, existence of more than one personality in the individual implies separate entities. Although in theory, a multiple personality dissociates in trance to call upon parts of oneself, i.e. personalities or 'configurations' of consciousness (Kluft, 1988: 51; Putnam, 1989: 103) which have developed as a result of repeated dissociation in earlier life, for the individual these parts or reconfigurations (alters) develop to virtually take on a life of their own.

This book proposes that the psychobiological mechanism and the phenomenology of MPD and possession both in the West and in Bali are similar if not the same; MPD alters are viewed as psychological entities equivalent to Balinese possessions. From the point of view of process, they are similar. MPD patients and possessed Balinese report similar experiences: some other entity or part of the self that to them has a real existence takes over. The two states may also serve the same ends in terms of the healthy expression of feelings and behaviours not otherwise permitted by the individual's ego or conscious state.

However, the thought content of the two conditions differs and it is important to recognize that the particular cause of and motivation for the 'like-kind' possession take-over in the two cultures differ. In the West, the multiple personality person's motivation to dissociate generally appears to be anxiety, fear, or avoidance of intolerable stress, terror, or distress stemming from reverberating traumatic experiences of early childhood, particularly sexual abuse. In Bali, the possessed one is motivated to dissociate by strong, positive, cultural sanctions to receive the privilege and to enhance family and community. As a consequence of these causal and motivational differences, it could be expected that the behaviour and/or symptomatologies of the conditions in the two cultures would differ in many ways.

Based on the findings presented in the foregoing chapters, the authors propose to expand the self-hypnosis theory of the process of MPD (Bliss, 1984a) to the following: self-hypnosis or trance with the possession process. The term self-hypnosis is used in the sense specified by Bliss (1984a): a rapid, usually unpremeditated withdrawal into a trance, a dissociation. This theory combines readily with the PTSD theory of MPD (D. Spiegel, 1984).

The concept of possessions as comparable to MPD alters need not be negated or confused by Western psychological concepts of MPD, including that of 'dissociated components of a single personality' as argued by Ross (1990). He viewed MPD patients as having only one personality, as they are only one person in one body and pointed out that 'the term personality is simply a convenient, historically sanctioned label for the dissociated states characteristic of the disorder'. The Balinese view possession as an aspect of their individual world of self.

It could be argued that the use of the concept of possession for understanding the alter states of MPD could be counter-productive if it implies that a supernatural outside-of-self entity (i.e. not a part of the individual) has taken over the individual, since the long-term goal in the treatment of MPD is to help the patients deal with alters as parts of themselves in a unified personality. Perhaps the important concept for the MPD patients to develop is that they dissociate into apparent separate entities, which periodically take over their behaviour and bodies, without viewing them as having an existence outside of their true personhood or personality. Trance-mediumship is a suitable model of MPD in this respect because trance-mediumship is a positive and useful process of possession (take-over) and, furthermore, it incorporates self-control. It can also be harnessed and utilized for the good of the individual, the family, and the community.

It is recognized that advancing the concept of MPD as a process of trance with possession carries the risk of confusing MPD with possession disorder. The two conditions are different clinically but share the same mechanism of dissociation. There are as yet insufficient clinical experiences and case reports of possession disorder in the West to enable clear differentiation from MPD, except in classical cases of each condition. Two helpful generalizations are: (1) in contrast to MPD, possession disorders are of shorter duration; and (2) once the possession leaves the person, it does not usually recur.

For most Westerners, the term 'possession' conjures up in the mind certain characteristics, especially an intruding malevolent spirit. Unfortunately, this idea can be misleading in terms of MPD. However, there does not seem to be a simple, better term for the possession-like phenomenon of MPD. Basic clinical elements of MPD and possession are the takeover phenomena with changes in identity, but this awkward and lengthy terminology would be limiting if it were to be used for the shorthand labelling of the mechanism of MPD.

Although a case has been made here to view MPD and possession as a similar psychobiological process, it remains to be proven. A conceivable way to do this is by neuropsychophysiological study (Braun, 1983; Putnam, 1984; Putnam, Zahn, and Post, 1990). Preliminary attempts have been made by utilizing concepts of state dependent learning to explain creation of alters, switching, and psychophysiologic characteristics of MPD (Braun, 1984a). MPD subjects have shown distinct physiologic differences across alter states (Putnam, Zahn, and Post, 1990). Coons's (1988) review of the literature on electroencephalographic (EEG) studies of MPD indicated that changes in alpha rhythm probably reflect 'the degree of arousal and tension across different personality states'. The EEGs (alpha, beta, and theta waves) of channellers while in trance and 'possessed' by an entity are distinctly and, statistically, significantly different compared with EEGs of persons in hypnosis (Hughes and Melville, 1990), who have not shown any clear-cut changes from the normal or non-hypnotic state (Putnam, 1991). This supports the concept that the trance-possession state is a neurophysiological state qualitatively distinct from simple hypnosis. Evoked potential measurements on EEG were found to be different for alters of MPD patients (Putnam, 1984). It would be desirable to do EEG studies on Balinese in trance-possession states but to pursue these at present presents technical and cultural problems. It must be recognized that all physiological studies so far have not been replicated and EEGs are not yet reliable indicators of MPD. Further research will be required to confirm and interpret EEG findings (Coons, 1988). Advances in biobehavioural research including the neurotransmitters (Demetrack et al., 1990) may eventually add to basic explanations.

Therapeutic Implications of MPD as a Trance-possession Process

A final consideration is the hypothetical and/or practical, therapeutic, and clinical implications of the relationship between possession and MPD. The treatment of MPD patients is a highly arduous and taxing endeavour for both therapist and patient. Many therapists are unwilling to undertake it, and those who do so continually seek to upgrade and add to their skills. When trance-possession of normal individuals is viewed as a psychobiological process like that of MPD patients, new questions may be asked about this disorder which can lead to a better understanding of it, both in terms of etiology and therapy.

It is possible to generalize that a knowledge of the possession state of the Balinese, including the helping and controlling techniques of the persons who assist possessed persons, can help therapists in several ways: (1) gain a sharper focus on a number of the characteristic patterns which are exhibited by MPD patients; (2) provide a perspective that alerts therapists to things they have not yet seen because they have not thought of them; and (3) suggest ideas for a therapist's demeanour and armamentarium for managing switches of difficult-to-control MPD alters. There are several issues that therapists should bear in mind:

1. It is necessary for the therapist to ask the patient specific questions which will identify the alter state(s) of MPD and differentiate it from possession disorder, other dissociative disorders, syndromes, or psychoses.
2. The instantaneous, as well as the more gradual, switching from one state to another by possessed Balinese and MPDs helps

therapists appreciate and gain insight into the underlying psychophysiology.

3. The involuntariness and lack of control, sometimes with associated bewilderment of both the possessed Balinese and MPD patient, helps the therapist understand the phenomenon of take-over of the body and the patient's inability to switch at will.
4. It is useful to appreciate the realness of the experience of both possessions and alters of MPD and their power to influence the behaviour and feelings of the person.
5. There is the concept of a shared body.
6. The patient has a range of degrees of consciousness in the presence and activities of a possession and/or alter(s).
7. The patient exhibits degrees of amnesia, ranging from partial to complete, and there are possibilities for the therapist to enhance recall.
8. There is a need for psychosocial support and understanding and sometimes positive physical assistance and restraint, especially when a possession or an alter is threatening or violent.
9. There is a need to believe in possessions and alters, to trust that they will disappear, and to maintain one's optimism about a favourable outcome.
10. It is necessary for therapists and persons who assist possessed persons or alters to be friendly, strong, unafraid, and respectful of them in these states whether they are co-operative or physically uncontrolled and violent. It is helpful to the patient when the therapist shows an understanding of the possession or alter by not reacting to his or her threatening behaviour with fear or anxiety. In the management of acute and crisis conditions of MPD patients, Kluft (1989) emphasized that it is important for the staff to be supportive, consistent, predictable, and [firm within] set limits. These techniques are vividly and graphically evident in the Balinese who help persons in ceremonial trance-possession. In addition to all this, the 'assisting' Balinese offer the possessed persons firm control and guidance, which prevent them from going wildly out of control or hurting themselves. It is illuminating to see the 'assisting' Balinese maintain such control and not be led into traps by the possessed individual. The potential for such problems as splitting of staff (e.g. staff taking opposite sides in response to patients' complaints about staff behaviour), sexual seduction by the patient,[30] or failure to predict serious

consequences by alters is amply demonstrated in mental health personnel's management of MPD patients (Watkins and Watkins, 1984).

11. There is a need for therapists to acquire and use timely effective state-terminating techniques, including hypnotherapy and Amytal interview, to switch the patient's self-destructive, threatening, violent, and socially decompensating alters.
12. It is useful to bear in mind both the psychosocial benefits and hazards of dissociative states for the possessed person and the MPD patient (Watkins and Watkins, 1984). For possessed Balinese and MPD patients, the dissociative state often has a secondary gain (e.g. personal attention). While some patients view dissociation as a coping mechanism, they can also stop using it and utilize other less problematic mechanisms, as seen with successfully treated MPD and other dissociative disorders (Goodman, 1988: 85).

The concept that possession, as described in this book, and MPD are equivalent in terms of process has other therapeutic implications. MPD patients frequently lament that for years doctors and therapists, as well as family and friends, did not recognize the true nature of their problem and did not understand them. This is no wonder in view of the puzzling behaviour they usually present and the scepticism, misapprehensions, and confusion surrounding the disorder (Ross, 1990). These distressed patients desperately want their hapless plight to be understood by someone, especially mental health professionals. The therapist may acquire an increased degree of understanding of the process of MPD by acquiring a knowledge of and familiarity with the allied normal process of trance-possession. Such an understanding will be sensed and appreciated by the patient and help build his trust and confidence in the therapist, thereby strengthening the therapeutic alliance.

General basic long-term aims of the treatment of MPD are to help the patient develop an awareness and acceptance that he/she is fundamentally one personality, just as he/she is one body, by enabling he/she to resolve conflicts and to gain control of precipitating and associated feelings so that they no longer result in the uncontrolled dissociation of the dysfunctional alter(s) (Beahrs, 1982; Bliss, 1986; Kluft, 1984a; Putnam, 1989). To accomplish these goals, a therapist generally helps the patient abreact (re-experience) painful, often repressed, unconscious memories and deal with psychological issues that are avoided or coped with by dissociating. Such objectives are not necessarily inconsistent with a conceptualization of MPD as a possession-like phenomenon. In the long term, there is the 'devilish' problem of the chronic use of self-hypnosis: it is a long-practised entrenched habit and old habits are hard to break (E. L. Bliss, personal communication).

MPD patients may require acute hospitalization because of self-mutilation, suicide threats or attempts, or aggressive antisocial behaviour. Some patients have a history of 50 or more such hospitalizations of relatively brief duration over a period of a number of years. It is generally their alters that cause the crises and they may be precipitated by perceived rejection, often seemingly slight, such as neglect by a family member or the absence of their therapist due to vacation. In these instances, a short-term goal is to stabilize the patient so that he/she is no longer suicidal and self-mutilating. A number of hypnotherapy techniques have been explicated, such as putting the alter 'to sleep' and calling forth protective alters (Kluft, 1989). Generally, the patients must switch out of their threatening alters and facilitating this is a short-term therapeutic goal. Under these conditions, therapists may utilize the Balinese concepts of a strong network of social support and co-operation with the patient and possession (alters), and unswerving expectation of the switch.

The phenomenon of Balinese switching out of possession states may have a parallel in MPD switching. The following vignette of an MPD patient is illustrative. A 45-year-old woman with a history of multiple hospital admissions because of suicide attempts and self-mutilation was admitted to the in-patient psychiatric unit because of suicide ideation. After one day of hospital service, the alter had left her and she seemed ready for discharge. However, she suddenly relapsed with anxiety and suicide ideation caused by another alter taking over; this continued unabated for four days in spite of support, encouragement, and psychotherapy. Switching was finally accomplished by an Amytal interview conducted jointly by the patient's regular psychotherapist (from outside the hospital) and Jensen serving as the hospital psychiatrist administering the Amytal. The psychotherapeutic interview under the influence of Amytal[31] succeeded in relieving her of the 'possession' by the threatening alter, and allowed her to switch back to her usual personality, permitting resumption of her usual state and discharge from the hospital the following day.

Selected patients may find it helpful in understanding their condition by conceptualizing their alter personalities as possession-like processes in some respects (i.e. valued, respected, or even frightening entities that take over their body/mind).[32] It is important to caution that this approach would be advisable only with patients for whom the term 'possessed' connotes a positive concept and for whom it does not have a negative or frightening connotation, as it has for many Westerners and particularly for MPDs who have suffered in Satanic cults. The next step would be to help the patient, possibly by suggestion, to accept such inside-based entities or 'possessions' (i.e. alter personalities) as split off parts of himself/herself and as potentially reintegratable parts or components of his/her whole self. The ultimate realistic and optimistic aim of psychotherapy is to help the patient reconstitute a single personality, or alternatively to bring about co-operation among the conflictual or destructive entities.

In the following case, a psychotherapist or hypnotherapist might conceivably utilize the concept of MPD as a benign type of possession phenomenon to develop the patient's insight. An MPD patient related part of her experience this way:

> All my life I knew I lost time and it seemed like I was watching [myself] from afar and I experienced the arguments [of the alters] but I didn't know they were entities. I didn't know I was a multiple personality. Almost all of my alters have come to realize it by now although there are still a few sceptics. This idea [of entities] made sense and explained all that I couldn't explain all my life. No one helped me understand it. I came to this view by myself.

The issue of responsibility for one's behaviour has conceptual and therapeutic significance for possession and MPD. Both the normal possession and abnormal (disorder) states of the Balinese and the alters of MPD are characterized by a relative lack of personal control (involuntariness) of the switch into or out of the states and by denial of personal responsibility for behaviour in the state. Non-disorder possession in Bali is a socially responsible action, while MPD in the West is not. In Bali, and other societies in which possession occurs as a socially integrated act, it is controlled and supported by the family and the community. It is also highly acceptable and valued and it works very well for society and the individual. MPD has not been integrated into society. Patients generally receive too little support from their family, friends, and community. It is not an acceptable or valued behaviour, and it is often incapacitating to the individual. A perspective on Balinese possession suggests that it would be useful in the management of MPD for the patient, families, mental health workers, clergymen, social agencies, and society in general to accept and assume greater responsibility, as well as to develop techniques, for supporting and assisting patients in the control of their dissociative states and behaviours. MPD patients need a consistent, reliable resource network, ancillary to therapy, preferably with an in-patient facility safety net. This network would further help individual MPD patients develop ways to take personal responsibility for their states in a manner analogous to the Balinese trance-medium, i.e. creatively and without guilt or blame.

The case of a 39-year-old woman with MPD illustrates the need for a positive, therapeutic, family and community support network for the patient. In the course of over 100 hospitalizations, mostly for self-mutilation or suicide attempts, her pastor was generally tolerant of her, her son tried to help but felt frustrated, a counsellor told her that it was all her fault, suicide prevention crisis workers asked her about her suicidal impulses and referred her to the usual sources of help, the clinic psychiatrist did not believe that she had MPD, and the mental hospitals and psychiatry clinics diagnosed her as a combination of borderline personality disorder, dysthymic disorder, and adjustment disorder, for which she had been prescribed neuroleptics and antidepressants, none of which helped. None of her friends or relatives were helpful, and nobody really understood her plight, pain, frustration, and need to understand what was really happening to her. She was unable to find anyone in the mental health system who could understand her. Her recent experience with psychiatric care in which she was diagnosed and managed as a case of MPD was highly reassuring to her and consequently she sought out therapists who understood MPD, and resources in her community which could provide support, particularly at times of anxiety and suicidal crises. Consequently, she began to trust others and be more open rather than withdraw into herself and conceal her alter states.

Another area of possible application of the non-Western possession concept pertains to MPD patients' potential for self-control of dissociation. Kluft (1989) has pointed out the therapeutic value in helping MPD patients develop a sense of control over themselves, including their alters which may 'run away' with them. Extrapolating from the Balinese trance-medium phenomenon, the therapist may introduce the concept of termination when contacting and exploring each alter's personality with the patient, especially in hypnotherapy. It is conceivable that by so doing the patient could be helped to develop control of dissociation tendencies by learning to self-terminate (i.e. switch off) the alter personalities as trance-mediums do in a state of possession. Such control would be helpful in reducing distress from alters and limiting episodes of psychosocial decompensation, including suicidality. This becomes of critical therapeutic importance because one of the serious problems of MPD patients is created by an alter who resists leaving (i.e. switching off) and threatens to torture or kill the patient.

The contagious quality of trance-possession may have implications for therapy. Trance by contagion was observed in a number of situations in Bali, including communal trance-possession (Chapter 4), dance (Chapter 5), and mass hysteria in schoolchildren (Chapter 7). It afflicts a person or persons in immediate association with the possessed person, it is generally unexpected by the individual, and it is often dramatic. Given that MPD patients' switch to an alter personality is a dissociative mechanism or trance-possession phenomenon, and that dissociation is a normal psychological mechanism of Westerners, it could be expected that there is the potential for contagion. It is conceivable that Western staff and therapists working with MPD patients are at risk for dissociating and experiencing self-hypnosis when dealing directly with the MPD patients and that this could contribute to various problems in therapy, such as staff splitting (e.g. the adoption of potential polar views of certain staff as being good or bad therapists or as being right or wrong in behaviour), failure to protect patients adequately against threatening alters, 'over-involvement' expressed in the form of unusual or excessive contact outside office hours, and submission to alters' sexual seduction. Such phenomena could be termed counter-dissociation or counter-trance. In a parallel phenomenon, the great hypnotherapist Milton Erikson discovered that he inadvertently underwent self-hypnosis while he treated patients with hypnosis. Subsequently he cultivated this phenomenon for positive use in therapy: 'When there is a critical issue with a patient [in trance] and I don't want to miss any of the clues, I go into trance.' (Erikson, 1977: 42.)

The foregoing implications of Balinese possession states for treatment of MPD patients do not imply a full range of the principles, techniques, or concepts that have been developed for successful therapy with MPD: these have been presented by skilled psychotherapists such as Bliss (1986); Bowers et al. (1971); Braun (1980, 1984a, 1986); Coons (1986); Fine (1991); Kluft (1984a, 1989, 1991a, 1991b); Putnam (1989); Turkus (1991); and Watkins and Watkins (1984). However, a number of the many principles and techniques cited by these authors are consistent with those brought forth and thrown into a fresh or highlighted perspective by the data presented on the Balinese possession phenomenon. Perhaps these data can serve to emphasize issues such as contagion and the network of family-community-society support.

Trance-suicide

The data presented in this book led to the conclusion that the Balinese generally attempt suicide while in a state of trance-possession. This finding has implications for evaluating, understanding, and treating Balinese and Western patients who have suicidal thoughts or who make suicide attempts. It behoves all mental health clinicians to be alert to the possibility of this process in the patient and get a precise history in order to recognize dissociation or exclude it in diagnosis. This means possessing an awareness of the disorder and giving careful thought in diagnosis to the possibility that the suicide patient may be suffering from MPD, possession disorder, borderline personality, PTSD, and psychogenic amnesia. Failure of the clinician to conceptualize dissociative suicide attempts correctly would diminish the effectiveness of psychotherapy aimed at the symptoms. In clinical practice it has been evident to the authors that Balinese and American patients who have made trance suicide attempts are relieved and reassured by a better understanding of the process itself. Some suicide attempters who have adjustment disorder with depressed mood appear to have dissociated during the acute phase of suicidal ideation and the attempt. The DES may be useful in supporting the diagnosis. Psychotherapy for suicide attempts would take on very different objectives in the case in which trance or dissociation is critical as contrasted with a case in which the suicide attempt is related to depression, adjustment disorder, or other psychiatric diagnoses most commonly associated with suicidality in the West. No one has yet studied a large series of attempted suicides to see how many have heightened dissociation ability or higher degrees of hypnotic susceptibility and/or who went into trance states during suicide attempts. Such fresh investigations are merited.

The phenomenon of trance-suicide may broaden one popular concept of hypnosis. It is generally believed that under hypnosis (trance) the subjects will not do anything that they would not do in their usual state; that is, their morals and self-protective instincts prevail. The Balinese cases of attempted suicide which occur in a trance state would appear to be an exception to this rule. It may be that on the unconscious level the suicide attempter wanted to do it in a manner similar to the alter of an MPD. MPD patients who describe suicide attempts and self-mutilation behaviour by alters also claim they have no conscious desire to carry out these actions.

Trance-possession and Mental Health

The investigations of Balinese trance-possession presented in this book have shown that these phenomena, both normal and abnormal, permeate, and are more entrenched in, the culture than heretofore suspected or documented. They are present in individuals, musicians, dancers, healers, and probably many other sectors or groups not yet investigated. This concurs with the opinion of Bateson and Mead (1942) and Belo (1960) that the Balinese and their culture are particularly disposed to trance. For substantiation, it will be desirable to conduct objective tests of hypnotic susceptibility on Balinese populations for comparison with Western data.

The emotionally expressive, often violent, socially uncontrolled behaviour which occurs in trance-possession but which is not permitted in everyday social life, followed by states of peace and calm lasting 1–3 days, supports the long-held belief that trance is a factor in the mental health of the Balinese (Belo, 1960). Preliminary data presented here support such a hypothesis and merit further study.

In a discussion of observations of trance and possession in non-Western societies, Whittkower (1970) stated:

> Trance and possession states have undoubtedly an adaptive function culturally as well as individually. Their individual psychological effects consist of drive release, ego support, problem solution, relief from superego pressures, and atonement. There can be no doubt in anybody's mind that trance and possession states in the countries in which they play a part of religious rituals have an important distress-relieving, integrative, adaptive function. As far as mental illness is concerned, they may be of prophylactic value. An increase in mental illness may have to be expected when, as a result of culture change, they have ceased to exist.

Kiev (1968) noted similar psychotherapeutic aspects of possession in Haitians.

Whether or not spontaneous trance and trance-possession experiences not associated with a religious group are positive for the mental health of Westerners is questionable. Channellers appear to derive personal benefit from such experiences and probably Western trance-mediums do too. However, Westerners reporting UFO experiences, which appear to be unrecognized dissociation or trance states, sometimes with amnesia, are often quite distressed by them and/are subject to social disapproval by society (Gordon, 1991). The content of reported UFO experiences often involves sexual abuse. These facets point to the critical roles played by the differences in causation, cultural context, and cultural relevance in Western trance experiences and Balinese experiences.

The data regarding the treatment of patients by Balinese traditional healers indicate that their techniques, which involve trance and possession of the healers themselves, resemble, in a number of respects, psychotherapy as practised in the West, and that their treatments are of considerable value in overcoming both the physical and mental problems of individuals and their families. It is also clear why the Balinese generally consult traditional healers before they seek care from psychiatrists using Western techniques and why, after treatment by Western methods, they continue to use the services of the traditional healers. The work of trance-mediums dealing with bereavement appears to be highly efficient and efficacious, possibly more so than Western psychotherapy techniques utilized for these problems in the Balinese. This does not imply that traditional healers' techniques would be more effective in the treatment of all or even most psychiatric disorders; certainly, in the case of psychoses, psychotropic medications are clearly the most effective.

The common history of *balian* (and shamans) experiencing severe illnesses, some of which appear to have been psychoses, just prior to becoming *balian*, or the grave concern that they might be punished by God or die if they did not respond to God's or the gods' direction, followed by their subsequent good health after becoming *balian*, indicates that the utilization of trance-possession has a highly therapeutic function to the *balian* as individuals. They are restored to a more sustained or higher level of mental health than would otherwise have been the case without it.

The data presented in this book documented, to some extent, the efficacy of the traditional healer's treatments in a number of case histories although this was not a primary aim of the study. The study was not limited to Balinese clients as was shown by the case histories of several Westerners treated by *balian*. Most of the Westerners observed and interviewed had a strong belief in the power of the healer and great confidence in his or her methods. It appears that the 'psychological set' of beliefs is a crucial factor in *balian* healing for both Balinese and Westerners.

* * *

In this chapter, the authors have indicated the roles of trance-possession in Balinese society, advanced a theory of possession, set forth specific diagnostic criteria for possession, and specified factors useful to differentiate trance-possession from mental conditions manifesting similar phenomena, including hallucinations. Although possession has been little considered in Western psychiatric literature and has not been in its nomenclature, it deserves to be professionally recognized. Dissociation is the correct term for the process but it is non-specific. The term 'intracorporal influence' is suggested as a potential psychological/psychiatric descriptive term. Trance and possession disorders are being recognized and are likely to be more clearly specified in the latest revisions of psychiatric classifications of diagnoses.

Similarities drawn between MPD in the West and possession in Bali show that the two states are phenomenologically similar in many respects. However, they differ in cause, motivation, and each culture's acceptance, appreciation, and control of the behaviour. A new theory of MPD is proposed: self-hypnosis or trance with a possession process. It extends and combines the extant MPD theories of self-hypnosis and post-traumatic stress disorder, generally secondary to child abuse. The apparent absence of MPD in the Balinese is related to the rarity of child abuse and neglect in the culture. Differences in the manifest behaviours, beliefs, and/or symptoms of the alter personality state of MPD in Westerners and the possession state in the Balinese are related to differences in the normal personality structure in the two types of culture: what is called unitary in Westerners and non-unitary in the Balinese. Non-unitary refers to the inclusion in the personality of supernatural elements such as spirits which are manifest in Balinese identity and personhood or personality. This type of spirit is readily accessible to the Balinese and provides the culturally approved and valued entities utilized in the possession state. Western unitary personality is conceptualized as an entity separate from the supernatural and a unit from which an individual can separate, split off, or dissociate into identified entities or alters as in the case of MPD.

A proposed theoretical view of MPD as representing a similar psychobiological process to that of Balinese possession has implications for the management and psychotherapy of MPD, including a clearer understanding of the mechanism of symptoms, a better patient insight, more efficient staff management of MPD symptoms and behaviour of alter personalities, improved techniques for assisting patients to acquire the ability to terminate alter states, an awareness of the need for a broader, community-wide support network, and a realization of the counter-therapeutic potential for dissociation contagion by the therapist and his staff.

Trance-possession suicide attempts revealed in the Balinese may open up new perspectives on and psychosocial analyses for diagnosis, psychological treatment, and prevention of suicide involving dissociation in both Balinese and Westerners.

There is evidence for positive mental health functions of trance and possession in the Balinese. The analyses suggest directions for further investigation in Bali, the West, and other cultures.

1. This book concentrates on the psychological aspects of trance-possession. In contrast, anthropologists (Connor, 1986) tend to focus on the ideological aspects of trance in the culture.

2. Briefly, depersonalization is defined as a condition in which one experiences feelings of unreality or strangeness concerning either the environment, the self, or both (APA, 1984: 28).

3. 'The symptom of derealization is defined as a sense that one's surroundings are unreal. Derealization may involve a feeling that one's home or workplace is unfamiliar, or a sense that friends or relatives are strange, unfamiliar, or unreal.' (Steinberg, 1991b.)

4. Connor (1986) pointed out that the communications of *balian* in trance are generally ambiguous.

5. Depth of trance is a recognized phenomenon but has not yet been reliably measured (Hilgard, 1977; Tart, 1972).

6. An example of possible 'creative' possession was that of the famous ventriloquist Edgar Bergen. Jean Houston reported that Bergen stated that he had no idea of what his dummy, Charlie McCarthy, would answer in response to his questions or statements to him (Charlie). It was as if Bergen was possessed by Charlie who spoke through him and he would have a dialogue with that possession.

7. Psychiatry (APA, 1984) defines the unconscious as 'that part of the mind or mental functioning of which the content is only rarely subject to awareness. It is a repository for data that have never been conscious (primary repression) or that may have become conscious briefly and later repressed (secondary repression).'

The psychiatrist C. O. Young concluded after studying cases of mediumship that discarnate spirit entities were likely constructions from within the unconscious but gave no explanation of how the unconscious constructed the entities (Hastings, 1991: 175).

8. Dissociation is defined by psychiatry as a 'defense mechanism operating unconsciously, through which emotional significance and affect are separated and detached from an idea, situation, or object' (APA, 1984). Thoughts and feelings are not associated or integrated with the stream of consciousness the way that they normally are.

9. E. L. Bliss (personal communication) argued that changing dissociation to self-hypnotic states would have an experimental advantage since one might use hypnotizability scales to study subsets of conditions to see whether high hypnotizability correlated with such things as hallucinations, religious experiences, suicidal efforts, and acute psychotic episodes in some people.

10. Connor (1986: 279), an anthropologist, regards 'possession' in terms of function and meaning as follows: 'It expresses attitudes to problems of dominance-subordination, equality and inequality, and agency and causality in human affairs.' In other words, for the Balinese people and the *balian*, possession is, in Connor's view, an ideology.

11. Briefly, depersonalization is defined as 'feelings of unreality or strangeness concerning either the environment, the self, or both' (APA, 1984: 28).

12. The *Comprehensive Textbook of Psychiatry III* (Kaplan, Freedman, and Saddock, 1980) mentions possession only in connection with biblical accounts (p. 21), practices of healing in the Middle Ages (p. 38), a 'folk cultural concept' widely used to explain altered states of consciousness (p. 497), voodoo especially as practised in Haiti (p. 497), and demonic possession believed by Catholic charismatics (p. 498).

13. Exorcism of demonic possession in Westerners by religious persons has been described by Goodman (1981, 1988). The procedure involves persuasion and ritual and sometimes physically painful violence to the possessed person in the belief that the demon is treacherous and must be dealt with harshly. The ritualistic aspect and painful aspects of these exorcisms have parallels in *balian* techniques to drive out evil spirits for the purpose of curing illnesses. For example, in some cases the *balian* administers pressure on the finger, which produces severe pain (see Chapter 3).

14. *ICD-10* is the tenth edition of the *International Classification of Diseases* used by psychiatrists in a large part of the world. It proposes to specify trance and possession disorders as follows: 'Disorders in which there is a temporary loss of sense of personal identity and full awareness of surroundings: in some instances, the individual acts as if taken over by another personality, deity, or "force".' Attention and awareness may be limited to only one or two aspects of the immediate environment, postures, and utterances. Only trance disorders which are involuntary or unwanted and which intrude into the ordinary activities by occurring outside (or [by] being a prolongation of) religious and other culturally accepted situations should be included here.

Trance disorders occurring during the course of schizophrenic or acute psychoses with hallucinations or delusions or multiple personality should not be included here nor should this category be used if the trance disorder is judged to be closely associated with any physical disorder (such as temporal lobe epilepsy or head injury) or with psychoactive substance intoxication.

It should be noted that this definition is applicable to disorders of trance with possession and does not pertain to the same phenomena in normal people. In the case of the Balinese, the possession disorders involve combined trance and possession.

15. The classification system *DSM-III-R* (APA, 1987), published by the American Psychiatric Association, has been influential in psychiatry and psychology in the United States, Europe, and widely throughout the world. *DSM-IV*, due for publication

in 1993, may include trance and possession disorder under the category of dissociative disorders. The draft form is as follows:

A. Either (1) or (2):
   (1) trance, i.e. temporary alteration in the state of consciousness, as evidenced by two of the following:
      (a) loss of customary sense of personal identity;
      (b) narrowing of awareness of immediate surroundings, or unusually narrow and selective focusing on environmental stimuli;
      (c) stereotyped behaviors or movements that are experienced as being beyond one's control.
   (2) possession, i.e. conviction that the individual has been taken over by a spirit, power, deity, or other person.

B. The trance or possession state is not authorized as a normal part of a collective cultural or religious practice.

C. The trance or possession state causes significant impairment in social or occupational functioning, or causes marked distress.

D. Not occurring exclusively during the course of a psychotic disorder (including Mood Disorder With Psychotic Features and Brief Reactive Psychosis) or Multiple Personality Disorder, and is not due to a Substance-induced Disorder (e.g. Substance Intoxication) or a Secondary Dissociative Disorder.

Saxena and Prasad (1989) recommended that possession disorder be recognized as a subcategory of atypical dissociative disorder. Two new categories have been proposed by Steinberg (1991b). The first, *transient dissociative disturbance*, would include 'culturally patterned dissociative syndromes' (Spiegel and Cardeña, 1991: 375) such as involuntary possession states, which result in distress or dysfunction. In Bali this could include *bebainan*, *kasurupan*, *amok*, and possibly trance-suicide. The second category, *brief reactive dissociative disorder* (D. Spiegel, 1991), specifies a definite precipitant traumatic event. So far no dissociative disorders of this latter type have been identified in Bali but it seems likely the occurrence will be reported in the near future. Some cases of trance-suicide (Chapter 7) and the non-pathologic condition of 'hidden by the evil spirit' (Chapter 2) may possibly be precipitated by a stressful event.

16. Multiple personalities are also not thought disordered during periods when alters are not manifest. They make good sense during those periods.

17. The concept of possession and MPD may be confused. For example, Allison (1980) reported a case of MPD where the subject was also considered to be possessed by a demon, which was exorcised by hypnosis. Conceivably this was a case of dual diagnosis, both MPD and possession disorder. Another such example was the case of Karen Kingston (Pelton, 1977), a teenage girl who reportedly had 13 demons exorcised by a Baptist evangelist over a three-day period. Handwriting analysis in this case indicated that the demons were distinct personalities. However, in the absence of long-term follow-up of this case, it is not possible to be sure whether these possessions have disappeared completely or could have reappeared as other alters of MPD.

18. It is notable that MPD has been found to occur in 35 per cent of exotic dancers (Ross et al., 1990).

19. In general, *balian* commonly believe that madness is a punishment given by the gods for a mistake or that it is due to one's karma from another life. They may interpret religious hallucinations as divine will (Connor, 1984).

20. This could be an illusion rather than a hallucination. An illusion is a

misinterpretation of a real stimulus whereas a hallucination is an experience of the senses not based on realistic stimuli.

21. The terminology of MPD and the patients themselves often indicate separate personalities. Actually, in terms of psychodynamics, alter personalities are dissociated components of a single personality. Ross (1990) has pointed out that 'personality is simply a convenient, historically sanctioned label for the dissociated states characteristic of this disorder'.

22. An example of a case of multiple personality in an individual who was not identified as a patient and did not know herself that she had MPD is a 35-year-old divorced woman, who, while chatting socially with Jensen at a workshop on shamanism in 1992, mentioned that she was often troubled by, in her words, a 'possession' of her grandmother who takes over her and chastises her. This sensation happens at intervals and its onset is uncontrollable. She readily acknowledged that in recent years she had struggled considerably over her anguish at being abused as a child between 4 and 8 years of age. Jensen explained her 'possession' phenomenon to her in terms of the classical characteristics of multiple personality disorder. She agreed that she could have a multiple personality and felt enlightened. The next day when Jensen enquired of her how she felt about the idea of MPD, she reported that she was reluctant to think of herself as MPD because it might imply to others that she was crazy. After further explanation of MPD and reassurance, she said that the concept of MPD as an explanation of her experience was useful to her because it helped her understand what was happening to her, something that was distressing and puzzling before. She volunteered that she would like to come to peaceful terms with the possessions in the future. She requested to complete the DES, which Jensen mentioned to her on the previous day. Her score on the DES was 25, consistent with scores of MPD patients.

23. The personality disorders include paranoid, schizoid, schizotypal, antisocial, borderline, narcissistic, avoidant, dependent, obsessive compulsive, passive aggressive, and not otherwise specified disorders.

24. Janet used the term 'déagrégation', translated into dissociation; he never recognized self-hypnotic states.

25. 'Occult' means 'hidden' or 'concealed.' Occultism basically involves a belief that: (1) there are hidden or unseen forces in the universe; (2) these forces exist whether we acknowledge them or not; (3) these forces operate according to well-defined laws; (4) there is thus an overall *meaning* inherent in the universe; and (5) the purpose of life has to do with fathoming that meaning and getting in tune with those forces (Crabtree, 1985: 232).

26. Possession by the *tromba* spirit in Madagascar (Sharp, 1990: 344) was described similarly: '... each *tromba* spirit has a very distinct personality and history as well as associated behaviors, styles of dress, food preference, and complicated taboos, all of which are identifiable to the trained observer once the medium has gone into trance.'

27. Based on a review of historical cases of possession and assessment of MPD, Crabtree (1985: 261) concluded that 'possession involves the invasion of a person by an entity from the outside' and 'multiple personality involves the spontaneous emergence of a personality manufactured within'. This is not entirely consistent with the data of possession in Balinese, which shows that possessions may be experienced as either an outside entity taking over or a nondescript power not exclusively derived from outside the individual. Furthermore some MPD patients may experience alters as external gods, spirits, or devils. Hence, the outside/inside quality of these phenomena is not a hard-and-fast rule.

28. There are as yet no generally accepted Western scientific explanations of such psychic phenomena.

29. Both in Bali and in the West, other dissociative disorders manifested by paralysis, amnesia, and fugue may also last for months and sometimes years.

30. It is well known that unethical sexual involvement of psychotherapists occurs most commonly with patients with borderline personality disorders, in which splitting of affects is a predominate symptom. A case of unethical sexual involvement by a prominent psychiatrist with an MPD patient was reported in *Psychiatric News* (March 1992).

31. Amytal is a fast-acting barbiturate (sedative) administered intravenously under highly controlled conditions, which relaxes patients and facilitates their expression of feelings and conflicts.

32. Similarly, depersonalization disorders and associated panic/anxiety have been successfully treated by a process of 'symbolic healing—that is changing the meanings associated in the minds of the patients so it is congruent, understandable, and acceptable within the cognitive and culture syntonic myths, beliefs, and concepts of the society or group' (Castillo, 1990).

Glossary

Only key terms and those used fairly frequently in the text are listed here.

alter — one of the 'personalities' of an MPD

amnesia — a specific or significant segment of time that is unavailable to memory

amok — an episode of dissociation in which the individual suddenly becomes uncontrollably violent; *amok* is precipitated by peak stress and amnesia may exist for the period of the attack

arak — distilled palm wine, white in colour, containing about 50 per cent of alcohol

ASC — altered state of consciousness

atman — the eternal soul

balian — a traditional healer

balian apun — a traditional healer who uses techniques of massage

balian kebal — a traditional healer who specializes in the use of magic paraphernalia such as an amulet

balian taksu — a traditional healer who acts as a trance-medium to communicate with gods, spirits, or ancestors

balian usada — a traditional healer who bases his or her powers on reading *lontar*

banjar — the organizational unit of a village whose tasks relate to religion, customs, and government

Barong — a lion, dragon, or pig-like figure which features prominently in Balinese dramas and ceremonies, especially during *galungan*; at the village temple it symbolizes God and protects the people

bebai — a malignant spirit and its material representation

bebainan — a culture-related dissociative disorder typical of Bali; a trance-possession disorder which the Balinese believed to be caused by evil spirit possession

bebutan — Balinese who experience trance-possession by evil spirits in ceremonies at Jimbaran, and who may

	perform kris-stabbing in such states; also the name of an extremely evil spirit
berem	rice wine, containing about 4 per cent of alcohol
channeller	Western advisers, healers, or counsellors who employ ASC and may function as trance-mediums
dadia	the clan system
depersonalization	feelings of unreality or strangeness concerning the self, the environment, or both; a state of feeling separate, apart, or detached from oneself
derealization	a sensation or perception of the surrounding environment (e.g. persons or things) being unreal or changed from usual; a feeling of detachment from one's environment; derealization may be accompanied by feelings of unreality concerning the environment
DES	the Dissociative Experiences Scale which measures the proportion of time that one engages in common dissociative behaviours
desa	a village
dissociation	a psychological mechanism, 'defence', or state of consciousness in which thoughts, affects, or actions are expressed and performed outside, or split off from, the usual stream of consciousness, i.e. they are not associated or integrated with other information as would normally be the case
DSM	Diagnostic and Statistical Manual of Mental Disorders
dupa	incense smoke
EEG	electroencephalogram; a brainwave recording
engkebang memedi	a dissociative condition which the Balinese call 'hidden by the evil spirit'
galungan	the ceremony held every 210 days, celebrating human victory of good deeds over bad
gamelan	traditional orchestra or music from Balinese xylophone-like instruments, drums, gongs, and flutes
gender	a xylophone-like traditional Balinese musical instrument used in shadow plays
gong orchestra	orchestra with gong instruments
hallucination	a sensory perception usually auditory or visual in the absence of actual external stimuli
hypnotizability	the degree to which one is hypnotizable
ICD	*International Classification of Diseases* (*ICD-9* is the ninth edition. *ICD-10*, published in 1992, is the latest edition.)
jaran	a hobby-horse used in a fire dance

kaja	direction towards the sacred mountain
kalinggihan	a trance involving possession by a god
karauhan	trance-possession
karma	the result of deeds, good and bad, accumulated throughout one's life or in previous lives
kasurupan	possession by a god or an evil spirit
katakson	a trance involving possession by a god; similar to *kalinggihan*
kawitan	the temple of the family clan
kecak	a chorus of men for a popular dance called the 'monkey dance' performed for both Balinese and tourists
kelod	direction towards the sea; direction associated with the unclean and evil spirit activity
keris	kris; a dagger or short sword
kreasi baru	literally, new creation; a new arrangement of gamelan which nevertheless retains the basic traditional pattern
kuningan	the ceremony held on the tenth day after *galungan*
latah	a condition akin to hysteria in which the afflicted person may exhibit shock, laugh uncontrollably, or utter obscene words; sometimes called a culture-bound syndrome, *latah* usually occurs among Malaysians, Indonesians, and Balinese
leak	a person who can change his or her spirit into other forms to disturb or harm people or cause mysterious events; witch-like spirits, creatures, or phenomena that are transformations of real people
lek	feeling of embarrassment or shame, particularly when interacting with a person of a higher status
lontar	ancient Balinese sacred 'books' inscribed on palm leaves
mantra	holy chanting to call the gods
MPD	Multiple Personality Disorder; a person suffering from this
musik kontemporer	contemporary or currently new music
neuroleptic	a class of antipsychotic medications, including 'major tranquilizers' with brand names such as Haldol, Prolixin, Thorazine, and Navane
ngaben	the death ceremonies, including cremation
ngambul	sulking quietly or alone
ngramang sawang	a state of non-thinking or no emotions; a state of 'absent' thinking or emotions characterized by an absence of thoughts, a staring or vacant-like facial expression; and inactivity; it is a dissociative behaviour

ngurek	act of self-stabbing with a kris
nyepi	a day of quiet and peace celebrating the new year
pedanda	a high priest from the Brahmana caste
pemangku	a priest of the temple with less authority than a high priest
pengadeg dasaran	a term meaning 'god uses the body', by which *balian* trance-mediums prefer to be called
pejati	an offering for an infant's birthday ceremony at six months of age
possession	a state of consciousness usually characterized by perception of a force, power, spirit, god, or person taking over and acting through the individual; also used to denote the entity in possession
psychotropic	medications that have primary effects on the mind, especially on the mood, emotions, and psychological functions
PTSD	post-traumatic stress disorder, one of the dissociative disorders
pura	a temple for the extended family, *banjar*, or village
puri	a palace of former kings or a house of the second and third castes
pusuh	the flowering end of the banana stalk
Rangda	a classic witch in dramas and ceremonies, as well as a symbol of a goddess
roh-jahat	evil spirits
sakti	strong spiritual power of a person
Sang Hyang Jaran	the dance of a man with a hobby-horse in a trance-possession state
Sang Hyang Dedari	the 'little girl trance-dance' in which pre-pubertal girls dance in trance-possession
sate	roast pork and other meat on a skewer
schizophrenia	a large group of mental disorders usually manifesting characteristically abnormal forms of language and communication, thought, perception, affect, and behaviour of more than 6 months' duration
shamans	a general term for traditional healers in diverse cultures who advise, treat illness, and occasionally act as trance-mediums
taksu	possession of a body by a god; an inner power conferred by the gods; a place of special power
tirta	holy water
trance	a non-usual state of consciousness usually characterized by changes in perceptions, cognition, or sensation; synonymous with a hypnotic state, it involves dissociation

Bibliography

Adityanjee, G. S. P. and Khandelwal, S. K. (1989), 'Current Status of Multiple Personality Disorder in India', *American Journal of Psychiatry*, 146: 1607–10.

Allison, R. B. (1980), *Minds in Many Pieces*, New York: Rawson Wade.

____ (1992), 'The Possession Syndrome: Myth, Magic and Multiplicity', Paper presented at the Annual Meeting of the Society for Anthropology of Consciousness, San Rafael, California.

Anon. (1992), 'One Addict's Experience with Ibogaine', *Psychiatric News*, 7 February, p. 9.

APA (American Psychiatric Association) (1984), *Psychiatric Glossary*, Washington, DC.

____ (1987), *Diagnostic and Statistical Manual of Mental Disorders*, cited in the text as *DSM-III-R*, Washington, DC.

'APA Deputy Director Resigns after Licence Suspended', *Psychiatric News*, 20 March 1992, p. 1.

Araki, S. and Murata K. (1981), 'Suicide in Japan: Socioeconomic Effects on Its Secular and Seasonal Trends', *Suicide and Life-threatening Behavior*, 17: 64–71.

Arboleda-Florez, J. (1985), 'Amok', in R. C. Simmons and C. H. Hughes (eds.), *The Culture-bound Syndromes*, Boston: D. Reidel Publishing Co.

Bach-y-Rita, G. (1974), 'Habitual Violence and Self-mutilation', *American Journal of Psychiatry*, 131: 1018–20.

Bandem, I. M. (1990), *The State and Development of Balinese Art*, Denpasar: Sikola Tinggi Serri Indonesia.

Bandem, I. M. and deBoer, F. E. (1981), *Kaja and Kelod: Balinese Dance in Transition*, Kuala Lumpur: Oxford University Press.

Barlow, D. H. (1988), *Anxiety and Its Disorders*, New York: Guilford Press.

Bateson, G. and Mead, M. (1942), *Balinese Character: A Photographic Analysis*, New York: Transactions of the New York Academy of Sciences.

Beahrs, J. O. (1982), *Utility and Multiplicity*, New York: Brunner-Mazell.

Beattie, J. (1964), *Other Cultures*, New York: Free Press of Glencoe.

Belo, J. (1953), *Bali Temple Festival*, Seattle: University of Washington Press.

____ (1960), *Trance in Bali*, New York: Columbia University Press.

Benedict, R. (1923), *The Concept of the Guardian Spirit in North America*, Menasha, Wisconsin: American Anthropological Association.

Benson, H. et al. (1990), 'Three Case Reports of the Metabolic and Electroencelphalographic Changes during Advanced Buddhist Meditation Techniques', *Behavioral Medicine*, 16: 90–5.

Bernstein, E. M. and Putnam, F. W. (1986), 'Development, Reliability, and Validity of a Dissociation Scale', *Journal of Nervous and Mental Disease*, 174: 727–35.

Berwick, P. R. and Douglas, R. R. (1977), 'Hypnosis, Exorcism and Healing: A Case Report', *American Journal of Clinical Hypnosis*, 20: 146–8.

Bhatia, S. C. et al. (1987), 'High-risk Suicide Factors across Cultures', *International Journal of Psychiatry*, 33: 226–36.

Blacker, K. and Wong, N. (1963), 'Four Cases of Autocastration', *Archives of General Psychiatry*, 8: 169–76.

Bliss, E. L. (1980), 'Multiple Personalities: A Report of 14 Cases with Implications for Schizophrenia and Hysteria', *Archives of General Psychiatry*, 37: 1388–97.

—— (1983), 'Multiple Personality, Related Disorders and Hypnosis', *American Journal of Clinical Hypnosis*, 26: 114–23.

—— (1984a), 'Spontaneous Self-hypnosis in Multiple Personality Disorder', *Psychiatric Clinics of North America*, 7: 135–48.

—— (1984b), 'A Symptom Profile of Patients with Multiple Personalities—with MMPI Results', *Journal of Nervous and Mental Disorders*, 172: 197–202.

—— (1986), *Multiple Personality, Allied Disorders and Hypnosis*, New York: Oxford University Press.

Boon, J. A. (1977), *The Anthropological Romance of Bali, 1597–1972*, Cambridge: Cambridge University Press.

Bourguignon, E. (1965), 'The Self, the Behavioral Environment, and the Theory of Spirit Possession', in M. E. Spiro (ed.), *Context and Meaning in Cultural Anthropology*, New York: Free Press of Glencoe.

—— (1968), 'World Distribution and Patterns of Possession States', in R. Prince (ed.), *Trance and Possession States*, Montreal: R. M. Bucke Memorial Society, pp. 3–34.

—— (1973), *Religion, Altered States of Consciousness and Social Change*, Columbus: Ohio State University Press.

—— (1976), 'Possession and Trance in Cross-cultural Studies of Mental Health', in W. P. Lebra (ed.), *Culture-bound Syndromes, Ethnopsychiatry, and Alternative Therapies*, Honolulu: University of Hawaii Press.

Bower, G. H. (1981), 'Mood and Memory', *American Psychologist*, 36: 129–48.

Bowers, M. K. (1961), 'Hypnotic Aspects of Haitian Voodoo', *International Journal of Clinical and Experimental Hypnosis*, 9: 269–82.

Bowers, M. K. et al. (1971), 'Therapy of Multiple Personality', *International Journal of Clinical and Experimental Hypnosis*, 19: 57–65.

Braid, J. (1899), *Neurohypnology; or the Rationale of Nervous Sleep*, London: John Churchill.

Braun, B. G. (1980), 'Hypnosis for Multiple Personalities', in H. J. Wain (ed.), *Clinical Hypnosis in Medicine*, Chicago: Year Book Medical Publishers.

____ (1983), 'Psychophysiologic Phenomena in Multiple Personality and Hypnosis', *American Journal of Clinical Hypnosis*, 26: 124–37.

____ (1984a), 'Towards a Theory of Multiple Personality and Other Dissociative Phenomena', *Psychiatric Clinics of North America*, 7: 171–94.

____ (1984b), 'Hypnosis Creates Multiple Personality: Myth or Reality', *International Journal of Clinical and Experimental Hypnosis*, 32: 191–7.

____ (1984c), 'Uses of Hypnosis with Multiple Personality', *Psychiatric Annals*, 14: 34–40.

____ (1986), 'Issues in the Psychotherapy of Multiple Personality', in B. G. Braun (ed.), *Treatment of Multiple Personality Disorder*, Washington, DC: American Psychiatric Press, pp. 1–28.

Bremner, J. D. et al. (1992), 'Dissociation and Post Traumatic Stress Disorder in Vietnam Combat Veterans', *American Journal of Psychiatry*, 149: 328–32.

Breuer, J. and Freud, S. (1955), 'Studies on Hysteria', in J. Strachey (ed.), *The Standard Edition of the Complete Works of Sigmund Freud*, London: Hogarth Press.

Brown, D. P. and Fromm, E. (1986), *Hypnotherapy and Hypnoanalysis*, Hillsdale: Lawrence Erlbaumm Associates, Inc.

Campbell, J. (1975), *The Portable Jung*, New York: Viking Press.

Cardeña, E. (1989), 'The Varieties of Possession Experience', *Association for the Anthropological Study of Consciousness Quarterly*, 5: 1–17.

Cardeña, E. and Spiegel, D. (1991), 'Suggestibility, Absorption and Dissociation: An Integrative Model of Hypnosis,' in J. F. Schumaker (ed.), *Human Suggestibility: Advances in Theory, Research and Application*, New York: Routledge, pp. 93–107.

Carlson, E. B. and Rosser-Hogan, R. (1991), 'Trauma Experiences, Post Traumatic Stress, Dissociation, and Depression in Cambodian Refugees', *American Journal of Psychiatry*, 148: 1548–51.

Carr, J. E. and Tan, E. K. (1976), 'In Search of the True Amok: Amok as Viewed within the Malay Culture', *American Journal of Psychiatry*, 133: 1295–9.

Castillo, R. J. (1990), 'Depersonalization and Meditation', *Psychiatry*, 53: 158–68.

Chaudhuri, H. (1974), 'Meditation: Dangers and Rewards,' in J. White (ed.), *What is Meditation?*, Garden City: Anchor Press/Doubleday.

Clark, W. H. (1977), 'Parapsychology and Religion', in A. B. Wolman (ed.), *Handbook of Parapsychology*, New York: Van Nostrand Reinhold Co., pp. 769–79.

Clifford, H. C. (1898), *Studies in Brown Humanity; Being Scrawls and Smudges in Sepia, White, and Yellow*, London: G. Richards.

Collinder, B. (1949), *The Lapps*, New York: Greenwood Press.

Connor, L. H. (1982), 'Ships of Fools and Vessels of the Divine: Mental Hospital and Madness: A Case Study', *Social Science Medicine*, 16: 783–94.

____ (1984), 'The Unbounded Self: Balinese Therapy in Theory and Practice', in A. J. Marcella and G. M. White (eds.), *Cultural Conceptions of Mental Health and Therapy*, Dordrecht: D. Reidel Publishing Company, pp. 251–67.

____ (1986), 'Balinese Healing', in L. H. Connor, P. Asch, and T. Asch (eds.), *Jero Topokan: Balinese Healer, an Ethnographic Film Monograph*, Cambridge: Cambridge University Press, pp. 59–80.

Connor, L. H.; Asch, P.; and Asch, T. (eds.) (1986), *Jero Topokan: Balinese Healer, an Ethnographic Film Monograph*, Cambridge: Cambridge University Press.

Coons, P. M. (1986), 'Treatment Progress in 20 Patients with Multiple Personality Disorder', *Journal of Nervous and Mental Disorders*, 174: 715–21.

____ (1988), 'Psychophysiologic Aspects of Multiple Personality Disorder', *Dissociation*, 1: 47–53.

Coons, P. M.; Bowman, E. S.; and Milstein, V. (1988), 'Multiple Personality Disorder: A Clinical Investigation of 50 Cases', *Journal of Nervous and Mental Disorders*, 176: 519–27.

Covarrubias, M. (1937), *Island of Bali*, New York: Alfred A. Knopf; reprinted Singapore: Oxford University Press, 1987.

Crabtree, A. (1985), 'Two Approaches to Multiple Man—The Occult and Psychological', in A. Crabtree (ed.), *Multiple Man*, New York: Praeger Publishers, pp. 239–40.

Czaplicka, M. A. (1914), *Aboriginal Siberia: A Study in Social Anthropology*, Oxford: Clarendon Press.

DeBerry, S. (1992), 'An Evaluation of Progressive Muscle Relaxation on Stress Related Symptoms in a Geriatric Population,' *International Journal of Aging & Human Development*, 14: 255–69.

DeBerry, S.; Davis, S.; and Reinhard, K. E. (1989), 'A Comparison of Meditation-relaxation and Cognitive/Behavioral Techniques for Reducing Anxiety and Depression in a Geriatric Population', *Journal of Geriatric Psychiatry*, 22(2): 231–47.

DeBoismont, B. A. (1855), *A History of Dreams, Visions, Apparitions, Ecstasy, Magnetism, and Somnambulism*, Philadelphia: Lindsay & Blâkiston.

Deikman, A. J. (1963), 'Experimental Meditation', *Journal of Nervous and Mental Disease*, 136: 329–43.

Delmonte, M. M. (1989), 'Meditation, the Unconscious, and Psychosomatic Disorders', *International Journal of Psychosomatics*, 36(1–4): 45–52.

Demetrack, M. A. et al. (1990), 'Relation of Clinical Variables to Dissociative Phenomena in Eating Disorders', *American Journal of Psychiatry*, 147: 1184–8.

Devereaux, G. (1956), 'Normal and Abnormal: The Key Problem in Psychiatric Anthropology', in J. B. Casagrand and T. Gladwin (eds.), *Some Uses of Anthropology: Theoretical and Applied*, Washington, DC: Anthropological Society of Washington.

—— (1961), 'Shamans as Neurotics', *American Anthropologist*, 63: 1088–90.

De Zoete, B. and Spies, W. (1970), 'Dance and Drama in Bali', in J. Belo (ed.), *Traditional Balinese Culture*, New York: Columbia University Press.

Diekstra, R. F. (1989), 'Suicide and the Attempted Suicide: An International Perspective', *Acta Psychiatrica Scandinavia, Supplement*, 354: 1–24.

Dillbeck, M. C. et al. (1989), 'Test of a Field Model of Consciousness and Social Change: The Transcendental Meditation and TM-Siddhi Program and Decreased Urban Crime', *Journal of Mind and Behavior*, 9(4): 231–52.

Dixon, J. C. (1963), 'Depersonalization Phenomena in a Sample Population of College Students', *British Journal of Psychiatry*, 109: 371–5.

Elaide, M. (1966), *Shamanism: Archaic Techniques of Ecstasy* (translated by W. R. Trask), Princeton: Princeton University Press.

Ellenberger, H. F. (1970), *The Discovery of the Unconscious*, New York: Basic Books.

Erikson, M. H. (1970), 'Hypnosis: Its Renaissance as a Treatment Modality', *American Journal of Clinical Hypnosis*, 13: 71–89.

—— (1977), 'Auto Hypnotic Experiences of Milton H. Erikson', *American Journal of Clinical Hypnosis*, 20: 36–68.

Favazza, A. R. (1989), 'Why Patients Mutilate Themselves', *Hospital Community Psychiatry*, 40: 137–45.

Favazza, A. R. and Conterio, K. (1988), 'The Plight of Chronic Self-mutilators', *Community Mental Health Journal*, 24: 22–30.

—— (1989), 'Female Habitual Self-mutilators', *Acta Psychiatrica Scandinavia*, 79: 283–9.

Fine, C. C. (1991), 'Treatment Stabilization and Crisis Prevention', *Psychiatric Clinics of North American*, 14: 661–75.

Fink, O. (1991), 'The Comorbidity of Multiple Personality Disorder and DSM-III-R Axis II Disorders', *Psychiatric Clinics of North America*, 14: 547–66.

Fishbain, D. A. and Aldrich, T. E. (1985), 'Suicide Pacts: International Comparisons', *Journal of Clinical Psychiatry*, 46: 11–15.

Forman, W.; Mazek, R.; and Forman, B. (1983), *Bali: The Spirit Gate to Heaven*, London: Orbis Publishing.

Frankel, F. H. (1976), *Hypnosis: Trance as a Coping Mechanism*, New York: Plenum Medical Books.

—— (1990), 'Hypnotizability and Dissociation', *American Journal of Psychiatry*, 147: 823–9.

—— (1991), 'Dr. Frankel Replies' (letter), *American Journal of Psychiatry*, 148: 814–15.

Frazer, J. G. (1935), *The Golden Bough*, New York: Macmillan.

Freud, S. (1901), 'The Psychopathology of Everyday Life', in *The Standard Edition of the Complete Works of Sigmund Freud*, Vol. VI (1960), London: Hogarth Press, pp. 84–251.

—— (1950), 'A Neurosis of Demoniacal Possession in the Seventeenth

Century', in E. Jones (ed.), *Sigmund Freud, Collected Papers*, Vol. IV, London: Hogarth Press.

Frigerio, A. (1989), 'Levels of Possession Awareness in Afro-Brazilian Religions', *Association for the Anthropological Study of Consciousness Quarterly*, 5: 5–11.

Fromm, E. (1979), 'The Nature of Hypnosis and the Altered States of Consciousness: An Egopsychological Theory', in E. Fromm and R. E. Shor (eds.), *Hypnosis, Developments in Research, and New Perspectives*, 2nd edn., New York: Aldine-Atherton.

Fuchs, S. (1964), 'Magic Healing Techniques among the Balahis in Central India', in A. Kiev (ed.), *Magic, Faith, and Healing: Studies in Primitive Psychiatry Today*, New York: Free Press, pp. 121–37.

Gaddis, V. H. (1967), *Mysterious Fires and Lights*, New York: David McKay Company, Inc.

Gallup, G., Jr. (1975), 'Hypnosis in Animals', *New Scientist* (April 10): 68–70.

Gallup, G., Jr. and Maser, J. D. (1977), 'Tonic Immobility: Evolutionary Underpinings of Human Catalepsy and Catatonia', in J. D. Maser and Segelman (eds.), *Psychopathology Experimental Models*, New York: W. H. Freeman & Co.

Gardner, D. L. and Cowdry, R. W. (1985), 'Suicidal and Parasuicidal Behavior in Borderline Personality Disorder', *Psychiatric Clinics of North America*, 8: 389–403.

Gauld (1977), 'Discarnate Survival', in B. B. Wolman (ed.), *Handbook of Parapsychology*, New York: Van Nostrand Reinhold, pp. 577–630.

Geertz, C. (1966), *Person, Time and Conduct in Bali: An Essay in Cultural Analyses*, New Haven: Yale South-east Asia Studies.

Geertz, H. (1968), '*Latah* in Java: A Theoretical Paradox', *Indonesia*, 3: 93–104.

Geertz, H. and Geertz, C. (1975), *Kinship in Bali*, Chicago: University of Chicago Press.

Gill, M. M. and Brenman, M. (1961), *Hypnosis and Related States*, New York: International University Press.

Gilmour, A. (1902), '*Latah* among South African Natives', *Scottish Medical Journal*, 10: 18–20.

Goodman, F. D. (1972), *Speaking in Tongues: A Cross-cultural Study of Glossolalia*, Chicago: University of Chicago Press.

____ (1981), *The Exorcism of Anneliese Michel*, New York: Doubleday.

____ (1988), *How about Demons? Possession and Exorcism in the Modern World*, Bloomington and Indianapolis: Indiana University Press.

____ (1990), 'A Trance Dance with Masks', *Drama Review*, 34: 102–14.

Gordon, J. F. (1991), 'Close Encounters of the Fourth Kind', *San Francisco Chronicle*, 22 September, pp. 7–11.

Graff, H. and Mallin, R. (1967), 'The Syndrome of the Wrist Cutter', *American Journal of Psychiatry*, 124: 36–42.

Grunebaum, H. U. and Klerman, G. L. (1967), 'Wrist Slashing', *American Journal of Psychiatry*, 124: 527–34.

Gudjonsson, G. H. and Haward, L. R. C. (1982), 'Case Reports and Hysterical Amnesia as an Alternative to Suicide', *Medicine, Science and Law*, 22: 68–72.

Haberman, M. A. (1986), 'Spontaneous Trance or Dissociation: A Suicide Attempt in a Schizophrenic Vietnam Veteran', *American Journal of Clinical Hypnosis*, 28: 177–82.

Halifax, J. (1992), 'The Psychotherapist as Shaman: Methods for Madness', Workshop at Esalon Institute, Big Sur, California, 4–16 February.

Hansen, C. (1969), *Witchcraft at Salem*, New York: Times Mirror.

Harrary, K. (1992), 'The Truth about Jonestown', *Psychology Today*, March/April: 62–88.

Hastings, A. (1991), *With the Tongues of Men and Angels: A Study of Channeling*, Chicago: Holt Rinehart & Winston, Inc.

Hendin, H. and Haas, A. P. (1991), 'Suicide and Guilt as Manifestations of PTSD in Vietnam Combat Veterans', *American Journal of Psychiatry*, 148: 586–91.

Henney, J. H. (1973), 'The Shakers of St. Vincent', in E. Bourguignon (ed.), *Religion, Altered States of Consciousness and Social Change*, Columbus: Ohio State University Press.

Herzog, H. A. (1978), 'Immobility in Intraspecific Encounters: Cockfights and the Evolution of "Animal Hypnosis"', *Psychological Record*, 28: 543–8.

Hilgard, E. R. (1965), *Hypnotic Susceptibility*, New York: Harcourt, Brace & World.

—— (1977), *Divided Consciousness: Multiple Controls in Human Thought and Action*, New York: John Wiley & Sons.

Hilgard, J. R. (1970), *Personality and Hypnosis: A Study of Imaginative Involvement*, 2nd edn., Chicago: University of Chicago Press.

Hollan, D. (1990), 'Indigent Suicide in the Pacific: An Example from the Toraja Highlands of Indonesia', *Culture, Medicine and Psychiatry*, 14: 365–79.

Holmes, D. S. (1990), 'The Evidence for Repression: An Examination of Sixty Years of Research', in J. L. Singer (ed.), *Repression and Dissociation*, Chicago: University of Chicago Press, pp. 85–119.

Hooykaas, C. (1977), *A Balinese Temple Festival*, The Hague: Martinus Nijhoff.

Hughes, D. J. (1989), 'Blending with Another: An Analysis of Trance Channeling in the United States', MA thesis, University of California, Los Angeles.

Hughes, D. J. and Melville, N. J. (1990), 'Changes in Brain Wave Activity during Trance Channeling: A Pilot Study', *Journal of Transpersonal Psychology*, 22: 175–89.

James, W. (1890), *The Principles of Psychology*, London: Macmillan.

Janet, P. (1898), *Nevroses et idees fixes*, 2 vols., Paris: Alcan.

Jensen, G. D. and Suryani, L. K. (1992), *The Balinese People: A Reinvestigation of Character*, Singapore: Oxford University Press.

Jilck, W. G. (1982), *Indian Healing: Shamanistic Ceremonialism in Pacific Northwest Today*, Blaine, Washington: Hancock House Publishers, Ltd.

Jones, E. (1953), *The Life and Work of Sigmund Freud*, New York: Basic Books.

Jung, C. G. (1977), *Psychology and the Occult*, Princeton: Princeton University Press.

Kaplan, H. E.; Freedman, A. M.; and Saddock, B. J. (eds.) (1980), *Comprehensive Textbook of Psychiatry III*, 3rd edn., Baltimore: Williams & Wilkins.

Kelly, G. A. (1955), *The Psychology of Personal Constructs*, New York: Norton.

Kennedy, R. B. (1976), 'Self-induced Depersonalization Syndrome', *American Journal of Psychiatry*, 133: 1326–8.

Kenny, M. G. (1981), 'Multiple Personality and Spirit Possession', *Psychiatry*, 44: 339–68.

—— (1985), 'Paradox Lost: The *Latah* Problem Revisited', in Ronald C. Simons and C. C. Hughes (eds.), *The Culture-bound Syndromes*, Baltimore: Williams & Wilkins, pp. 63–76.

Kiev, A. (1961a), 'Folk Psychiatry in Haiti', *Journal of Nervous and Mental Disorders*, 132: 160–265.

—— (1961b), 'Spirit Possession in Haiti', *American Journal of Psychiatry*, 118: 133–8.

—— (1968), 'The Therapeutic Value of Spirit Possession in Haiti', in R. Prince (ed.), *Trance and Possession States*, Montreal: R. M. Bucke Memorial Society, pp. 143–8.

Kihlstrom, J. F. and Hoyt, J. P. (1990), *Repression, Association and Hypnosis,* n.p., pp. 181–208.

Kim, E. and Ainslie, G. (1990), 'Another Case of Self-cutting after Combat Stress', *American Journal of Psychiatry*, 147: 1572–3.

Klemm, W. R. (1966), 'Electroencephalographic-behavioral Dissociations during Animal Hypnosis', *Electroencephalography and Clinical Neurophysiology*, 21: 365–72.

Klemperer, E. (1965), 'Post Ego States Emerging in Hypnoanalysis', *International Journal of Clinical and Experimental Hypnosis*, 13: 112–20.

Klimo, J. (1987), *Channeling: Investigations on Receiving Information from Paranormal Sources*, Los Angeles: Jeremy Tarcher, Inc.

Kluft, R. P. (1983), 'Hypnotherapeutic Crisis Intervention in Multiple Personality', *American Journal of Clinical Hypnosis*, 26: 73–83.

—— (1984a), 'Treatment of Multiple Personality Disorder', *Psychiatric Clinics of North America*, 7: 9–31.

—— (1984b), 'An Introduction to Multiple Personality Disorder', *Psychiatric Annals*, 14: 19–24.

—— (1984c), 'Multiple Personality in Childhood', *Psychiatric Clinics of North America*, 7: 121–34.

—— (1985), 'The Natural History of Multiple Personality Disorder', in R. P. Kluft (ed.), *Childhood Antecedents of Multiple Personality*, Washington, DC: American Psychiatric Press, pp. 197–238.

—— (1987a), 'First-rank Symptoms as a Diagnostic Clue to Multiple Personality Disorder', *American Journal of Psychiatry*, 144: 293–5.

—— (1987b), 'Making the Diagnosis of Multiple Personality', in F. F. Flach (ed.), *Diagnostics and Psychopathology*, New York: W. W. Norton, pp. 207–25.

—— (1988), 'The Phenomenology and Treatment of Extremely Complex Multiple Personality Disorder', *Dissociation*, 1: 47–58.

—— (1989), 'Playing for Time: Temporizing Techniques in the Treatment of Multiple Personality Disorder', *Journal of Clinical Hypnosis*, 32: 90–7.

—— (1991a), 'Multiple Personality Disorder', in A. Tasman and S. M. Goldfinger (eds.), *Review of Psychiatry*, Vol. 10, Washington, DC: American Psychiatric Association Press.

—— (1991b), 'Hospital Treatment of Multiple Personality Disorder: An Overview', *Psychiatric Clinics of North America*, 14: 695–719.

—— (1991c), 'Clinical Presentations of Multiple Personality Disorder', *Psychiatric Clinics of North America*, 14: 605–29.

Kokoszka, A. (1990), 'Axiological Aspects of Comparing Psychotherapy and Meditation', *International Journal of Psychosomatics*, 37: 78–81.

Krause, G. (1988), *Bali, 1912*, Wellington: January Books.

Krippner, S. (1987), 'Cross-cultural Approaches to Multiple Personality Disorder Practices of Brazilian Spiritism', *Ethos*, 15: 273–95.

Kris, E. (1952), *Psychoanalytic Explorations in Art*, New York: International University Press.

Kroeber, A. L. (1952), 'Psychosis or Social Sanction', in A. L. Kroeber (ed.) *The Nature of Culture*, Chicago: University of Chicago Press, pp. 310–19.

Kunkle, E. C. (1967), 'The *Jumpers* of Maine: A Reappraisal', *Archives of Internal Medicine*, 119: 355–8.

Kutz, I. K.; Borysenko, J. Z.; and Benson, H. (1985), 'Meditation and Psychotherapy: A Rationale for the Integration of Dynamic Psychotherapy, the Relaxation Response, and Mindfulness Meditation', *American Journal of Psychiatry*, 142: 1–8.

Langness, L. (1976), 'Hysterical Psychoses and Possession', in W. P. Lebra (ed.), *Culture-bound Syndromes, Ethnopsychiatry and Alternative Therapies*, Honolulu: University of Hawaii Press.

Lebra, W. P. (ed.) (1976), *Culture-bound Syndromes, Ethnopsychiatry and Alternative Therapies*, Honolulu: University of Hawaii Press.

Leff, J. (1981), *Psychiatry around the Globe*, New York: Marcel Dekker, Inc.

Leibenluft, E.; Gardner, D. L.; and Cowdry, R. W. (1987), 'The Inner Experience of the Borderline Self-mutilator', *Journal of Personality Disorders*, 1: 317–24.

Leimena, S. L. and Thong, D. H. (1983), 'Pengobatan Tradisional di Bali: Suatu Laporan', in Setyonegoro and W. M. Roan (eds.), *Traditional Healing Practices*, Jakarta: Directorate of Mental Health, pp. 160–206.

Levy, J. and Wachtel, P. (1978), 'Depersonalization: An Effort at Clarification', *American Journal of Psychoanalysis*, 38: 291–300.

Lewis, I. M. (1971), *Ecstatic Religion: An Anthropological Study of Spirit Possession*, Baltimore: Penguin Books.

Li, Y. (1976), 'Shamanism in Taiwan: An Anthropological Inquiry', in W. P. Lebra (ed.), *Culture-bound Syndromes, Ethnopsychiatry and Alternative Therapies*, Honolulu: University of Hawaii Press.

Linton, R. (1956), *Culture and Mental Disorders*, Springfield: Charles C. Thomas Publishers.

Liu, G. L. et al. (1990), 'Changes in Brainstem and Cortical Auditory Potentials during Qi-Gong Meditation,' *American Journal of Chinese Medicine*, 18(3–4): 95–103.

Loewenstein, R. J. (1991), 'Office Mental Status Examination for Complex Chronic Dissociative Symptoms and Multiple Personality Disorder', *Psychiatric Clinics of North America*, 14: 567–604.

Ludwig, A. M. (1983), 'The Psychobiological Functions of Dissociation', *American Journal of Clinical Hypnosis*, 26: 93–9.

Ludwig, A. M.; Brandsma, J. M.; and Wilbur, C. B. (1972), 'The Objective Study of a Multiple Personality', *Archives of General Psychiatry*, 26: 298–310.

MacKinnon, R. P. (1980), 'Psychiatric History and Mental Status Examination', in H. E. Kaplan, A. M. Freedman, and D. S. Saddock (eds.), *Comprehensive Textbook of Psychiatry III*, 3rd edn., Baltimore: Williams & Wilkins.

Magarey, C. J. (1988), 'Aspects of the Psychological Management of Breast Cancer', *Medical Journal of Australia*, 148: 239–42.

Maniam, T. (1988), 'Suicide and Parasuicide in a Hill Resort in Malaysia', *British Journal of Psychiatry*, 153: 222–5.

Martin, M. (1976), *Hostage to the Devil: The Possession and Exorcism of Five Living Americans*, New York: Reader's Digest Press.

Martinez-Tuboas, A. (1989), 'Preliminary Observations on MPD in Puerto Rico', *Dissociation*, 2: 120–31.

Masters, W. H. and Johnson, V. E. (1970), *Human Sexual Inadequacy*, Boston: Little, Brown & Co.

Mayer-Gross, W. (1935), 'On Depersonalization', *British Journal of Medical Psychology*, 15: 103–26.

McDougal, W. (1926), *Outline of Abnormal Psychology*, New York: Charles Scribner's Sons.

McPhee, C. (1946), *A House in Bali*, New York: J. D. Day Co.; issued as an Oxford University Press paperback, 1979; reprinted Singapore: Oxford University Press, 1986.

—— (1970), 'Children and Music in Bali', in J. Belo (ed.), *Traditional Balinese Culture*, New York: Columbia University Press.

Meares, A. (1978), 'Vivid Visualization and Dim Visual Awareness in the Regression of Cancer in Meditation', *Journal of the American Society of Psychosomatic Dentistry and Medicine*, 25(3): 85–8.

Metraux, A. (1959), *Voodoo in Haiti*, London: Andre Deutsch.

Mills, P. J. et al. (1990), 'Beta-adrenergic Receptor Sensitivity in Subjects Practicing Transcendental Meditation', *Journal of Psychosomatic Research*, 34: 19–33.

Moerdowo, R. M. (1973), *Ceremonies in Bali*, Jakarta: Bhrataru.

Moll, A. (1902), *Hypnotism*, New York: Charles Scribner's Sons.

Morgan, A. H. (1973), 'The Heritability of Hypnotic Susceptibility in Twins', *Journal of Abnormal Psychology*, 82: 55–61.

Morgan, A. H. and Hilgard, J. R. (1978–9), 'The Stanford Hypnotic Clinical Scale for Children', *American Journal of Clinical Hypnosis*, 21: 148–55.

Mueser, K. T. and Butler, R. W. (1987), 'Auditory Hallucinations in Combat-related Chronic Posttraumatic Stress Disorder, *American Journal of Psychiatry*, 144: 299–302.

Murphy, H. B. M. (1976), 'Notes for a Theory on *Latah*', in W. P. Lebra (ed.), *Culture-bound Syndromes, Ethnopsychiatry and Alternative Therapies*, Honolulu: University of Hawaii Press.

____ (1982), *Comparative Psychiatry: The International and Intercultural Distribution of Mental Illness*, Berlin: Springer-Verlag.

Myers, D. and Grant, G. (1970), 'A Study of Depersonalization in Students', *British Journal of Psychiatry*, 12: 59–65.

Naher, A. (1962), 'A Physiological Explanation of Unusual Behavior in Ceremonies Involving Drums', *Human Biology*, 34: 153–6.

Nakagawa, H. (1973), '*Imu* of the *Ainu*' [in Japanese], Lecture privately published honouring the retirement of H. Nakagawa, Sapporo, Japan: Sapporo Medical College.

Nemiah, J. C. (1980), 'Dissociative Disorders', in H. E. Kaplan, A. M. Freedman, and D. S. Saddock (eds.), *Comprehensive Textbook of Psychiatry III*, 3rd edn., Baltimore: Williams & Wilkins, pp. 1544–61.

Nissen, M. J. et al. (1988), 'Memory and Awareness in a Patient with Multiple Personality Disorder', *Brain Cognition*, 8: 117–34.

Noll, R. (1989), 'What Has Really Been Learned about Shamanism?', *Journal of Psychoactive Drugs*, 21: 47–50.

Oesterreich, T. K. (1974), *Possession and Exorcism*, New York: Causeway Books.

Ogata, S. N. et al. (1990), 'Childhood Sexual and Physical Abuse in Adult Patients with Borderline Personality Disorder', *American Journal of Psychiatry*, 147: 1008–13.

Orne, M. T. (1959), 'The Nature of Hypnosis: Artifact and Essence', *Journal of Abnormal and Social Psychology*, 58: 277–99.

Orne, M. T.; Dinges; P. F.; and Orne, D. C. (1984), 'On the Differential Diagnosis of Multiple Personality in the Forensic Context, *International Journal of Clinical Hypnosis*, 22: 118–69.

Pattison, E. M. and Kahan, J. (1983), 'The Deliberate Self-harm Syndrome', *American Journal of Psychiatry*, 140: 867–72.

Pattison, E. M. and Wintrob, R. M. (1981), 'Possession and Exorcism in Contemporary America', *Journal of Operational Psychiatry*, 12: 13–20.

Pelton, R. (1977), *The Devil and Karen Kingston*, New York: Pocket Books.

Pitman, R. K. (1990), 'Self-mutilation in Combat-related PTSD', *American Journal of Psychiatry,* 147: 123–4.

Powell, H. (1930), *The Last Paradise*, New York: Jonathan Cape & Harrison Smith, Inc.

Prince, M. (1909), 'The Psychological Principles and Field of Psychotherapy', in N. G. Hale (ed.) (1975), *Morton Prince, Psychotherapy and Multiple Personality, Selected Essays*, Cambridge, Mass.: Harvard University Press, pp. 113–26.

Prince, R. (1968), 'Can the EEG Be Used in the Study of Possession States?' in R. Prince (ed.) *Trance and Possession States*, Montreal: R. M. Bucke Memorial Society.

Putnam, F.W. (1984), 'The Psychophysiologic Investigation of Multiple Personality Disorder', *Psychiatric Clinics of North America*, 7: 31–9.

____ (1985), 'Dissociation in Response to Extreme Trauma', in R. P. Kluft (ed.), *The Childhood Antecedents of Multiple Personality*, Washington, DC: American Psychiatric Press.

____ (1988), 'The Switch Process in Multiple Personality Disorder and Other State-change Disorders', *Dissociation*, 1: 24–32.

____ (1989), *Diagnosis and Treatment of Multiple Personality Disorder*, New York: Garfield Press.

____ (1991), 'Dissociative Phenomena', in A. Tasman and S. M. Goldfinger (eds.), *Review of Psychiatry*, Vol. 10, Washington, DC: American Psychiatric Association Press.

Putnam, F. W. et al. (1986), 'The Clinical Phenomenology of Multiple Personality Disorder: A Review of 100 Recent Cases', *Journal of Clinical Psychiatry*, 47: 285–93.

Putnam, F. W.; Zahn, T.; and Post, R. (1990), 'Differential Autonomic Nervous System Activity in Multiple Personality Disorder', *Psychiatry Research*, 31: 251–60.

Puysegur, A. M. J. (1784), 'Chastenet de Memoires pour Servir a l'Histoire et a l'Establishment du Magnetisme Animal', cited by H. F. Ellenberger (1970), *The Discovery of the Unconscious*, New York: Basic Books.

Ramseyer, U. (1986), *The Art and Culture of Bali*, Singapore: Oxford University Press.

Ravenscroft, K. (1965), 'Voodoo Possession: A Natural Experiment in Hypnosis', *International Journal of Clinical Experimental Hypnosis*, 13: 157–82.

Rosenthal, R. J. et al. (1972), 'Wrist-cutting Syndrome: The Meaning of a Gesture', *American Journal of Psychiatry*, 128: 1363–8.

Ross, C. A. (1989), *Multiple Personality Disorder: Diagnoses, Clinical Features, and Treatment*, New York: John Wiley & Sons.

—— (1990), 'Twelve Cognitive Errors about Multiple Personality Disorder', *American Journal of Psychotherapy*, XLIV: 348–61.

Ross, C. A. and Norton, G. R. (1989), 'Suicide and Parasuicide in Multiple Personality Disorder', *Psychiatry*, 52: 365–71.

Ross, C. A.; Joshi, S.; and Currie, R. (1990), 'Dissociative Experiences in the General Population', *American Journal of Psychiatry*, 147: 1547–56.

Ross, C. A.; Norton, G. R.; and Wozney, K. (1989), 'Multiple Personality Disorder: An Analysis of 236 Cases', *Canadian Journal of Psychiatry*, 34: 413–18.

Ross, C. A. et al. (1989), 'Differences between Multiple Personality Disorder and Other Diagnostic Groups on Structured Interview', *Journal of Nervous and Mental Disorders*, 177: 487–91.

Ross, C. A. et al. (1990), 'Dissociation and Abuse among Multiple-personality Patients, Prostitutes, and Exotic Dancers', *Hospital and Community Psychiatry*, 41: 328–30.

Ross, C. A. et al. (1991), 'The Frequency of Multiple Personality Disorder among Psychiatric Inpatients', *American Journal of Psychiatry*, 148: 1717–20.

Rouget, G. (1985), *Music and Trance*, Chicago: University of Chicago Press.

Roy, A. (1985), 'Suicide: A Multidetermined Act', *Psychiatric Clinics of North America*, 8(2): 243–50.

Russell, D. (1983), 'The Incidence and Prevalence of Interfamilial and Extrafamilial Sexual Abuse in Female Children', *Child Abuse and Neglect*, 7: 133–46.

Sanders, B. and Giolas, M. H. (1991), 'Dissociation and Childhood Trauma in Psychologically Disturbed Adolescents', *American Journal of Psychiatry*, 148: 50–4.

Sargent, W. (1974), *The Mind Possessed*, Philadelphia: J. B. Lippincott.

Saxena, S. (1987), 'Simple Dissociative Disorder: A Subcategory in DSM-III-R?', *American Journal of Psychiatry*, 144: 524–5.

Saxena, S. and Prasad, K. V. S. R. (1989), 'DSM-III Subclassification of Dissociative Disorders Applied to Psychiatric Outpatients in India', *American Journal of Psychiatry*, 146: 261–2.

Schneidman, E. S. (1987), 'A Psychological Approach to Suicide', in G. R. Vander Bos and B. K. Bryant (eds.), *Cataclysms, Crises, and Catastrophes: Psychology in Action*, Washington, DC: American Psychiatric Association.

Schneidman, E. S. and Farberow, N. (1960), 'A Socio-psychological Study of Suicide', in H. David and J. Brengelmann (eds.), *Perspectives in Personality Research*, New York: Springer Publishing Co.

Schwartz, G. E. (1983), 'Disregulatory Theory and Disease: Applications to the Repression/Cerebral Disconnection Cardiovascular Disorder Hypothesis', *International Review of Applied Psychology*, 32: 95–118.

Sedman, G. (1966), 'Depersonalization in a Group of Normal Subjects', *British Journal of Psychiatry*, 109: 376–9.

Sharp, L. A. (1990), 'Possessed and Dispossessed Youth: Spirit Possession of Schoolchildren in Northwest Madagascar', *Culture, Medicine and Psychiatry*, 14: 339–64.

Shirokogoroff, S. M. (1935), *The Psychomental Complex of the Tungus*, London: Kegan Paul, French & Trubner.

Shor, R. E.; Orne, M. T.; and O'Connell, D. N. (1962), 'Validation and Cross-validation of a Scale of Self-reported Personal Experiences Which Predicts Hypnotizability', *Journal of Psychology*, 53: 55–75.

Silberman, E. K. et al. (1985), 'Dissociative States in Multiple Personality Disorder: A Quantitative Study', *Psychiatry Research*, 15: 253–60.

Silverman, J. (1967), 'Shamans and Acute Schizophrenia', *American Anthropologist*, 69: 21–31.

Simons, R. C. (1985a), 'Introduction: The Startle Matching Taxon', in R. C. Simons and C. C. Hughes (eds.), *The Culture-bound Syndromes*, Boston: D. Reidel Publishing Co.

—— (1985b), 'The Resolution of the *Latah* Paradox', in R. C. Simons and C. C. Hughes (eds.), *The Culture-bound Syndromes*, Boston: D. Reidel Publishing Co., pp. 43–62.

—— (1985c), 'Sorting the Culture-bound Syndromes', in R. C. Simons and C. C. Hughes (eds.), *The Culture-bound Syndromes*, Boston: D. Reidel Publishing Co., pp. 25–38.

Simpson, C. A. and Porter, G. L. (1981), 'Self-mutilization in Children and Adolescents', *Bulletin of the Menninger Clinic*, 45: 428–38.

Smith, D. H. and Hackathorn, L. (1982), 'Some Social and Psychological Factors Related to Suicide in Primitive Societies: A Cross-cultural Comparative Study', *Suicide and Life-threatening Behavior*, 12: 195–211.

Soskis, D. A. (1986), *Teaching Self-hypnosis: An Introductory Guide For Clinicians*, New York: W. W. Norton.

Spiegel, D. (1984), 'Multiple Personality as a Post-traumatic Stress Disorder', *Psychiatric Clinics of North America*, 7: 101–11.

—— (1990), 'Hypnosis, Dissociation and Trauma: Hidden and Overt Observers', in J. Singer (ed.), *Repression and Dissociation*, Chicago: University of Chicago Press, pp. 121–42.

—— (1991), 'Dissociation and Trauma', *Psychiatric Clinics of North America*, 14: 261–75.

Spiegel, D. and Cardeña, E. (1991), 'Disintegrated Experience: The Dissociative Disorders Revisited', *Journal of Abnormal Psychology*, 100: 366–78.

Spiegel, D.; Hunt, T.; and Dondershine, H. E. (1988), 'Dissociation and Hypnotizability in Posttraumatic Stress Disorder, *American Journal of Psychiatry*, 145: 301–5.

Spiegel, H. (1963), 'The Dissociation-association Continuum', *Journal of Nervous and Mental Disorders*, 136: 374–8.

Steinberg, M. (1990), 'Transcultural Issues in Psychiatry; The *Atague* and Multiple Personality Disorder', *Dissociation*, 3: 287–9.

Steinberg, M. (1991a), 'The Spectrum of Depersonalization: Assessment and Treatment', in A. Tasman (ed.), *Psychiatric Update,* Washington, DC: American Psychiatric Press.

____ (1991b), 'Systematizing Dissociation: Symptomatology and Diagnostic Assessment', Paper presented at the Dissociation Workshop for the Research Network in Mind–Body Interactions, Stanford, California.

Steinberg, M.; Howland, F.; and Cicchetti, D. (1986), 'The Structured Clinical Interview for DSM-III-R Dissociative Disorders', in B. Braun (ed.), *Proceedings of the International Conference on Multiple Personality and Dissociative States*, Chicago: Rush Presbyterian Hospital.

Steinberg, M.; Rounsaville, B.; and Cicchetti, D. (1990), 'The Structured Clinical Interview for DSM-III-R Dissociative Disorders: Preliminary Report on a New Diagnostic Instrument', *American Journal of Psychiatry*, 147: 76–82.

Steinbrook, E. (1952), 'Some Characteristics of the Psychopathology of Schizophrenic Behavior in Bahrain Society', *American Journal of Psychiatry*, 109: 330–5.

Stengel, E. (1941), 'On the Etiology of Fugue States', *Journal of Mental Science*, 87: 572–9.

Stevenson, R. L. (1928), *A Child's Garden of Verses*, London: Henry Altemeurs Co.

____ (1937), *Dr. Jekyll and Mr. Hyde*, New York: Bantam Books.

Stone, M. H. (1987), 'A Psychodynamic Approach: Some Thoughts on the Dynamics and Therapy of Self-mutilating Borderlinc Patients', *Journal of Personality Disorders*, 1: 347–9.

Suryani, L. K. (1978), 'Percobaan Bunuh Diri yang Dirawat di RSU Wangaya 1968–1976', *Majalah Kedokteran Udayana*, 24: 109.

____ (1984), 'Culture and Mental Disorder: The Case of *Bebainan* in Bali', *Culture, Medicine and Psychiatry*, 8: 95–113.

____ (1992), 'Traditional Healers in Bali, the Relationship with Psychiatrists', Paper presented at the Third International Ayurvedie Conference, Denpasar, Bali, 4 September.

Suryani, L. K. and Jensen, G. D. (1991), 'Psychiatrist, Traditional Healer and Culture Integrated in Clinical Practice in Bali', *Medical Anthropology*, 13: 301–14.

Sutcliffe, J. P. and Jones, J. (1962), 'Personal Identity, Multiple Personality and Hypnosis', *International Journal of Clinical and Experimental Hypnosis*, 10: 231–69.

Takahashi, Y. (1988), '*Aokigahara-jukai*: Suicide and Amnesia in Mt. Fuji's Black Forest', *Suicide and Life-threatening Behavior*, 18: 164–75.

____ (1989), 'A Clinical Study of Generalized Amnesia', *Saishin Shinkeigaku Zasshi*, 91: 260–93.

Tart, C. T. (1972), 'Measuring the Depth of an Altered State of Consciousness, with Particular Reference to Self-repeat Scales of

Hypnotic Depth', in E. Fromm and R. E. Shor (eds.), *Hypnosis: Research Developments and Perspectives*, Chicago: Aldine-Atherton, pp. 169–83.

Tellegen, A. and Atkinson, G. (1974), 'Openness to Absorbing and Self-altering Experiences ("Absorption"), a Trait Related to Hypnotic Susceptibility', *Journal of Abnormal Psychology*, 83: 268–77.

Terr, L. C. (1991), 'Childhood Trances: An Outline and Overview', *American Journal of Psychiatry*, 148: 10–20.

Travis, F. T. and Orme-Johnson, D. W. (1989), 'Field Model of Consciousness: EEG Coherence Changes as Indicators of Field Effects', *International Journal of Neuroscience*, 49: 203–4.

Triman, P. et al. (1978), 'Effek Fistiologik and Psikologik dara Meditasi', *JIWA*, 11 (4): 73–95.

Trueman, D. (1984), 'Anxiety and Depersonalization and Derealization Experiences', *Psychological Report*, 54: 91–6.

Tseng, W. (1976), 'Folk Psychotherapy in Taiwan', in W. P. Lebra (ed.), *Culture-bound Syndromes, Ethnopsychiatry and Alternative Therapies*, Honolulu: University of Hawaii Press.

Tsoi, W. F. (1970), 'Attempted Suicides', *Singapore Medical Journal*, 11: 258–63.

Tsoi, W. F. and Kok, L. P. (1982), 'Suicide Behavior in Singapore in the Year 1980', *Singapore Medical Journal*, 23: 29.

Tsoi, W. F. and Kua, E. H. (1987), 'Suicide Following Parasuicide in Singapore', *British Journal of Psychiatry*, 151: 543–5.

Turkus, J. A. (1991), 'Psychotherapy and Case Management for Multiple Personality Disorder: Synthesis for Continuity of Care', *Psychiatric Clinics of North America*, 14: 649–60.

Valentine, T. (1973), *Psychic Surgery*, Chicago: Henry Regnery.

van der Castle, R. L. (1977), 'Parapsychology and Anthropology', in A. B. Wolman, *Handbook of Parapsychology*, New York: Van Nostrand Reinhold.

van der Kolk, B. S. and van der Hart, O. (1989), 'Pierre Janet and the Breakdown of Adaptation in Psychological Trauma', *American Journal of Psychiatry*, 146: 1530–40.

van der Kolk, B. S.; Perry, J. C.; and Herman, J. L. (1991), 'Childhood Origins of Self-destructive Behavior', *American Journal of Psychiatry*, 148: 1665–71.

van Lawick-Goodall, J. (1967), 'My Friends the Wild Chimpanzees', Washington, DC: National Geographic Society.

Varma, L. P.; Srivastava, D. K.; and Sahay, R. N. (1970), 'Possession Syndrome', *Indian Journal of Psychiatry*, 12: 58–69.

Veith, I. (1977), 'Four Thousand Years of Hysteria', in M. J. Horowitz (ed.), *Hysterical Personality*, New York: Jason Aronson, Inc.

Walker, S. S. (1972), *Ceremonial Spirit Possession in Africa and Afro-American*, Leiden: E. J. Brill.

Wallace, A. F. C. (1959), 'Cultural Determinants of Responses to Hallucinatory Experiences', *Archives of General Psychiatry*, 1: 59–60.

____ (1966), *Religion: An Anthropological View*, New York: Random House, Inc.

Wallace, R. (1990), *The Agony of Lewis Carroll*, Melrose, Massachusetts: Gemini Press.

Wallanau, L. B. and Gallup, G. G., Jr. (1977), 'A Serotonergic, Mid-brain Raphe Model of Tonic Immobility', *Biobehavioral Reviews*, 1: 35–43.

Walsh, R. N. (1990), *The Spirit of Shamanism*, Los Angeles: Jeremy P. Tarcher, Inc.

Watkins, J. G. and Watkins, H. H. (1979), 'The Theory and Practice of Ego-State Therapy', in H. Greyson (ed.), *Short Term Approaches to Psychotherapy*, New York: National Institute for the Psychotherapies and Human Sciences Press, Chapter 11.

____ (1984), 'Hazards to the Therapist in the Treatment of Multiple Personalities', *Psychiatric Clinics of North America*, 7: 111–19.

Weck, W. (1937), *Pengetahuan tentang Penyembuhan dan Pekerti Rakyat di Bali*, Stuttgart: Ferdinand Enke.

Weingartner, H. (1978), 'Human State Dependent Learning', in B. T. Ho, D. W. Richards, and D. C. Chute (eds.), *Drug Discrimination and State Dependent Learning*, New York: Academic Press, pp. 361–82.

West, L. J. (1967), 'Dissociative Reaction', in A. M. Freedman and H. E. Kaplan (eds.), *Comprehensive Textbook of Psychiatry*, 2nd edn., Baltimore: Williams & Wilkins, pp. 825–99.

Whittkower, E. D. (1970), 'Trance and Possession States', *International Journal of Social Psychiatry*, 16: 153–60.

Wick, J. A. (1941), 'Modern Spirit Dancing of Northern Puget Sound', Manuscript, University of Washington Library.

Wilbur, C. G. (1984), 'Multiple Personality and Child Abuse: An Overview', *Psychiatric Clinics of North America*, 7: 3–7.

WHO (1992), *Classification of Mental and Behavioral Disorders: Clinical Descriptions and Diagnostic Guidelines*, cited in the text as *ICD-10* (*International Classification of Diseases*, 10th edn.), Geneva, pp. 156–7.

Yap, P. M. (1960), 'The Possession Syndrome: A Comparison of Hong Kong and French Findings', *Journal of Mental Science*, 106: 114–37.

____ (1969), 'The Culture-bound Reactive Syndromes', in W. Caudell and T. Lin (eds.), *Mental Health Research in Asia and Pacific*, Honolulu: East–West Center Press.

Index

Figures in italics refer to Plate numbers.

ADITYANJEE, G. S. P., 216
Ahli kebatinan, 146
Ainslie, G., 138
Aldrich, T. E., 136
Allison, R. B., 157, 182
Altered states of consciousness (ASC), 1, 3, 28–32, 45, 86, 160, 169, 170, 171, 180; and suicide, 134–40; *see also* Hypnosis; Meditation; Trance; Trance-possession; Yoga
American Psychiatric Association (APA), 20, 129, 173, 185, 191, 197–8, 233–4
Amnesia, 37, 39, 52, 64, 94, 98, 106, 172, 186, 204, 206, 208, 215, 223, 231
Amok, 44–5, 143–6, 172
Amytal interviews, 130, 158, 225
Andersen, Hans Christian, 21
Arboledo-Florez, J., 44
Asch, P., 70–1, 87
Asch, T., 70–1, 87
Atkinson, G., 140, 177

BACH-Y-RITA, G., 142
Balance, 16–18
Bali: ceremonies, 11–15; communal organization, 7; geography, 6; history, 1, 3, 6; occupations, 7; population, 6; religion, 6, 8–9, 11–18; social systems, 8–10; *see also* Balinese; Hindu–Dharma beliefs
Balian, 17–18, 40, 49–51, 154–5, 189–90, 214–15, 231, 235, *28–43*; *apun*, 49, 77–8; and *bebai*, 146; ceremonial trance, 104; comparison with shaman, 83–4; *kebal*, 50; *matuun*, 15; *taksu*, 49–71, 86–7, 177; *usada*, 49, 71–4, 78–82, *39*; use of incense, 28
Balinese: caste, 9; character, 2, 217; culture, 2, 3, 4, 6–18; household, *1–2*; religion, 2, 3, 7, 8–9, 15–18, *1–23*
Bandem, I. M., 3, 16
Banjar, 7–8
Barkin, Elaine, 128
Barlow, D. H., 179
Barong, 1, 14, 96, 98–104, 107–8, 195, *21*
Bateson, G., 1, 3, 13, 38, 95, 109, 206, 209, 230
Beahrs, J. O., 224
Bebai, 146–8, 150
Bebainan, 78–82, 144–52, 173, 182
Bebutan, 101
Belo, J., 1–3, 5, 11, 14, 38, 50, 95, 97, 106, 108–9, 111, 117, 166, 206–8, 230
Benedict, R., 34
Benson, H., 162–3
Bergen, Edgar, 233
Bernstein, E. M., 20, 22–3, 142, 177, 205, 216
Berwick, P. R., 186
Bhatia, S. C., 136
Blacker, K., 182, 187
Black magic, 78–82, 146–7
Bliss, E. L., 129, 172–3, 177, 197–8, 203, 205–7, 209–11, 216, 220, 224–5, 228, 234
Boma, 78
Bona: dances, 110–11
Bone removal, 75–7

Boon, J. A., 11
Borysenko, J. Z., 162
Bourguignon, E., 31, 33–5, 40, 171, 191
Bower, G. H., 204
Bowers, M. K., 228
Bowman, E. S., 198, 206
Braid, J., 205
Brandsma, J. M., 204
Braun, R. G., 198, 221, 228
Brenman, N., 191, 206
Breuer, J., 200–2
Brown, D. P., 22, 28–9, 127, 177, 191
Burman-Hall, Linda, 128
Butler, R. W., 138

CAMPBELL, J., 180
Cardeña, E., 20, 35–7, 47, 172, 235
Carlson, E. B., 23
Carr, J. E., 145
Carroll, Lewis, 21
Caste system, 9
Castillo, R. J., 162, 185–6, 237
Ceremonies, 2, 11–15, *9–12*, *14–18*; family, 105–6; Jimbaran, 98–104, 174, *44–45*, *50*; Kesiman, 95–8, 175, *47*; Timbrah, 89–95, *46*, *48–49*
Channellers, 85, 230–1
Charcot, Jean-Martin, 2, 199
Chaudhuri, H., 160
Child abuse, 203–6, 216, 232
Chimpanzees, 32
Cicchetti, D., 28, 216
Clark, W. H., 186
Clifford, H. C., 47
Cock-fights, 31, 95, *8*
Collinder, B., 47
Connor, L. H., 16–17, 68, 70–1, 87, 135, 166, 188, 217, 233, 235
Conterio, K., 143
Coons, P. M., 198, 206, 211, 222, 228
Covarrubius, M., 2, 9, 11, 47
Cowdry, R. W., 143
Crabtree, A., 181–3, 198, 200, 202–3, 236
Currie, R., 23, 197
Czaplicka, M. A., 47

DANCE, 2, 11, 108–18; fire/hobby-horse, 111–13, *52*; *kecak*, 113–15, *53*; little girl trance-possession, 3, 109–11, *51*

Davis, S., 161
DeBerry, S., 161
DeBoer, F. E., 16
DeBoismont, B. A., 203
Deikman, A. J., 162
Delmonte, M. M., 161
Demetrack, M. A., 222
Depersonalization, 21, 172, 178, 180, 185–6, 233–4
Derealization, 172, 233
Desa, 7–8
Devale, Sue, 128
Devereaux, G., 186, 195, 212
De Zoete, B., 2, 107
Diagnostic and Statistical Manual of Mental Disorders, 178, 181, 185, 198, 215, 234–5
Diekstra, R. F., 136
Dillbeck, M. C., 163
Dinges, P. F., 177
Dissociation, 20–3, 32, 45, 232, 234; continua, 177–9; disorders, 5, 27–8, 45, 129–30, 138–9, 158, 178, 196–7
Dissociative disorders, 4, 5, 27, 45, 129–59, 172, 178; *amok*, 44, 143–6, 172, 186; *bebainan*, 44, 146–52, 174, 182, 196; diagnostic instruments, 216; dizziness, 216; 'hidden by the evil spirit', 23–4; *kasurupan*, 44, 152–6, 182, 205; *latah*, 24–7, 47; *ngramang sawang*, 22; survival value, 22; theory, 32
Dissociative Experiences Scale (DES), 23, 142–3, 216, 229
Dixon, J. C., 186
Dondershine, H. E., 20, 138, 173, 177
Douglas, R. R., 186
DSM-III-R, see Diagnostic and Statistical Manual of Mental Disorders
DSM-IV, see Diagnostic and Statistical Manual of Mental Disorders

ELAIDE, M., 88
Electroencephalography (EEG), 221–2
Ellenberger, H. F., 33, 203
Engkebang memedi, 23–4, 45
Erikson, M. H., 2, 228
Evil spirits, 40, 78–82, 146, 174, 182, 186–7
Exorcism, 4, 159, 176, 234

FARBEROW, N., 135
Favazza, A. R., 143
Fine, C. C., 228
Fink, O., 198
Fire-walking, 38
Fishbain, D. A., 136
Forman, B., 38
Forman, W., 38
Frankel, F. H., 20, 28, 33, 178–9
Frazer, J. G., 209
Freedman, A. M., 43, 234
Freud, Sigmund, 2, 5, 33, 35, 46, 199, 201–2
Frigerio, A., 35–7
Fromm, E., 22, 28–9, 127, 177, 191
Fuchs, S., 83
Fugue, 24, 47, 139

GADDIS, V. H., 38
Gallup, G., 31–2
Galungan ceremony, 98–104, *12*
Gamelan, 7, 14, 103, 105, 119–28, 153; effects on composers, 123–5; effects on players, 121–3, *54–55*; types of, 120
Gardner, D. L., 143
Gauld, 65
Geertz, C., 15, 217
Geertz, H., 15, 24
Gegean, 26
Gill, M. M., 191, 206
Gilmour, A., 47
Gong orchestra, 90–1, 96–7
Goodman, F. D., 30, 35, 87, 157, 175, 206, 224, 234
Gordon, J. F., 44, 231
Graff, H., 143
Grant, C., 22
Grunebaum, H. U., 143
'Guardian spirit complex', 34
Gudjonsson, G. H., 139

HAAS, A. P., 138
Haberman, M. A., 138
Hackathorn, L., 136
Halifax, J., 83
Hallucenogenic plants/drugs, 28, 47
Hallucinations, 190–1, 235–6
Hansen, C., 3, 181
Harrary, K., 137
Hastings, A., 47, 85, 175, 233
Haward, L. R. C., 139
Healing meditation, 76
Health care, 9
Hendin, H., 138
Henney, J. H., 173, 175
Herzog, H. A., 31
'Hidden by the evil spirit', *see Engkebang memedi*
Hilgard, E. R., 21, 29, 32, 46, 201, 206, 233
Hindu–Dharma beliefs, 15–16, 18, 172, *6–7, 13*
Hindu high priest, *see Pedanda*
Hollan, D., 131, 136
Holmes, D. S., 33
Hooykaas, C., 11
Howland, F., 28
Hughes, D. J., 85, 221
Hunt, T., 20, 138, 173, 177
Hypnosis, 1, 2, 3, 19, 28–33, 44–5, 106, 129, 173, 174, 208, 229–30; and brain changes, 31; and MPD, 206–11; self-hypnosis, 31, 205–6, 215–16, 232
Hypnotherapy, 2, 130, 167–70, 182

IBOGAINE, 47
ICD-10, see International Classification of Diseases
Illness, 17
Illusion, 235–6
Ilmu pengiwa, see Black magic
International Classification of Diseases, 129, 151, 178, 181, 234
Isherwood, J., 82

JAMES, WILLIAM, 177, 180
Janet, Pierre, 35, 177, 191, 198–9, 236
Jensen, G. D., 2–4, 29, 76–7, 120, 141, 152, 181, 206, 209–10, 214–15, 217, 236; chimpanzee study, 32
Jilck, W. G., 34
Jimbaran: mass trance-possession, 98–105, 174, *17, 44–45*
Johnson, V. E., 22
Jones, E., 5
Jones, J., 205
Jones, Jim, 137
Joshi, S., 23, 197
Jung, Carl, 180

KAHAN, J., 143
Kaplan, H. E., 43, 234
Kasurupan, 152–6, 182
Kecak dance, 113–15, *53*
Kelly, G. A., 161
Kennedy, R. B., 162
Kenny, M. G., 24–5, 203
Kesiman: mass trance-possession, 95–8, 175, *47*
Khandelwal, S. K., 216
Kiev, A., 230
Kim, E., 138
Kleins, 233
Klemm, W. R., 31
Klemperer, E., 219
Klerman, G. L., 143
Kluft, R. P., 188, 197–8, 203, 206–10, 212, 216, 219, 223–5, 227–8
Kok, L. P., 131
Kokoszka, A., 161
Krause, G., 7
Krippner, S., 203, 211
Kris, E., 191
Kris stabbing, 96–8, 101, *50*
Kua, E. H., 130–1, 135–6
Kuningan ceremony, 89–95, 104
Kunkle, E. C., 47
Kutz, I. K., 162

LANGNESS, L., 171, 195
Latah, 24–7, 47, *24–27*
Leak, 40–5, 47
Leff, J., 88
Leibenluft, E., 143
Leimena, S. L., 17, 87
Lek, 217
Levy, J., 180, 186
Lewis, I. M., 173–4, 186
Li, Y., 83
Linton, R., 35–6, 175
Liu, G. L., 162
Loewenstein, R. J., 216
Lontar, 49, 71, 74–5, 78–9, *42*
Ludwig, A. M., 22, 177, 204

McDOUGAL, W., 202
MacKinnon, R. P., 191
McPhee, C., 14, 41, 119, 126, 128
Magarey, C. J., 161
Mallin, R., 143
Maniam, T., 130–1, 136
Maramis, W., 190
Martin, M., 157
Martinez-Tuboas, A., 197
Maser, J. D., 31
Massage, 49, 77–8
Masters, W. H., 22
Mayer-Gross, W., 28, 180
Mazek, R., 38
Mead, M., 1, 3, 13, 38, 95, 109, 206, 209, 230
Meares, A., 161
Meditation, 160–4, 170, *58*; field effects of, 30, 163; healing, 163–7, 170; neurophysiological changes in, 162–3; technique, 47–8
Melville, N. J., 221
Mental health, 18; and dissociation, 22; and trance-possession, 230–2
Metraux, A., 181
Mills, P. J., 162
Milstein, V., 198, 206
Moerdowo, R. M., 11
Moll, A., 205
Morgan, A. H., 47
Mueser, K. T., 138
Muller, C., 104
Multiple personality disorder (MPD), 3, 23, 28, 45, 129, 138, 142, 158, 171–2, 177–8, 183, 187, 188, 197, 235–6; and hypnosis, 206–11; in other cultures, 197; and personality, 217–19; and possession disorder, 221; therapy, 222–9; as trance-possession, 196–229, 232–3
Murphy, H. B. M., 47, 130
Myers, D., 22

NAKAGAWA, H., 47
Nemiah, J. C., 20, 129, 185
Ngramang sawang, 22
Nissen, M. J., 204
Noll, R., 172
Norton, R. P., 197, 203, 206, 208

OCCULTISM, 202–3, 236
O'Connell, D. N., 177
Oesterreich, T. K., 3, 33–4, 180
Ogata, S. N., 206
Orme-Johnson, D. W., 163

Orne, D. C., 177
Orne, M. T., 173, 177

Pattison, E. M., 143, 211
Pedanda, 146, 154
Pelton, R., 235
Pengadeg dasaran, 50
Porter, G. L., 143
Possession, 1, 3–4, 19, 33–40, 45–6, 152–6; disorders, 181–90, 221, 235; in other cultures, 33–7, 144–5, 156–8, 173–6, 180–1, 216, 230–1, 234, 236; professional recognition of, 179–81; theories, 191–6; *see also* Trance-possession
Post, R., 138, 221
Post-traumatic stress disorder (PTSD), 23, 28, 138, 142, 204
Poverty, 9
Powell, H., 7
Prasad, K. V. S. R., 172, 235
Prince, Morton, 177
Psychosis, 186–9
Psychotherapy, 2, 130, 166, 231
Putnam, F. W., 20, 22–3, 138, 142, 177–8, 197, 205–6, 208, 211, 216, 219, 221–2, 224, 228
Puysegur, A. M. J., 198

Ramseyer, U., 2
Rangda, 96–105, 107–9, 153, 173–4, 195, *19*
Ratu Gde Dalem Peed (RGDP), 62, 88
Ravenscroft, K., 203, 211
Reinhard, K. E., 161
Repression, 32–3
Rice-growing, 9–10, *3–5*
Rosenthal, D., 216
Rosenthal, R. J., 143
Ross, C. A., 23, 142, 197–8, 203, 206, 208–9, 219, 224, 235–6
Rosser-Hogan, R., 23
Rouget, G., 28, 127, 186, 195
Rounsaville, B., 28, 216
Roy, A., 143
Russell, D., 206

Saddock, B. J., 43, 234
Sahay, R. N., 216
Sang Hyang Dedari, 3, 109–11, 174, *51*
Sang Hyang Jaran, 111–13, *52*
Saraswati, 74
Sargent, W., 191
Saxena, S., 172, 235
Schneidman, E. S., 135–6, 139–40
Schwartz, G. E., 161
Sedman, G., 22
Seka, 9
Sekolah Tinggi Seni Indonesia (STSI), 121
Shaman, 30, 83–4, 87, 88, 231
Sharp, L. A., 156–7, 236
Shirokogoroff, S. M., 30
Shor, R. E., 177
Sibling spirits, 16, 218
Silberman, E. K., 204
Silverman, J., 186
Simons, R. C., 24–5
Simpson, C. A., 143
Smith, D. H., 136
Social systems, 8–11
Sorcery, *see* Black magic
Soskis, D. A., 29
Spiegel, D., 20, 47, 138, 173, 177–8, 203–5, 220, 235
Spies, W., 2, 107
Spiritualist, *see Ahli kebatinan*
Srivastava, D. K., 216
State-dependent learning, 203–4, 221
Steinberg, M., 27, 172, 180, 185–6, 197, 216, 235
Stengel, E., 139
Stevenson, Robert Louis, 21, 199–200
Stone, M. H., 143
Structured Clinical Interview for DSM-III-R Dissociative Disorders, 216
Subak, 9–10
Suicide: ASC and, 134–5, 137–8; mass, 137; religion and, 135; study, 130–6; and trance, 3, 130–43, 158, 172, 229–30, 233
Suryani, L. K., 2–4, 23, 29, 59, 66–8, 73–6, 86, 95, 120, 146, 181, 190, 197, 205–6, 209, 217; *amok* study, 144–5; as *balian*, 163–4; *bebainan* study, 147–52; hypnotherapist, 44, 47–8, 167–70; *kasurupan* study, 152–6; and *leak*, 42–3; meditation healing, 163, *58*; possession, 37, 117, 163–6, 172; as

psychotherapist, 166; suicide study, 131–6
Sutcliffe, J. P., 205

TAKAHASHI, Y., 138
Taksu, 50, 87, 218
Tan, E. K., 145
Tart, C. T., 233
Tellegen, A., 140, 177
Temples, 6, 13, 17, *2, 18–20, 22–23*
Terr, L. C., 204
Thong, D. H., 17, 60, 87, 144
Timbrah: mass trance-possession, 89–95, *46, 48–49*
Tourism, 110–11
Traditional healers, *see Balian*
Trance, 1, 3, 5, 28–33, 171; in animals, 31–2; depth of, 38, 178; in musicians, 123–8; in other cultures, 30, 230–1; and suicide, 136–43; trance-medium, *see Balian*: *taksu*
Trance-possession, 1, 38–40, 46, *30, 34–37, 45–57*; and amnesia, 39, 215; ceremonies, 2, 11; characteristics of, 172–7, 206–14; in dance and drama, 108–15, 174–5; individual, 115–18; mass ceremonies, 89–107, *44–50*; and mental health, 230–2; and MPD, 206–13; and religion, 172, 175; sex distribution, 176; in schoolchildren, 152–6, *56–57*; *see also Balian*
Trance-suicide, 3, 130–43, 158, 172, 229–30, 233
Travis, F. T., 163
Triman, P., 162
Trueman, D., 186
Tseng, W., 83
Tsoi, W. F., 130–1, 135–6
Turkus, J. A., 228
Turtle Island: ceremonial trance, 104

UNCONSCIOUS, 233
Unidentified flying objects (UFO), 43–4, 231

VALENTINE, T., 88
Van der Hart, O., 191
Van der Kolk, B. S., 142, 191
Van Lawick-Goodall, J., 32
Varma, L. P., 258

WACHTEL, P., 180, 186
Walker, S. S., 191
Wallace, R., 21
Wallanau, L. B., 32
Walsh, R. N., 88
Wangaya Hospital Department of Psychiatry, 132–3
Watkins, H. H., 219, 224, 228
Watkins, J. G., 219, 224, 228
Weck, W., 146
Weingartner, H., 203
West, L. J., 20
Whittkower, E. D., 44, 230
Wick, J. A., 34–5
Wilbur, C. G., 203–4
Wintrob, R. M., 211
Wong, N., 182, 187
World Health Organization (WHO), 27, 129, 151, 158, 180–1
Wozney, K., 197, 203, 206, 208

YAP, P. M., 47, 108, 181, 183
Yoga, 169–70
Young, C. O., 233

ZAHN, T., 138, 221